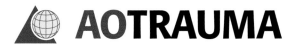

David A Volgas | Yves Harder

Manual of Soft-Tissue Management in Orthopaedic Trauma

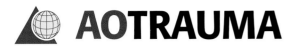

AOTRAUMA

David A Volgas | Yves Harder

Manual of Soft-Tissue Management in Orthopaedic Trauma

711 illustrations/figures, 14 videos, and 20 cases

The videos and animation in this book are only accessible on the internet:

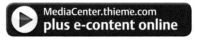

MediaCenter.thieme.com
plus e-content online

For more information see last page of this book.

Library of Congress Cataloging-in-Publication Data is available from the publisher.

Hazards

Great care has been taken to maintain the accuracy of the information contained in this publication. However, the publisher, and/or the distributor, and/or the editors, and/or the authors cannot be held responsible for errors or any consequences arising from the use of the information contained in this publication. Contributions published under the name of individual authors are statements and opinions solely of said authors and not of the publisher, and/or the distributor, and/or the AO Group.

The products, procedures, and therapies described in this work are hazardous and are therefore only to be applied by certified and trained medical professionals in environments specially designed for such procedures. No suggested test or procedure should be carried out unless, in the user's professional judgment, its risk is justified. Whoever applies products, procedures, and therapies shown or described in this work will do this at their own risk. Because of rapid advances in the medical sciences, AO recommends that independent verification of diagnosis, therapies, drugs, dosages, and operation methods should be made before any action is taken.

Although all advertising material which may be inserted into the work is expected to conform to ethical (medical) standards, inclusion in this publication does not constitute a guarantee or endorsement by the publisher regarding quality or value of such product or of the claims made of it by its manufacturer.

Legal restrictions

Copyright © 2011 by AO Foundation, Switzerland, Clavadelerstrasse 8, CH-7270 Davos Platz
Distribution by Georg Thieme Verlag, Rüdigerstrasse 14, DE-70469 Stuttgart and Thieme New York, 333 Seventh Avenue, US-New York, NY 10001

ISBN: 978-3-13-166371-9
e-ISBN: 978-3-13-166381-8

1 2 3 4 5 6

Preface

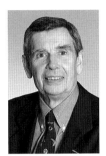

Thomas P Rüedi, MD, Professor, FACS
Founding and honorary member
of the AO Foundation

Is there really an interest in or a need for an AO Manual on the management of soft tissues? Especially in view of the fact that most fractures are being stabilized by so-called minimally invasive surgical techniques, which supposedly do less harm than conventional surgery? Even so, it is unfortunately often forgotten or at least neglected that "a fracture first and foremost is a soft-tissue injury, in which the bone happens to be broken". This simple statement actually seems to justify the publication of this textbook as a useful and valuable adjunct to the manuals on operative fracture fixation.

We can and do teach on a broad scale, both in theory and in practical workshops, how to apply nails, screws, plates, and other implants to the most complex fractures of almost any bare, synthetic bone or joint. However, there is as yet no way to simulate the often tricky reduction maneuvers, as they are encountered regularly in the operation room, nor can we teach how to assess, evaluate, and handle the injured soft tissues on realistic models or on an individual basis.

Although the founders of the AO—from the very beginning of their teaching—stressed the importance of preserving the vascularity of the soft tissues and bone, too much attention and emphasis was—and still is—addressed to the mechanical aspects of an anatomical reconstruction and absolute rigid fixation of a fracture. This has contributed to the tendency for approaches that are much too extensive, unnecessary exposures, and rough manipulation of the fracture fragments as well as careless stripping of periosteum. Neglecting the biology in general and, in particular, underestimating the vascularity of the soft parts and bone, has all too often resulted in necrotic bone, delayed healing or no healing at all, infection as well as other complications.

In open fractures the immediate debridement and surgical stabilization—as proposed and initiated by the AO more than 50 years ago—proved to be of great benefit for the recovery of the damaged soft tissues surrounding the fracture. However, careful assessment of the injury, correct timing and planning of the procedure followed by experienced surgery remain of crucial importance for the successful outcome for all fractures—open as well as closed. Furthermore, critical soft-tissue conditions, loss of skin, or large tissue defects demand special interest and much expertise in order to handle or cover the damaged area.

The goal of this manual on soft-tissue management in trauma of the extremities is to provide a scientific background, validated basic instructions, and practical hints by experts on how to handle the soft tissues and especially the skin. After correct debridement, only vital and healthy tissues providing an intact coverage are able to guarantee a safe barrier against infection or the basis to successfully fight a residual infection inside an injured limb. Similarly, an associated fracture will only be able to heal if the soft-tissue envelope is viable.

The two editors–David A Volgas, an American orthopaedic trauma surgeon with a special interest in soft-tissue surgery and Yves Harder, a Swiss plastic and reconstructive surgeon with a broad background in general surgery, trauma and research—have been able to convince a number of experts from around the world to contribute their knowledge and experience to this textbook, which is addressed mainly to those surgeons—young or older—involved and interested in the overall management of trauma of the locomotor system.

The first chapters of this book have been reserved for the principles of soft-tissue handling, the anatomy of the soft parts and bone as well as their healing patterns, the mechanisms of injury and the assessment and classification of the injury. Next, the focus is on treatment strategies as well as the stabilization and conditioning of the wound, followed by chapters that discuss the principles and techniques of wound closure and coverage including the most common local and regional flaps for extremity trauma. The use of free flaps and other less frequently applied flaps is mentioned, but not addressed in detail, as this should remain the domain of the specialists. Finally, postoperative care, as well as hazards and complications round off the content. In support of the text, illustrations, tables, and video clips have been produced and as a special feature, a number of instructive case reports are provided as examples of how to manage individual situations. Cases are presented progressively from those requiring simpler surgical skills to those that should only be carried out by a specialized surgeon familiar with reconstructive procedures, including microsurgery.

While this textbook is no substitute for what a skilled surgeon should be learning at the operation table, it is intended to help improve the understanding of the principles and philosophy of soft-tissue management in trauma.

Maienfeld, June 2011

Acknowledgments

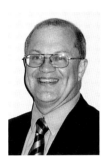

David A Volgas, MD, Associate Professor

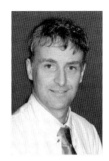

Yves Harder, MD, PD

From the time this project was first conceived, Thomas P Rüedi has been a facilitator, mentor, and friend, providing encouragement and support. Throughout his long career as a dexterous and dedicated surgeon with a special interest in trauma surgery and as a founding member of the AO Foundation, he has emphasized and taught the principles of soft-tissue handling to the residents and fellows fortunate enough to learn in his operating room. He helped bring this project to fruition, brought the editors together, and assisted with the refining and proofreading of chapters. His help has been invaluable and the editors would like to thank him heartily for his guidance throughout the project.

The editors also wish to express their gratitude to the many authors who wrote chapters, taking time away from their very busy clinical practices. We are convinced that this effort will significantly further the education of surgeons. We would also like to thank all surgeons who provided material such as photographs, or whose skills in the operating room helped us produce instructive learning material such as case reports. Dr Ladislav Nagy is one of them.

The AO team has provided resources, expertise, and opportunities, without which this book would not have been possible. Urs Rüetschi and Kathrin Lüssi have continued to support and put their faith in this book. Special thanks go to Sigrid Unterberg, who proved tireless in planning, managing, and advising this complex project. She was instrumental in overcoming obstacles whenever they arose. Thanks go to all illustrators, in particular Jecca Reichmuth as the main illustrator, Simone Monhart Wüthrich, and Susanne Stettler. Roger Kistler and Tom Wirth did a tremendous job in typesetting, while Carl Lau and Barbara Gernert helped with the proofreading. From the video team, Mike Laws has been most helpful in the production process, and Robin Greene generously lent us his voice to produce instructive learning material. Further thanks go to nougat GmbH, Basel.

Finally, the editors wish to thank Thieme for their assistance in publishing and distributing this book.

Zurich, August 2011

Contributors

Editors

David A Volgas, MD, Associate Professor
Department of Orthopaedic Surgery
University of Missouri
One Hospital Drive
DC053.00
US-Columbia, MO 65212

Yves Harder, MD, PD
Department of Plastic Surgery and Hand Surgery
Klinikum rechts der Isar
Technische Universität München
Ismaninger Straße 22
DE-81675 Munich

Editorial Advisor

Thomas P Rüedi, MD, Professor, FACS
Founding and honorary member of the AO Foundation
Im Brisig
CH-7304 Maienfeld

Authors

Sammy Al-Benna, MD, MB ChB, PGCNano, MRCS
Department of Plastic and Reconstructive Surgery
BG University Hospital Bergmannsheil
Ruhr University Bochum
Bürkle-de-la-Camp-Platz 1
DE-44789 Bochum

Christoph Andree, MD
Department of Plastic and Aesthetic Surgery
Sana Hospital Düsseldorf
Gräulingerstraße 120
DE-40625 Düsseldorf

Jeffrey Anglen, MD, FACS, FAAOS, Professor of
Orthopaedics
Indiana University School of Medicine
541 Clinical Drive, Suite 600
US-Indianapolis, IN 46202

Volker A Braunstein, MD
Surgical Hospital and Health Center
Ludwig-Maximilians-University
Nussbaumstraße 20
DE-80336 Munich

Angelo M Biraima, MD
Division of Plastic Surgery and Hand Surgery
Departement of Surgery
University Hospital Zurich
Rämistrasse 100
CH-8091 Zurich

Maurizio Calcagni, MD
Division of Plastic Surgery and Hand Surgery
Departement of Surgery
University Hospital Zurich
Rämistrasse 100
CH-8091 Zurich

Claudio Contaldo, MD, PD
Division of Plastic Surgery and Hand Surgery
Departement of Surgery
University Hospital Zurich
Rämistrasse 100
CH-8091 Zurich

John S Early, MD, Professor
University of Texas Southwestern Medical Center
Texas Orthopaedic Associates, L.L.P
8210 Walnut Hill Ln #130
US-Texas, TX 75231

Dominique Erni, MD, Professor
Plastic Surgery Erni
Küferweg 9
CH-6403 Küssnacht

Jian Farhadi, MD, PD
Department of Plastic Surgery
Guy's and St Thomas' Hospital
Westminster Bridge Road
UK-SE1 7EH London

James R Ficke, MD, Chairman
Department of Orthopaedics and Rehabilitation
Brooke Army Medical Center
3851 Roger Brooke Drive
US-Fort Sam Houston, TX 78234

Elmar Fritsche, MD
Department for Hand and Plastic Surgery
Cantonal Hospital Lucerne
CH-6016 Lucerne

Pietro Giovanoli, MD, Professor
Division of Plastic Surgery and Hand Surgery
Departement of Surgery
University Hospital Zurich
Rämistrasse 100
CH-8091 Zurich

Jörg Grünert, MD, Professor
Department of Hand, Plastic and
Reconstructive Surgery
Cantonal Hospital St Gallen
Rorschacherstrasse 95
CH-9010 St Gallen

Merlin Guggenheim, MD
Division of Plastic Surgery and Hand Surgery
Departement of Surgery
University Hospital Zürich
Rämistrasse 100
CH-8091 Zurich

Yves Harder, MD, PD
Department of Plastic Surgery and Hand Surgery
Klinikum rechts der Isar
Technische Universität München
Ismaninger Straße 22
DE-81675 Munich

William J Harrison, MD, Associate Professor,
MA (Oxon), FRCS
Countess of Chester Hospital
Liverpool Road
UK-CH2 1UL Chester

Urs Hug, MD
Department for Hand and Plastic Surgery
Cantonal Hospital Lucerne
CH-6016 Lucerne

Rafael Jakubietz, MD
Department of Trauma, Hand and Plastic Surgery
Julius-Maximilians-University
Oberdürrbacherstr. 6
DE-97080 Würzburg

Daniel F Kalbermatten, MD, PD, PhD, MPhil
Division of Plastic and Reconstructive Surgery
University Hospital Basel
Spitalstrasse 21
CH-4031 Basel

Stefan Langer, MD, Professor
Department of Plastic and Reconstructive Surgery
BG University Hospital Bergmannsheil
Bürkle-de-la-Camp-Platz 1
DE-44789 Bochum

L Scott Levin, MD, FACS, Paul B Magnuson
Professor of Bone and Joint Surgery,
Professor of Surgery Chairman
Department of Orthopaedic Surgery
Hospital of the University of Pennsylvania
3400 Spruce Street, 2 Silverstein
US-Philadelphia, PA 19104-4283

Douglas W Lundy, MD
Orthopaedic Surgery
61 Whitcher Street, Suite 1100
US-Marietta, GA 30060

Jörn A Lohmeyer, MD
Department of Plastic Surgery and Hand Surgery
Klinikum rechts der Isar
Technische Universität München
Ismaninger Straße 22
DE-81675 Munich

James N Long, MD, FACS, Associate Professor
Divison of Plastic, Reconstructive, Hand and
Microsurgery
University of Alabama
510 Twentieth Street South, FOT1152
US-Birmingham, AL 35294

Hans-Günther Machens, MD, Professor
Department of Plastic Surgery and Hand Surgery
Klinikum rechts der Isar
Technische Universität München
Ismaninger Straße 22
DE-81675 Munich

Stefan Milz, MD, Professor
Department of Anatomy
Ludwig-Maximilians-University
Pettenkoferstraße 11
DE-80336 Munich

Themistocles S Protopsaltis, MD, Assistant
Professor of Orthopaedic Surgery
School of Medicine
New York University
301 East 17th Street, Room 413
US-New York, NY 10003

Farid Rezaeian, MD
Department of Plastic Surgery and Hand Surgery
Klinikum rechts der Isar
Technische Universität München
Ismaninger Straße 22
DE-81675 Munich

Timo Schmid, MD
Department of Orthopaedic Surgery
University Hospital of Berne
CH-3010 Berne

Maxime Servaes, MD
Division of Plastic, Reconstructive and Aesthetic
Surgery
St Luc University Hospitals of Brussels
Avenue Hippocrate, 10
BE-1200 Brussels

James P Stannard, MD, Professor
Chairman, Orthopaedic Surgery Department
Missouri Orthopaedic Institute
University of Missouri
1100 Virginia Avenue, fourth floor
US-Columbia, MO 65212

Hans-Ulrich Steinau, MD, Professor
Department of Plastic and Reconstructive Surgery
BG University Hospital Bergmannsheil
Bürkle-de-la-Camp-Platz 1
DE-44789 Bochum

Lars Steinsträßer, MD, Professor, FACS
Department of Plastic and Reconstructive Surgery
BG University Hospital Bergmannsheil
Bürkle-de-la-Camp-Platz 1
DE-44789 Bochum

Ulrich Stöckle, MD, Professor
Department of Trauma Surgery
BG Trauma Hospital
University of Tübingen
Schnarrenbergstraße 95
DE-72076 Tübingen

Robert D Teasdall, MD, Professor
Department of Orthopaedic Surgery
Wake Forest University
Medical Center Boulevard
US-Winston-Salem, NC 27157

Esther Vögelin, MD, PD
Department of Plastic, Reconstructive and
Aesthetic Surgery
Inselspital Berne
Freiburgstrasse
CH-3010 Berne

David A Volgas, MD, Associate Professor
Department of Orthopaedic Surgery
University of Missouri
One Hospital Drive
DC053.00
US-Columbia, MO 65212

Reto Wettstein, MD
Division of Plastic, Reconstructive and Aesthetic
Surgery, Hand Surgery
Solothurn Hospitals and University Hospital Basel
Schöngrünstrasse 42
CH-4500 Solothurn

Mirjam Zweifel-Schlatter, MD
Plastic Surgery
Private Practice
Marktplatz 5
CH-4001 Basel

Abbreviations

ABI	ankle-brachial index	**MIF**	macrophage migration inhibitory factor
ATLS	advanced trauma life support	**MRI**	magnet resonance imaging
bFGF	basic fibroblast growth factor	**MRSA**	methicillin-resistant *Staphylococcus aureus*
BMI	body mass index	**MSC**	mesenchymal stem cell
CRP	C-reactive protein	**NISSSA**	nerve, ischemia, soft-tissue, skeletal, shock, and age score
CT	computed tomography		
DSA	digital subtraction angiography	**NPWT**	negative-pressure wound therapy
ED	emergency department	**ORIF**	open reduction and internal fixation
FDA	Food and Drug Administration	**PDGF**	platelet-derived growth factor
FGF-2	fibroblast growth factor-2	**PDS**	polydioxanone
FTSG	full-thickness skin graft	**PLA**	polylactic acid
GCS	Glasgow coma scale	**PMMA**	polymethyl methacrylate
HFS	Hanover fracture scale	**PMN**	polymorphonuclear leukocyte
HIT	heparin-induced thrombocytopenia	**pO2**	partial oxygen pressure
HPL	high-pressure lavage	**psi**	pounds per square inch (1 psi = 0.07 atmospheres)
IL	interleukin	**PU**	perfusion unit
INR	international normalized ratio	**SPARC**	secreted protein acidic and rich in cysteine
IV	intravenous	**SSRI**	serotonin reuptake inhibitor
LDF	laser Doppler flowmetry	**STSG**	split-thickness skin graft
LEAP	lower extremity assessment project	**TGF-β**	transforming growth factor β
LISS	less invasive stabilization system	**TNF-α**	tumor necrosis factor α
LMWH	low-molecular-weight heparin	**UFH**	unfractionated heparin
LPL	low-pressure lavage	**VAC®**	Vacuum Assisted Closure
LSI	limb salvage index	**VEGF**	vascular endothelial growth factor
MESS	mangled extremity severity score	**VRE**	vancomycin-resistant enterococcus

Table of contents

Table of contents

PRINCIPLES

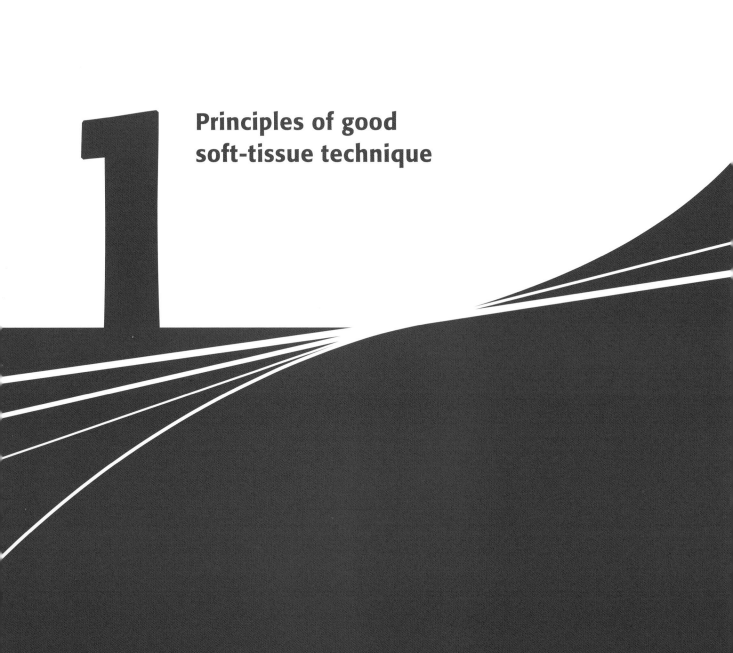

1

Principles of good soft-tissue technique

1.1 Importance of correct handling of soft tissues

Author James N Long

Fractures are nearly always associated with some degree of soft-tissue injury. Often they are merely soft-tissue injuries with an associated hard-tissue injury. While surgeons cannot change the amount of damage caused by the initial injury, they can, through skillful use of instruments and retraction, avoid further injury to these traumatized tissues. Conversely, in the quest to achieve anatomical restoration of a fracture, surgeons too often have ignored the iatrogenic injury caused by wide exposure of the fracture. Even more commonly, surgical assistants have caused further injury to tissues by careless application of retraction. However, extensive soft-tissue injury can also occur without a fracture, and incorrect

handling can eventually lead to functional impairment such as loss of range of motion and chronic pain.

Contributing to this problem is a tendency of surgeons to focus on the care of the fracture while in training. Soft-tissue techniques are not described in detail in classic textbooks and often senior surgeons delegate the surgical approach and debridement to junior members, thereby foregoing the opportunity to teach good soft-tissue handling. This chapter will teach the fundamentals of instrument handling and retraction. Suture techniques will be discussed in chapter 10.1.

1.2 Preparation for surgery

Author James N Long

1.2.1 Skin preparation

While there are several different solutions available for effective skin disinfection, it seems important that their application is carried out according to the specific instructions of the producer and the guidelines of the hospital. The solution must have completely dried before the skin is incised. In general, open wounds should be debrided of large foreign bodies such as dirt, large pieces of gravel and leaves prior to surgical prep because they have to be removed anyway and it is difficult to fully decontaminate them.

Superficial abrasions with embedded gravel, rocks or other foreign debris require special attention. The wound may be gently debrided prior to surgical scrub with a scrub brush of the type used to scrub the surgeon's hands. Care must be taken to ensure that no additional damage to the soft tissue is caused by overly aggressive, course debridement. The goal is to remove loose material, which might come free during the surgical scrub. However, in some cases, material has become embedded in the full thickness of the dermis and should be removed during the surgical debridement.

Iodine-containing preparations (ie, Betadine®, Braunol®) are relatively toxic to underlying soft tissues and thus are often avoided in cases of open wounds. They also impair osteogenesis and should not be used on exposed bone. Alcohol-based preparations can basically present a risk of

fire when electrocautery is used and the alcohol has not dried.

1.2.2 Use of the tourniquet

Tourniquets are often used in extremity surgery to reduce bleeding and to facilitate difficult preparation, for example when dissecting a flap, its pedicle or the recipient vessels. With careful intraoperative hemostasis, however, a tourniquet is not routinely required, particularly during the debridement procedure. Continuous assessment of punctate bleedings during debridement is essential to decide whether the tissues are viable or not. The prolonged application of a tourniquet may increase edema formation after its release due to reperfusion of the limb, exacerbating the edema, which will occur as a result of the fracture. This differs from elective surgery, where there is no preexisting edema or inflammation.

1.2.3 Planning incisions

The skin incision should provide the most adequate and least harmful exposure for the planned fixation of a specific fracture. It should be extensile, which is best done with straight incisions rather than curved ones. Most described approaches make use of Langer lines, sometimes also called cleavage lines. They are topological lines drawn on a map of the human body along which the skin has the least flexibility. They correspond to the natural orientation of collagen fibers in the dermis. These lines represent small folds in the skin, which allow stretching of the skin perpendicular to the lines. They can easily be seen by gently pinching the skin or by examining areas such as joints where they allow flexion and extension of the joint (**Fig 1.2-1a–b**). If a surgeon can choose where and in which direction to place an incision, he or she may decide to cut in the direction of Langer lines. Incisions made parallel to Langer lines may heal better and produce less scarring than those cutting across and thus minimize contracture and restriction of motion. The orientation of stab wounds relative to Langer lines

can have a considerable impact upon the presentation of the wound.

Ideally, the incision should not cross bone prominences such as the olecranon or medial malleolus, but rather gently curve around them to avoid having a scar on a potential pressure area. The surgeon should also take into consideration the possible need for later surgery, ie, secondary knee arthroplasty after a proximal tibial fracture or a secondary closure of a defect with a local or regional flap (chapter 10.4, 10.5).

If more than one incision is planned, care should be taken not to compromise the vascularity of the skin bridge. Generally, a skin bridge should be performed as wide as possible,

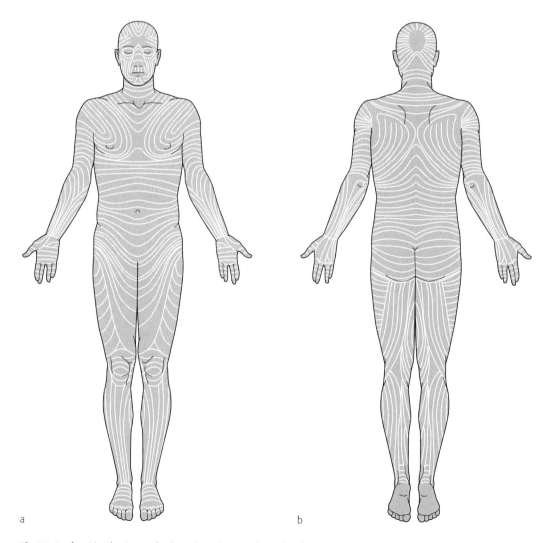

a   b

Fig 1.2-1a–b   Distribution and orientation of Langer lines (ie, cleavage lines) in the adult.
a   Anterior view.
b   Posterior view.

bearing in mind an adequate width-to-length ratio of the randomly perfused flap (chapter 10.3). This ratio will vary depending on the flap's location (eg, lower extremity versus upper extremity, thigh versus lower leg). The surgeon should be aware that swelling, bruising or internal degloving of the tissue between incisions are cause for concern. Also, the location of the incisions must be considered with regard to closure and the resulting scar. Skin which overlies bone prominences is less resistant to shear because there is less subcutaneous tissue. The resulting scar is often prone to hypersensitivity and tends to be unstable.

Surgeons may also be confronted with an old scar or skin graft near the site they would like to make a new incision. If the scar is more than 6 months old, surgeons may safely proceed to make a new incision where they deem necessary without regard for creating a nonviable skin bridge. Skin grafts may be incised as soon as they have completely taken (generally 6 weeks after application), though the graft should not be undermined.

A situation which often arises is the issue of a transverse laceration. This laceration compromises the skin distal to it because it disrupts the longitudinal blood flow within the fascia. However, usually there is also an associated fracture or tendon laceration. This requires extension of the wound to allow adequate exposure for inspection, debridement and eventually repair. Extension can be performed in two ways.

The surgeon may decide to extend in a Z-fashion (**Fig 1.2-2a**) or in a T-fashion (**Fig 1.2-2b**). The theoretical advantage of extending the incision perpendicular to the transverse incision is to reestablish blood flow by ingrowth of vessels adjacent to the zone of injury as the blood flow to the skin distal to the laceration is compromised. The distance from healthy skin to the edge of the incision is longer in a Z-incision than in a T-incision as shown in **Fig 1.2-2c–d**. Extension of the wound using a perpendicular incision is preferred. Acute angles should be avoided.

Despite the benefits of a minimally invasive approach [1], short incisions are not necessarily better than longer ones. Too much traction on the wound edges and extensive subcutaneous dissection can result in poor healing and scarring. Furthermore, the surgeon should be aware that stab incisions for placement of percutaneous screws may put nerves in jeopardy (eg, superficial fibular nerve). For the management of open fractures consult chapter 7.

Finally, it is generally agreed that the less time skin is open, the lower the risk of infection, especially in cases of trauma. However, this should not imply that a less than ideal reduction of the joint should be accepted for the sake of shorter operative time. Organizing an experienced team, not delegating the procedure to less-experienced colleagues, and moving purposefully through the case are ways to decrease operative time without compromising outcome.

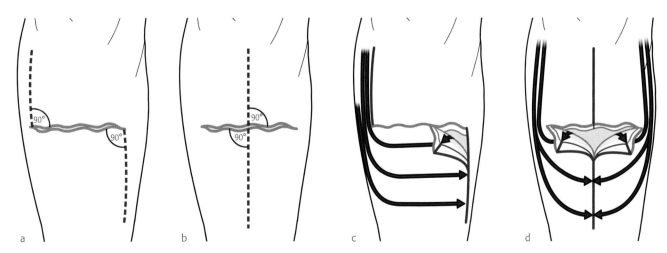

Fig 1.2-2a–d   Management of a transverse wound.
a   Transverse wound extended in a Z-fashion (red dotted line = planned incision).
b   Transverse wound extended in a double opposing T-fashion (red dotted line = planned incision).
c   Perfusion of a skin flap using a Z-like extension technique. Note that blood flow must traverse the entire zone of elevated skin flap (arrows).
d   Perfusion of a skin flap using a double-opposing T-like extension technique. Note that the distance, which must be perfused (arrows) to reach the incision, is halved in comparison to that in **Fig 1.2-2c**.

1.3 Intraoperative principles

Author   James N Long

1.3.1   Choice of instruments

Introduction

Instruments (**Video 1.3-1**) are an extension of the surgeon's hands used to manipulate the tissues, expose the surgical field or reduce and fix a fracture. They should be carefully chosen to minimize damage and tension to the skin and all other tissues, while providing adequate exposure for surgery. Each surgeon has a preference for which instrument to use in a given situation. However, there are some guidelines and caveats regarding instruments, which can be generalized.

Forceps or pick-ups

There are numerous types of forceps (**Fig 1.3-1a–g**) commonly used in orthopaedic surgery. Large forceps such as rat-tooth forceps are used for heavier tissue such as muscle fascia, bone fragments or tendon. Large forceps such as Ferris-Smith forceps are used for the heaviest tissues such as fascia lata and tendon insertions. Small forceps such as Adson forceps are used for skin and delicate tissues such as peritoneum or perineurium. DeBakey forceps are typically used when dissecting neurovascular structures. Smaller forceps apply less force to tissues than large forceps when used in appropriate tissues. Large, toothed forceps such as rat-tooth or Ferris-Smith forceps should not be used on skin.

Beside the different sizes for more delicate or heavier tissues, the structure of the teeth—smooth or sharp (V-groove)—will influence the amount of force or squeeze required to hold a specific tissue. Smooth-toothed forceps (Cushing, Adson-Brown) depend on compression force to grasp tissue and, therefore, will require more force to grasp than sharp-toothed forceps (rat-tooth, Ferris-Smith), which grasp by penetrating the tissue with their teeth. Large forceps such as Russian forceps are used primarily for placement of bone grafts, sponges, etc into a wound or defect, rather than for grasping.

Scissors

Scissors (**Fig 1.3-2a–f**) should be selected according to the tissue that is being separated or divided. They should be well maintained with a smooth action and should be regularly sharpened or replaced. Dull scissors will crush tissue rather than cleanly divide it and should be avoided, especially in traumatized tissue.

Small tenotomy and Reynolds scissors should be used exclusively to dissect delicate structures such as nerves or vessels, while large Metzenbaum scissors are appropriate for heavier tissues such as the fascia lata. A separate pair of scissors should be used to cut suture, because this will rapidly dull scissors.

Sharp-pointed scissors are typically used to divide tissue while blunt-pointed scissors are more often used to spread tissue.

Tissue clamps

Tissue clamps are similarly structured as forceps— with sharp teeth (Kocher, Mikulicz) or smooth (Pean)—and come in different dimensions. The most delicate clamps and forceps are designed for vascular surgery and called "nontraumatic" as they do not damage the vessel wall, which they gently occlude during vascular reanastomosis.

Retractors

There are many different types of retractors. Some have a ratchet device on the handle, which allows them to be self-retaining. Others are held by hand. Retractors are used to provide exposure of the target area such as a fracture.

Some retractors are smooth and depend on downward pressure on the retractor to contain the tissue they retract. Blunt retractors such as US-Army or Faraboeuf retractors (**Fig 1.3-3a–i**) are commonly used for retraction of small to moderately large tissue masses. Toothed or sharp retractors such as Kilner, McIndoe, or Volkmann hooks and retractors (**Fig 1.3-4a–d**) have hooks or sharp teeth, which bite into soft

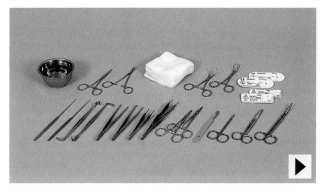

Video 1.3-1   Assortment of instruments needed for soft-tissue surgery.

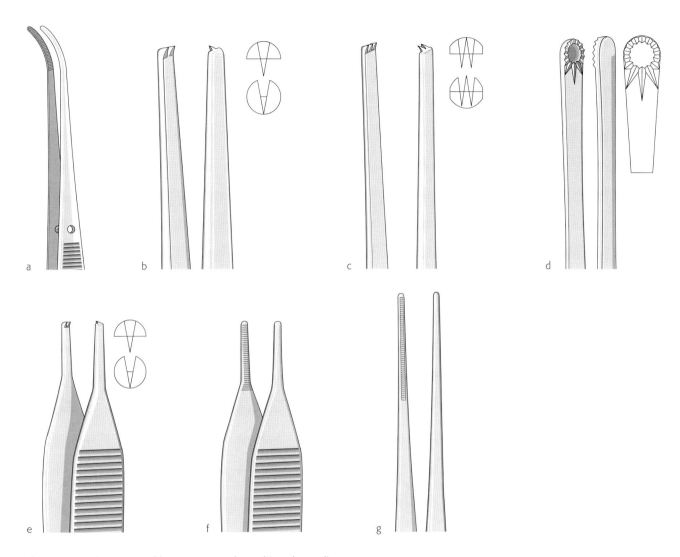

Fig 1.3-1a–g Assortment of forceps commonly used in orthopaedic surgery.
a Cushing forceps (straight or curved), available as noninsulated or insulated (electrocautery) forceps.
b Rat-tooth forceps.
c Ferris-Smith forceps.
d Russian forceps.
e Adson forceps (surgical forceps).
f Adson-Brown forceps (anatomical forceps).
g DeBakey forceps (vascular forceps).

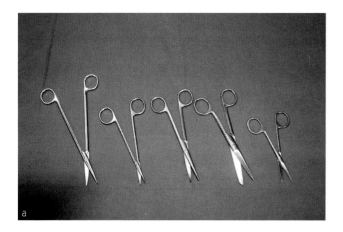

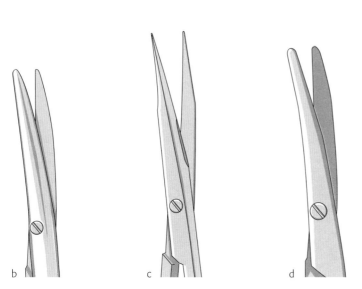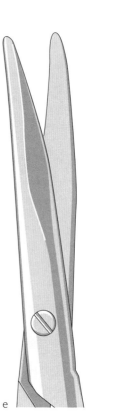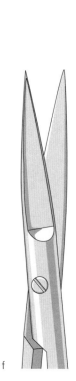

Fig 1.3-2a–f   Assortment of scissors commonly used in orthopaedic surgery.
a   Overview.
b   Tönnis-Adson scissors.
c   Reynolds scissors.
d   Metzenbaum scissors (curved).
e   Mayo scissors (straight).
f   Sharp-pointed small scissors that may be used for sutures.

tissue to retract skin (Kilner, McIndoe) or subcutaneous and muscle tissues (Volkmann). They are potentially more damaging to soft tissue but may require less retraction force. Retractors such as Hibbs retractors are a hybrid between the two, with a broad, smooth blade and small teeth at the base of the blade.

Self-retaining retractors (**Fig 1.3-5a–c**) also come in sharp or blunt varieties. These retractors are used when the surgeon requires another set of hands. Some, such as Weitlaner retractors, distribute force across a large area and expose more underlying tissue, whereas others such as Gelpi retractors concentrate force in a narrow area.

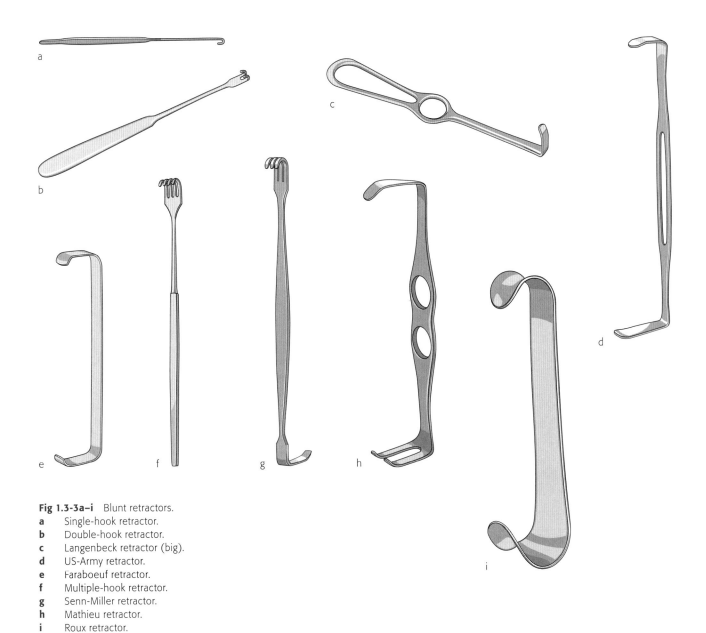

Fig 1.3-3a–i Blunt retractors.
- **a** Single-hook retractor.
- **b** Double-hook retractor.
- **c** Langenbeck retractor (big).
- **d** US-Army retractor.
- **e** Faraboeuf retractor.
- **f** Multiple-hook retractor.
- **g** Senn-Miller retractor.
- **h** Mathieu retractor.
- **i** Roux retractor.

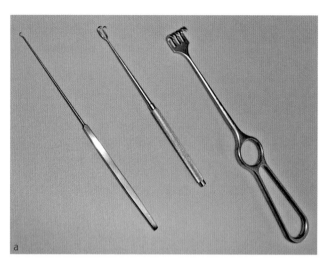
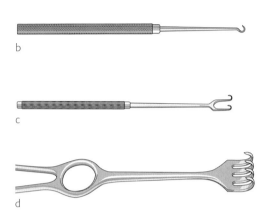

Fig 1.3-4a–d Assortment of sharp retractors commonly used in orthopaedic surgery.
a Overview.
b Kilner retractor (ie, single skin hook).
c McIndoe retractor (ie, double skin hook).
d Volkmann retractor (ie, multi-hook retractor).

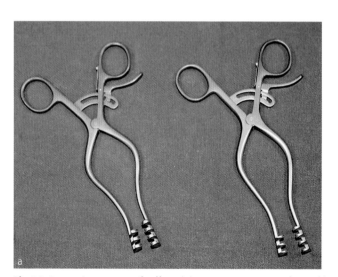
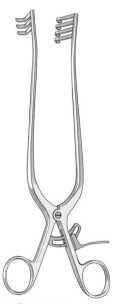
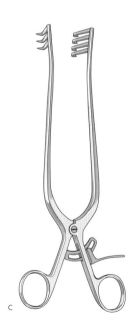

Fig 1.3-5a–c Assortment of self-retaining retractors commonly used in orthopaedic surgery.
a Overview.
b Weitlaner retractor (blunt).
c Weitlaner retractor (sharp).

Finally, lever retractors (**Fig 1.3-6a–d**) such as Hohmann, Bennett, and double-angle Schumacher retractors are designed to be placed around bones with leverage applied to retract tissue. They are commonly used when plating long bones or pelvic fractures.

1.3.2 Handling of instruments

Scalpel (Video 1.3-2)

For the skin incision, the scalpel blade must be new and sharp. It must be held perpendicular to the skin surface and incise the skin completely on the first pass of the blade, rather than making multiple small and partial incisions through the dermis. Large scalpels such as #10 and #21 are typically used for incision of the skin, while #10 and #15 blades are generally used for smaller incisions and dissection in deeper planes (**Fig 1.3-7a**). For most orthopaedic procedures, the scalpel is held as one would hold a pen, between the thumb and index finger (**Fig 1.3-7b**). Skiving and undermining of the skin must be done parsimoniously, as this compromises its vascularity and healing capacity (**Fig 1.3-7c**). The dip of the scalpel is not used, except when making stab incisions for percutaneous pins, screws, etc.

Depending on the surgeon's preference, scalpels may also be used for tissue dissection in deeper layers than the skin. A separate blade than that used for skin should be used, because cutting skin rapidly dulls the blade and, moreover, may potentially contaminate deeper structures due to the first cut through the skin. Sharp dissection with a scalpel tends to cause less tissue damage than sharp dissection by scissors, because the latter tend to locally crush tissue.

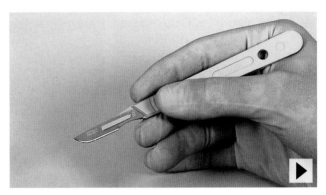

Video 1.3-2   Correct versus incorrect use of the scalpel.

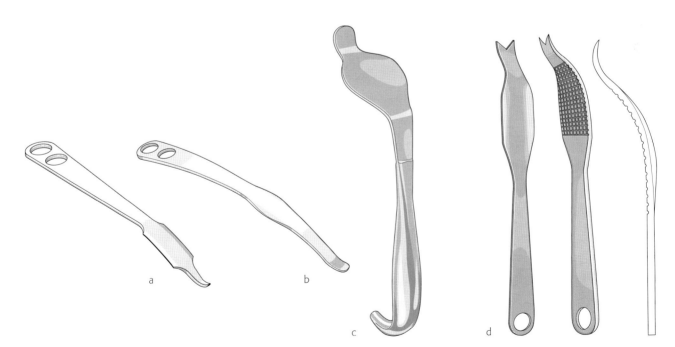

Fig 1.3-6a–d   Assortment of lever retractors commonly used in orthopaedic surgery.
a   Hohmann retractor (sharp).
b   Hohmann retractor (blunt).
c   Bennett retractor.
d   Schumacher retractor.

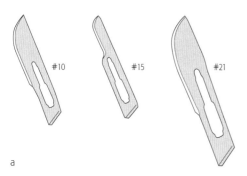

a

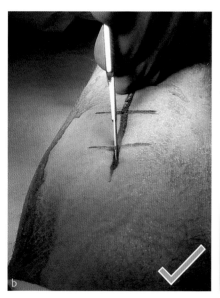

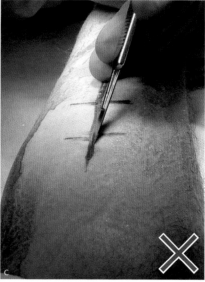

Fig 1.3-7a–c Use of the scalpel.
a Common blades: size #10 and #21 for skin incisions; size #10 and #15 for subcutaneous dissection.
b Hold the scalpel correctly between thumb and fingers like a pencil and make sure the blade stays perpendicular to the tissue.
c Incorrect use of the scalpel. Always avoid skiving (cutting obliquely to) the skin.

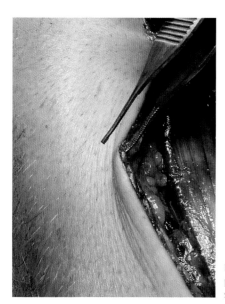

Fig 1.3-8 Use of forceps to lift skin for placement of sutures without grasping the skin edge.

Forceps or pick-ups (Video 1.3-3)

Forceps are used to lift or grasp tissue. All forceps require some pressure between the tips in order to grasp tissue. However, the surgeon must always be always mindful of the degree of pressure which is applied, since crushing of tissue may cause permanent injury. This is especially true in traumatized tissue. Use only enough force to not allow the tissue to slip. Toothed forceps can be used to lift tissue without pinching it (**Fig 1.3-8**). Use small forceps for skin and subcutaneous tissue. Large forceps can be used on heavy fascia. Forceps should also be routinely used to handle suture, rather than grasping the needle with the fingers, in order to avoid needle puncture injuries.

Scissors (Video 1.3-4)

In some cases, scissors will be used to cut through tissue, in others, for example in loose connective tissue, scissors may also be used for blunt dissection. Dissection by scissors should be in a vertical direction (**Fig 1.3-9a–b**) and should follow anatomical structures and cleavages. Longitudinal dissection along the course of nerves and vessels helps reduce injury to skin vessels and nerves. Horizontal dissection between dermal layers and subcutaneous layers or between muscle fascia and subcutaneous tissue should be avoided whenever possible. Similarly, muscles and tendons should not be cut unless inevitable. Muscle insertions to bone are often better released by tangential osteotomy than by tissue transection (ie, tip of trochanter or olecranon).

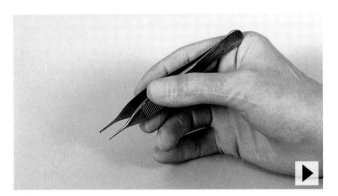

Video 1.3-3   Correct versus incorrect use of forceps.

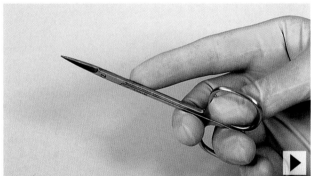

Video 1.3-4   Correct versus incorrect use of scissors.

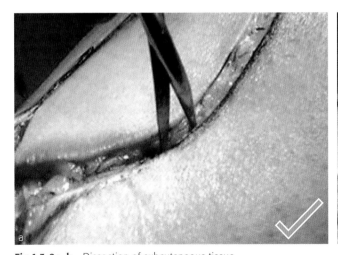

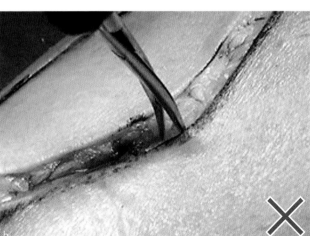

Fig 1.3-9a–b   Dissection of subcutaneous tissue.
a   Correct: dissection following the line of incision.
b   Incorrect: crosswise dissection within the incision.

Retractors (Video 1.3-5)

Using retractors, the surgeon needs to find a balance between adequate exposure and avoiding injury to the tissues under strain. Assistants should always be conscious of how much pressure is being applied to the already traumatized soft parts. When the surgeon is not actively working in the wound, retraction must generally be released in order to allow the tissues to relax and reperfuse. Great care should be taken not to place excessive traction on neurovascular structures.

Just as important as the pressure applied to retractors is the length of time in which they are actually retracting. When a retractor is being used, local microvascular ischemia is created because of direct pressure on capillaries. Therefore, when the surgeon does not need to view the area exposed by the retractor, its hold should be released.

Whenever possible, retractors should be placed as deeply as possible. Virtually never should retractors be placed between the epidermal and dermal layers of the skin. While the assistant(s) usually hold the retractor, it is the responsibility of the surgeon to bring the retractor into the correct position and to instruct and supervise its careful use.

Special care should be used when employing lever retractors. These retractors can provide a great deal of pressure on the soft tissues, yet are relatively easy for the assistant to hold. Thus, they tend to be retracted too much compared to other handheld retractors. Likewise, self-retaining retractors may also be dangerous because there is a tendency to forget releasing them once they are placed but are no longer needed. They may also be a tendency to forget them after being placed as widely spread as possible, although this may only be required during a small part of the procedure.

Sharp retractors are more likely to cause damage to adjacent neurovascular structures because their teeth are buried in tissue. They should be used with care around these structures.

When working without an assistant, a suture may be placed through the wound edge and then brought through adjacent skin to provide retraction.

1.3.3 Achieving hemostasis (Video 1.3-6)

Hemostasis is an important part of surgery. Poor hemostasis not only obscures the operative field but also may cause excessive intraoperative blood loss. It can also lead to wound complications due to hematoma, postoperative pain and infection. Meticulous hemostasis will considerably help to prevent hematoma formation and allow the wound to heal without the need to enzymatically degrade hemoglobin by-products and to deprive bacteria of a potential growth medium, which decreases the risk of infection [2]. Hemostasis may be achieved by the use of direct or indirect compression, electrocautery or vascular occlusion (ie, vessel ligation, vascular clip).

All students are taught to use direct pressure to control bleeding by clot formation. However, this may only be temporarily effective and makes it difficult to see the bleeding vessel in order to cauterize or ligate it. Therefore, local

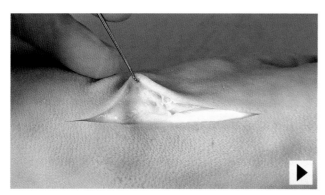

Video 1.3-5 Correct versus incorrect use of retractors.

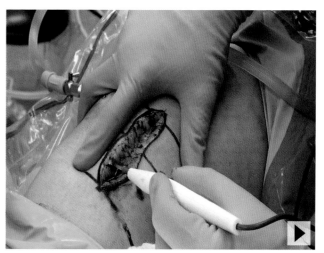

Video 1.3-6 Correct versus incorrect hemostasis techniques.

compression is more useful for emergency control of larger vessels, which are subsequently ligated or clipped. To control small bleeders, pressure is applied to the skin adjacent to the bleeding vessel. This allows the surgeon to identify and grasp the vascular stump selectively with an Adson forceps and cauterize it precisely. In deeper tissues, a sponge can first be applied to the bleeding area, which is then gently rolled away from the lacerated vessel to expose it. Although this seems intuitively obvious, it is often neglected and large areas of tissue are cauterized uncritically, inducing areas of tissue necrosis. Indirect pressure may be applied to the skin by using a self-retaining retractor, which—although not very elegant—may stop skin bleeders long enough to allow clot formation.

Bipolar electrocautery is used in areas where there is risk of damage to adjacent sensitive tissues, such as in hand surgery. Bipolar electrocautery is more precise because current only flows through the tissue between the electrodes. It does not have as wide an area of effect, though and typically uses lower current. For this reason, with larger vessels, it may not be as effective as tying off the vessel.

Care should also be taken to avoid inadvertent injury to the skin when the forceps are allowed to rest against the skin while electrocautery is applied. Furthermore, electrocautery should be precise, targeting only the individual vessel, rather than an entire area of tissue. As an alternative and for larger vessels ligation or clipping may be safer than electrocautery.

1.3.4 Removal of blood from the operative field
(Video 1.3-6)

Blood may be removed from the operative field either by absorptive sponge or by suction. When utilizing suction, it is important to note any bleeding vessels and cauterize actively bleeding vessels, rather than to continue to suction blood. Sponges can be used to apply direct pressure to small bleeding vessels long enough to stop bleeding. They should be used to blot rather than rub or swipe the tissue, in order to avoid knocking loose any clot, which may have formed.

References and further reading

[1]   **Helfet D, Suk M** (2004) Minimally invasive percutaneous plate osteosynthesis of fractures of the distal tibia. *Instr Course Lect;* 53: 471–475.

[2]   **Lorenz HP, Longaker MT** (2006) Wound healing: repair biology and wound and scar treatment. *Mathes SJ (ed), Plastic Surgery, Vol. 1.* 2nd ed. Philadelphia: Saunders Elsevier, 209–234.

2

Basic anatomical principles and functions of soft tissue and bone

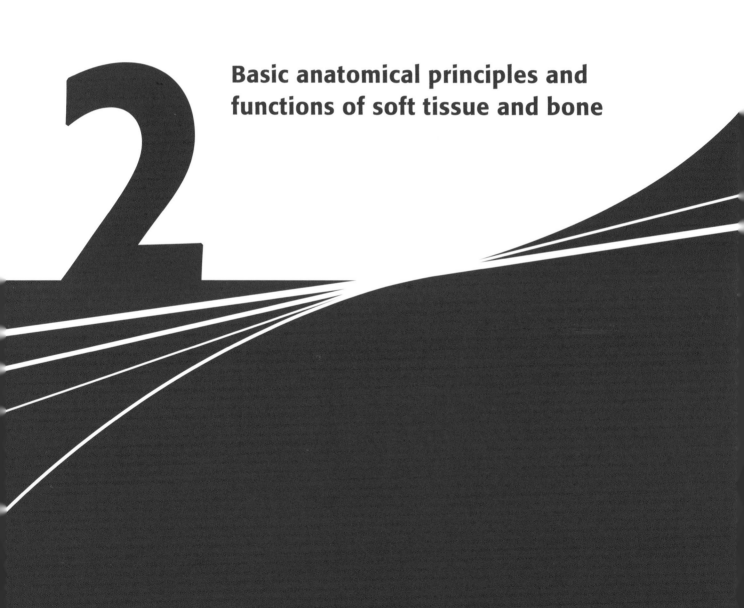

2.1 General anatomical considerations

Authors   Reto Wettstein, Dominique Erni

The musculoskeletal system may be considered as an inter-connected system of bones and muscles, which is responsible for locomotion. For detailed histomorphologic analysis, one would differentiate the following tissue units: skin, subcutaneous tissue, tendon-muscle and bone-joint. However, from a functional point of view, a distinction can plausibly be made between a skin-subcutaneous and a bone-muscle unit.

Several physiological functions have been attributed to the skin-subcutaneous tissue unit, such as a mechanical barrier function, preventing the invasion of bacteria and the infiltration of chemicals, homeostatic and thermostatic regulation, motion, respectively gliding as well as cushioning, eg, by palmar and plantar fat pads. Adipose tissue is specifically involved in energy and vitamin storage, serves endocrine functions, and functions as a stem cell reservoir.

The bone-muscle unit has been studied intensively for its biomechanical properties (stability, motion/movement, force transmission). The two functional subunits—bone and muscle—are interconnected, and their anatomical position is maintained by the fascial system. Neurovascular structures support their function, except in cartilaginous tissue.

The following texts illustrate the specifics of both, the soft tissues and the bone, starting out with the fascial system. Special emphasis is on the basic knowledge and the description of the vascular anatomy, a prerequisite for surgeons dealing with soft-tissue injuries and defects.

2.2 Fascial system: a connective tissue framework

Authors   Reto Wettstein, Dominique Erni

2.2.1   Introduction

The core of the continuous fascial system, which penetrates and permeates all tissue layers, is formed by bone and periosteum. The fascial system forms a 3-D scaffold responsible for the compartmentalization of the muscle-tendon unit and the differentiation of the subcutaneous tissue into a superficial and a deep layer before it merges into the reticular dermis. The dimensions and strength of these connective-tissue bands and their attachment to the dermis determine the mobility of the skin relative to the underlying structures and, thus, its stability. The main function of the fascial system lies in the maintenance of structural integrity, ie, the support and protection of the soft-tissue envelope. In case of trauma, the fascial tissue plays an essential role in tissue repair as this framework—rich in vessels—can provide a well-vascularized tissue matrix, allowing for rapid regeneration.

The fascial framework is a continuous syncytium of dense fibrous and loose areolar connective tissue, comparable to the walls of a honeycomb. The neurovascular elements are embedded in this connective tissue and follow the framework that serves as a scaffold down to the microscopic level. If the connective tissue is rigid and tear resistant, such as in intermuscular septa, periosteum, or deep fascia, (ie, muscle fascia), the neurovascular structures run beside or along it. If the connective tissue is loose, the vessels and nerves run within it as in the superficial fascia of the skin (**Fig 2.2-1**). Occasionally neurovascular structures and tendons are found in fibrous sheaths or canals within bone, providing stability and protection against bowstringing of tendons. Loose areolar tissue within these tunnels allows the arteries to pulsate and the veins to dilate.

From a pathophysiological point of view, the fascial system can form an anatomical barrier to tumor growth and infiltration. It can also be a site of potential inflammation (eg, plantar fasciitis) or infection (eg, panniculitis, cellulitis, fasciitis,) allowing them to spread (eg, necrotizing fasciitis). Furthermore, the fascial system may constitute a strong limitation in posttraumatic and postischemic swelling, initiating a cascade, which leads to the clinical picture of compartment syndrome.

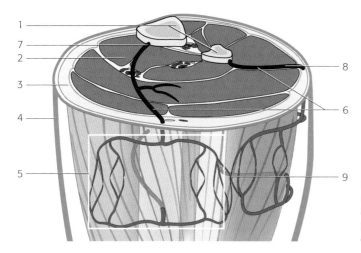

Fig 2.2-1 3-D tissue segment schematically showing bone (1), muscle (2), subcutaneous tissue (3), and skin (4) with its angiosomes (5) originating from source vessels (6) that either perforate muscles (7) or run within septa (8). Angiosomes are interconnected by choke vessels and anastomoses (9).

The knowledge of the vascular anatomy integrated within this fascial system is a prerequisite for any surgeon who intends to adequately deal with soft-tissue trauma or major flap surgery.

This vascular system is differentiated into:
- vascular axes and source vessels
- vascular arrangement
- vascular plexuses
- microcirculation
- venous drainage.

This is essential in order to illustrate the different levels of blood flow from the heart to the muscle, subcutaneous tissue, and skin as well as backflow in the venous system, and to appreciate the vascular organization within these tissues, especially the physiologically most active zones for the exchange of metabolites, ie, the microcirculation.

2.2.2 Vascular axes and source vessels

Starting at the level of the groin and axilla, respectively, the arborization of the major arteries and veins provides source vessels for different flaps that can be isolated for specific indications. The anatomical details of the vascular tree, in particular the one of the lower extremity, is described in chapter 10.3.

2.2.3 Vascular arrangement

Arterial injection studies of source vessels (segmental and distributing arteries) have proven the existence of 3-D units consisting of skin and underlying deep tissue, forming vascular territories [1, 2]. These are called angiosomes (**Fig 2.2-1, 2.2-2a–b**). On the next level embedded within such vascular territories, the blood supply to the skin is provided by two main sources:
- a direct cutaneous vascular system
- a musculocutaneous vascular network [3].

The cutaneous vascular system runs through structures such as fascia or septa of muscles. The musculocutaneous vascular network consists of three types of vessels:
- **segmental arteries,** which are a direct extension of the aorta. They generally run beneath the muscles and are accompanied by a single large vein and often by a peripheral nerve [4].
- **perforating vessels,** passing through septa or muscles (true muscle perforators). They serve as connections from segmental vessels to the cutaneous circulation. These vessels or perforators form ramifications to supply the muscles with blood [5].
- **cutaneous vessels** consisting of musculocutaneous arteries which run perpendicular to the skin surface, and direct cutaneous vessels, which run parallel to the skin. The latter can be divided into a fascial, subcutaneous, and cutaneous plexus (**Fig 2.2-3**).

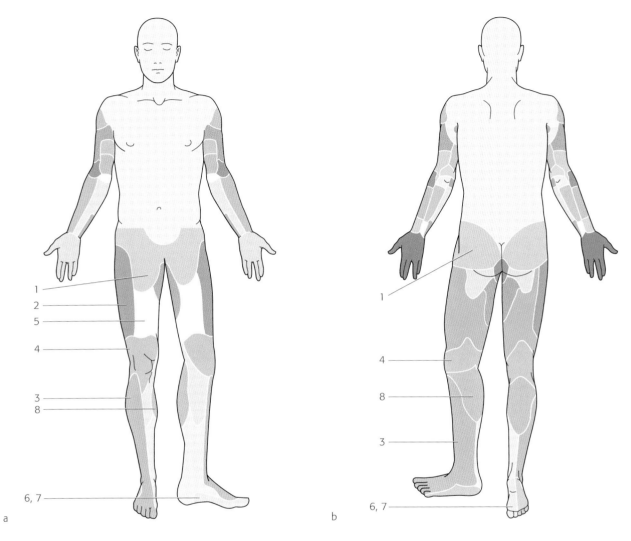

Fig 2.2-2a–b   Angiosomes of the body's extremities and their importance for flap surgery.
a   Anterior view
b   Posterior view.
   1 Groin flap (superficial iliac circumflex artery).
   2 Anterolateral thigh flap (descending or horizontal branch originating from the lateral circumflex femoral artery).
   3 Lateral supramalleolar flap (lateral malleolar artery originating from the fibular artery).
   4 Saphenous flap (terminal branch of the descending genicular artery).
   5 Distal medial thigh flap (medial collateral artery originating from the popliteal artery).
   6 Medial foot flap (cutaneous branch originating from the medial plantar artery).
   7 Medial plantar artery flap, the so-called instep flap (medial plantar artery).
   8 Sural artery flap (sural artery with reversed flow).

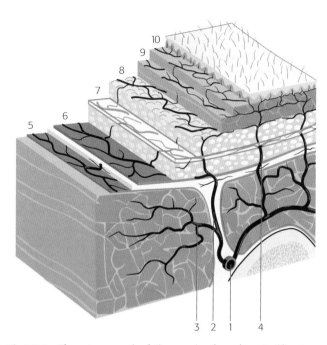

Fig 2.2-3 The cutaneous circulation passing through septa (direct cutaneous system) or perforating muscles (musculocutaneous system). Subdivision into horizontal plexuses. The segmental artery (1) splits into the septocutaneous (2), muscular (3), and musculocutaneous (4) branches. The septocutaneous and musculocutaneous vessels perforate the deep fascia (muscle fascia). The cutaneous vessels consist of perforating vessels (2, 4), of which only the vessels perforating the muscle are true perforators. After muscle perforation, these vessels continue to run perpendicular to the skin. These give rise to three horizontal arterial plexuses: the fascial plexus, which can be subfascial (5) and prefascial (6), the subcutaneous plexus within the superficial fascia of the skin (7), and the cutaneous plexus, which has three elements: a subdermal (8), dermal (9), and subepidermal (10) one.

Interconnections exist at all levels between adjacent vascular territories and can be true anastomosis or choke vessels (**Fig 2.2-1**). Bidirectional perfusion via vascular connections between adjacent angiosomes may occur, depending on local pressure changes. Thus, compensation is possible in case one branch should be occluded, which permits the transfer of more than one angiosome on a single pedicle, based on its source vessel respectively. In general, the anatomical territory of each tissue in the adjacent angiosome can be included without endangering distal flap perfusion. It is of the utmost importance to know these safe anatomical boundaries of tissue in each layer that can be transferred separately or combined as a composite flap.

2.2.4 Vascular plexuses

Beside connecting superficial with deep structures, fascial frameworks present also a horizontal orientation, and so do their accompanying vascular plexuses. The deep muscle fascia is well vascularized with a pre- and subfascial plexus. In contrast, subcutaneous tissue is relatively poorly vascularized with the exception of the superficial fascial layer. Even more superficially, a subdermal, dermal, and subepidermal plexus guarantee an appropriate perfusion of the skin (**Fig 2.2-3**).

2.2.5 Microcirculation

The vascular network between arteries and veins, ie, arterioles, capillaries and venules, forms the zone of the vascular system where most of the tissue oxygenation, nutrition, and metabolite exchange occurs. Insufficient arterial inflow pressure, venous outflow obstruction due to trauma, vascular insufficiency, inadequate surgical tissue manipulation (ie, incision, undermining), hematoma, seroma, and kinking of the pedicle can jeopardize microcirculatory tissue perfusion in zones furthest from the source vessels. This may lead to ischemic tissue damage, resulting in delayed wound healing, dehiscence and necrosis (**Fig 2.2-4a–b**). This, in turn, increases the risk of infection, which will further aggravate the situation. Maintenance of tissue perfusion in critical situations (**Fig 2.2-4c–e**) by hemodilution or pharmacological substances has been investigated intensively as has preoperative tissue protection, ie, tissue preconditioning [6, 7].

2.2.6 Venous drainage system

There are two systems of perforating veins. Communicating veins are large veins that pierce the deep fascia and connect the superficial venous plexus to the deep venous system. Concomitant veins are small, usually paired, and accompany the cutaneous arterial perforators often present within the fascial system. Another important distinction lies in the distribution of valves. Oscillating, avalvular veins permit the bidirectional flow usually found in smaller, horizontally organized veins, whereas the bigger veins mentioned above are equipped with valves that direct venous return toward the heart. Insufficiency of the venous outflow can be detrimental to the delicate equilibrium of the arteriovenous blood flow. Venous stasis can lead to edema formation and increases the risk of infection, wound-healing disorders, and tissue necrosis.

2.2.7 Innervation

Cutaneous nerves, like the arteries, pierce the deep fascia at certain fixed skin sites and follow the connective tissue framework. For muscle innervation, the nerve enters the tissue at the neurovascular hilum of the muscle and follows the intramuscular connective tissue to reach the muscle bundles. Usually, nerves take the shortest extra- and intramuscular routes compatible with the function of each muscle. Tendon innervation is largely, if not entirely, afferent.

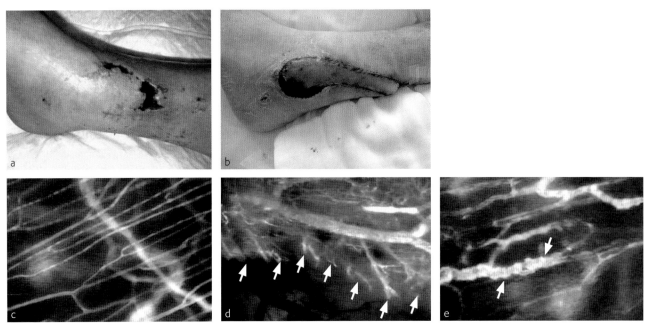

Fig 2.2-4a–e Microcirculation and necrosis.
a Partial flap necrosis of the distal area of a local skin flap.
b Partial flap necrosis of a regional fasciocutaneous sural artery flap.
c–e Images taken on an in vivo mouse model.
c Normal anatomy of capillaries arranged in parallel.
d Tissue necrosis with perfused tissue demarcated by adjacent nonperfused tissue (arrows).
e Microvascular remodeling (ie, dilation, tortuosity) of perfused capillaries (arrows) sustaining acute persistent ischemia.

2.3 Skin and subcutaneous tissue

Authors   Reto Wettstein, Dominique Erni

2.3.1 Skin composition

The skin is kept in place by the fascial framework mentioned before, as can be observed in bodybuilders, where septal, periosteal or muscle fascia attachments that form grooves and dimples become visible. Extensions of the fascial system blend with the collagen fibrils of the reticular dermis. The extracellular matrix of the reticular and papillary dermis, composed mainly of collagen, provides the strength of the dermis. The subcutaneous tissue is formed by adipose cells embedded in lobules within the fascial network and which, in most parts of the body, is divided into a superficial and deep layer by the superficial fascia or so-called Scarpa fascia in the abdomen and Colles fascia in the perineum [8]. In the distal parts of the extremities there is no distinct subcutaneous fascia [9], instead, a barely visible, attenuated fibrous membrane can be found, separating a single layer of subcutaneous fat from the underlying muscle fascia.

In the palmar region of the hand and, respectively the plantar region of the foot, highly specialized tissues are found. In these zones, especially in the foot, which are subjected to shear force, torsion and compression, the skin and subcutaneous tissue present specific features, as an adaptation to bipedal locomotion. The characteristics of plantar skin are as follows: a significantly thicker stratum corneum of 2–4 mm in contrast to 0.04 mm elsewhere, with the presence of a stratum lucidum visible under the light microscope. There are no pilosebaceous units and apocrine sweat glands but an abundance of eccrine sweat glands and, therefore, there are no oily secretions, which would compromise gait. Firm, fibrous septae bind the skin that has a deeper dermal papillary layer with pronounced friction ridges, to the underlying tissues. In addition, a rich supply of sensitive receptors is present. The heel pad functions as a cushion between bone and the overlying skin in order to provide an even distribution of the pressure and to prevent ulcer formation. Loculi of adipose tissue are contained in compartments bound by fibrous septa, which extend from the skin to the calcaneus and the plantar aponeurosis. Although these fat-filled compartments are deformed under compression, the dense fibrous septa prevent an escape of fat tissue from any compartment. The numerous elastic fibers in these loculi assure the return to their original shape.

2.3.2 Clinical implications

The surgical relevance of skin and subcutaneous tissue anatomy is basically defined by the vascular supply and the mechanical strength provided by the different components for wound closure. In healthy, nontraumatized tissue, closure of a single surgical incision does not cause any problems. Contusion, bruising, extensive tissue mobilization, posttraumatic and operative swelling, hematoma or seroma formation as well as underlying diseases such as diabetes mellitus, arteriosclerosis or venous thrombosis can change the balance and cause healing disorders (chapter 4.4). To prevent complications, tissue mobilization should be restricted to an absolute minimum, hemostasis should be optimal, and tissue handling must be gentle (chapter 1). Over bone prominences and in the lower leg, skin perfusion can be critical in comparison with other locations. Multiple, especially parallel incisions should be avoided or carefully planned and the anatomical principles outlined above must be respected in order not to disturb vascularity, thereby risking subsequent necrosis of the soft-tissue cover and skin. In traumatic injuries the amount and extent of tissue damage is often difficult to judge initially and may only become evident after a few days (chapter 5.1, 10.3). Devascularization and contamination increase the risk of infection, which will further compromise wound healing. In cases of soft-tissue defects, a thorough assessment of the wound ground with evaluation of viable tissue and exposure is necessary. In such case debridement (chapter 7.1) of poorly vascularized structures and irrigation (chapter 7.2) of contaminated wounds is essential for further treatment.

From the principles outlined above, it becomes evident that the fascial structures provide mechanical stability and are the ones capable of withstanding any tension associated with wound closure. At the level of the deep muscle fascia, primary closure is indicated in cases of extensive incisions in order to prevent bulging or herniation of the muscle. However, the risk of compartment syndrome must be taken into consideration, and a mesh patch may be useful if a fascial defect is to be covered primarily. The next layer that can resist tension in wound closure is the superficial fascia within the subcutaneous tissue, which should be sutured as selectively as possible in order to prevent necrosis of subcutaneous fat. In addition, an intact layer of adipose tissue between the deep fascia and the skin can prevent adhesion formation. Probably the most stable layer for wound closure is the dermis. Deep dermal stitches can align the wound edges so that an aesthetically attractive intradermal suture can be achieved with minimal tension and so that early removal (4–7 days) of the transdermal suture material is possible in order to prevent stepladder marks on the skin. Contour deformities due to insufficiency of the superficial fascia, adhesion, and stepladder marks are common complaints of the patient postoperatively if everything else went well.

2.4 Tendon and muscle

Authors   Reto Wettstein, Dominique Erni

Tendons, just like muscles and nerves, may be considered as specialized structures within a scaffold built by a reticular network of connective tissue—similar to the body-forming fascial system (chapter 2.2), with which it is interconnected—forming the endo-, peri-, and epimysium, the para-, epi-, and endotenon, and the endo-, epi-, and perineurium. This extracellular matrix framework defines tissue and organ architecture, separates cells and tissues into functional units, acts as storage and dissipative component for elastic energy, and serves as the substrate for cell adhesion, growth, and differentiation of a variety of cell types. Histologically, tendons are composed of an extracellular matrix network consisting of collagen fibrils, containing mainly type I collagen, the ground substance primarily composed of proteoglycans, glycosaminoglycans, and glycoproteins, and the cellular elements, mainly tenocytes and tenoblasts. Tendons have a relatively low metabolic rate and a well-developed anaerobic tolerance, which is important for situations of sustained mechanical stress. Correspondingly, they are poorly vascularized and have a slow healing capacity.

Tendons act as a buffer by absorbing external forces in order to limit muscle damage on the one hand, and by bundling and transmitting the force created by contractile proteins of the muscle to rigid bone levers on the other hand. Whereas fleshy muscle insertions do not induce any structural changes in bone, tendinous insertions produce distinct markings such as tubercles or ridges. In order to change the direction of forces (eg, pull), tendons are routed by retinacular fibrous sheaths (ie, pulleys). These sheaths serve as cover over bone prominences or grooves, which can be lined with fibrocartilage. Tendons vary in shape and size, may be flattened (eg, aponeurosis) or rounded, and are found at the origin or insertion of a muscle, or at tendinous intersections. Three zones can be distinguished in a tendon: the musculotendinous and the osteotendinous junctions with the actual tendon lying between the two. The musculotendinous junction is subjected to great mechanical stress, and muscle tears tend to occur at this level. The osteotendinous junction involves a gradual transition from tendon to fibrocartilage to lamellar bone. This prevents damage to the collagen fibers by bending, fraying, or shearing. The fibrocartilage can act as a "stretching brake" as the cartilage matrix prevents the tendon from narrowing, which normally occurs during stress.

The vascularization of tendons is not very well known and is variable. Vessels originating from the perimysium and periosteum (intrinsic vasculature), or the paratenon and mesotenon (extrinsic vasculature) can supply the three regions of the tendon. Blood perfusion of tendons is less at junctional sites (**Fig 2.4-1**), especially in fibrocartilaginous areas, and at sites of mechanical stress by friction, torsion, or compression. This partly explains the propensity of the tibialis posterior, supraspinatus, and Achilles tendon to rupture at specific sites.

Muscles, in contrast to tendons, have a comparatively high metabolic demand and are consequently well perfused with blood. As a general rule, muscle perfusion originates from relatively short, segmental vascular pedicles at sites of relative fixation, and from longer vessels if large gliding surfaces without fixations points are present. Skeletal muscles are almost exclusively formed by muscle cells wrapped in a muscle fascia system. Whole muscle groups are compartmentalized. Muscle tissue reacts to hyper- or hypoperfusion by edema formation, leading to a change in volume. As the fascial envelope forming the muscle compartments is not elastic at all, this will rapidly result in an increase of pressure within the muscle compartment (ie, compartment syndrome).

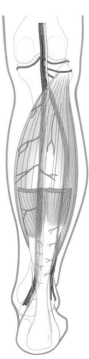

Fig 2.4-1   Muscles, tendons, major vessels, and nerves of the posterior and anterior muscle compartment in the lower leg. Note the sparse vascular supply at the musculotendinous junction.

2.5 Bone

Authors   Stefan Milz, Volker A Braunstein

2.5.1   Bone composition

Bone tissue derives from cells of mesenchymal origin. It provides mechanical support to the surrounding soft tissues, defines the shape of the body, and protects the central nervous system. Bone tissue can be formed directly by replacing dense connective tissue, eg, desmal ossification, or indirectly by replacing a preformed cartilaginous template, eg, chondral ossification. After initial bone formation the tissue undergoes remodeling. In the human body this results in a lamellar type of bone, which in certain parts of the body is characterized by a specific osteonal composition. Osteonal organization is typical for the compact bone of the cortical diaphyses, whereas the cancellous trabecular meshwork is characteristic for metaphyseal and epiphyseal regions of long bones. The level of structural organization is influenced by factors such as developmental stage, age, topographical localization, and prevailing mechanical stress. Structural organization and healing response of bone tissue differs considerably between species [10].

2.5.2   Periosteal blood supply

Bone tissue is highly vascularized and its blood supply follows characteristic patterns. The outer third of the cortical bone receives its blood supply from the periosteum and the overlying muscle vascularization (**Fig 2.5-1**). In addition, substantial intracortical anastomoses between the outer periosteal and the inner medullary microvessels exist [11, 12]. The fundamental importance of periosteal blood supply is reflected by observations in femora of guinea pigs, showing that between 70 and 80% of the arterial supply and 90–100% of the venous drainage depend on periosteal vessel function [13].

2.5.3   Endosteal blood supply

Diaphysis

In long tubular bones, the inner part of the cortex receives its blood supply from the inner vascular system, which is supplied via nutrient arteries that enter either through defined foramina at the diaphyses of long bones or via numerous small vascular branches near the epiphyses. Nerve fibers accompany the nutrient arteries and branch into the intracortical canal system before they finally reach the endosteum and the bone marrow cavity [14]. Many of these nerve fibers are immunoreactive for substance P and calcitonin gene-related peptide, and thus are likely to be related to pain reception [15]. The arteries supplying the bone marrow show a comparable reaction to vasoactive agents as arteries in other parts of the human body [16].

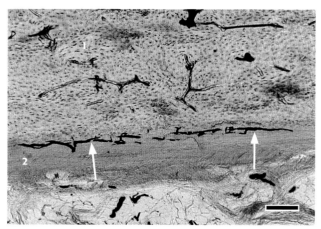

Fig 2.5-1 Periosteal blood supply in sheep bone demonstrated by india ink injection. The outer part of the cortical bone (1) receives its blood supply from vessels (arrows) running in the periosteum (2). Scale bar: 200 μm.

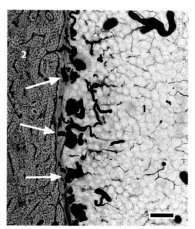

Fig 2.5-2 Endosteal vascular system in ground section of sheep bone demonstrated by india ink injection. Capillary sinuses coming from the medullary cavity (1) form an endosteal vascular system (arrows) near the cortical bone surface (2). Scale bar: 200 μm.

Nutrient vessels enter the diaphyseal cortex through one or multiple foramina, which are often located at the dorsal aspect of long bones, branch towards the proximal or distal end of the diaphysis and provide vascular supply for bone marrow and the inner two thirds of the cortical shell [17, 18]. In the medullary cavity, part of the venous sinuses unite to form a central vein, which drains through a nutrient foramen [19]. Additionally, capillary sinuses form an endosteal vascular system near the medullary cortical surface (**Fig 2.5-2**) with direct connections to the venous system in periosteum and muscle [19, 20].

Epiphysis

Vessels remaining from skeletal growth and development typically form the vascular supply to the epiphyseal bone regions [17, 21]. During growth, the human epiphyseal vascular system is only barely connected to the metaphyseal vascular system by transphyseal vessels [22]. Later in life when the trabecular plate, which represents the epiphyseal scar, is remodeled and the resulting porosity of the bone plate enhances the contact between the epiphyseal and metaphyseal marrow cavities, the connection may become closer [23]. Bones with lifelong persisting epiphyseal scars undergo a change in porosity of the epiphyseal bone plate, which is supposed to potentially seal off the metaphyseal region from the epiphyseal region. An MRI investigation revealed an increased incidence of avascular osteonecrosis of the femoral head in patients with apparently sealed-off epiphyseal scars [24]. Transphyseal vessels, which are more commonly observed in avian than in the human species, have been associated with the spreading of bacteria from metaphyseal to epiphyseal regions, resulting in osteomyelitis [25].

2.6 Regional variations in vascular anatomy

Authors   Reto Wettstein, Dominique Erni

2.6.1   General aspects

The pattern of blood supply may differ in the various areas of the body in such a way that may be relevant for the restoration of injured soft tissue. The thickness of the skin and subcutaneous tissue as well as the density of the vascular plexus within the fascial system are decisive for the choice of incisions, extent of mobilization of skin, and width-to-length ratio of flaps. The specific characteristics are described below.

2.6.2   Head and neck

This area provides the best perfused skin of the entire body. The arteries are usually accompanied by only one concomitant vein. Due to the close vicinity to the heart, arterial intraluminal pressure is higher than anywhere else in the body. The course of the arteries tends to be undulating. Venular valves are only rarely present, which makes venous outflow vulnerable to increased intrathoracic pressure. The subdermal vascular plexus is extremely well developed, which offers a wide range of choice in repositioning avulsed skin flaps, surgical undermining of wound edges, and the design of random-pattern skin flaps with regard to width-to-length ratio (chapter 10.3). Accordingly, the head and neck area has the highest tolerance against wound infection, unless the wound is contaminated with saliva. In addition, in wide areas of the face and neck, remnants of the original panniculus carnosus muscle can still be found in terms of the platysma muscle and the subcutaneous musculoaponeurotic system, which are located directly beneath the skin and provide an additional, highly vascularized layer of tissue.

2.6.3   Trunk

In the trunk, the pattern of soft-tissue vascularization is determined by the presence of muscles with large surfaces, eg, pectoralis major, latissimus dorsi, rectus abdominis muscle, which can all be used as carriers of cutaneous blood supply especially suited for musculocutaneous flaps. Furthermore, there are also subcutaneous vascular axes, such as the circumflex scapular, the intercostal, the superficial epigastric, and the superficial circumflex iliac artery. The vascularity of the skin is not as good as in the head and neck area, but better than in the lower extremities. The lower in the body, the thicker the vascular walls, and the higher the number of venous valves. Subcutaneous fat is thickest in the trunk, which, therefore, is the area most susceptible to fat necrosis and subsequent infection. On the other hand, this may be an advantage if voluminous tissue transfer is required.

2.6.4 Upper extremity

The upper extremity is well vascularized and thus almost as tolerant against traumatic or surgical lacerations as the head and neck area. This not only applies to the soft tissues but also for the skeletal structures. While the proximal part of the arm is supplied by a musculocutaneous perfusion system, in the distal forearm and the hand—with hardly any muscles—the skin is merely perfused via septal and subcutaneous vascular structures. Nevertheless, the hand belongs to the best perfused parts of the body. As in other acral structures, a high density of functional arteriovenous anastomoses is found in the palm of the hand and the fingers [26].

2.6.5 Lower extremity

The lower extremity shows the poorest vascular perfusion of the body. In addition, in humans the legs show a high susceptibility to vascular diseases such as peripheral artery occlusive disease, varices, or venous insufficiency with microcirculatory disorders, respectively edema formation. The more distal the localization, the more critical the situation. Due to the increased orthostatic pressure in the lower extremity, thickening of the vascular walls and shorter distances between venous valves are found. In the calf, the venous anatomy is characterized by a plexiform configuration of concomitant veins, which makes their dissection difficult. As in the upper extremities, there is no musculocutaneous skin perfusion in the distal third of the lower leg and foot, where the skin and fascial structures provide the only vascularized soft-tissue coverage of bones, tendons, vessels, and nerves [27, 28].

References and further reading

[1]   **Taylor GI, Palmer JH** (1987) The vascular territories (angiosomes) of the body: experimental study and clinical applications. *Br J Plast Surg;* 40(2): 113–141.

[2]   **Taylor GI, Gianoutsos MP, Morris SF** (1994) The neurovascular territories of the skin and muscles: anatomic study and clinical implications. *Plast Reconstr Surg;* 94(1):1–36.

[3]   **Daniel RK, Williams HB** (1973) The free transfer of skin flaps by microvascular anastomoses. An experimental study and a reappraisal. *Plast Reconstr Surg;* 52(1):16–31.

[4]   **Daniel RK, Williams HB** (1975) The anatomy and hemodynamics of the cutaneous circulation and their influence on skin flap design. *Grabb WC, Myers MB (eds), Skin Flaps.* 1st ed. Boston: Little Brown.

[5]   **Taylor GI** (2003) The angiosomes of the body and their supply to perforator flaps. *Clin Plast Surg;* 30(3):331–342.

[6]   **Erni D, Wettstein R, Schramm S, et al** (2003) Normovolemic hemodilution with Hb vesicle solution attenuates hypoxia in ischemic hamster flap tissue. *Am J Physiol Heart Circ Physiol;* 284(5):1702–1709.

[7]   **Harder Y, Amon M, Laschke MW, et al** (2008) An old dream revitalised: preconditioning strategies to protect surgical flaps from critical ischaemia and ischaemia-reperfusion injury. *J Plast Reconstr Aesthet Surg;* 61(5):503–511.

[8]   **Lockwood TE** (1991) Superficial fascial system (SFS) of the trunk and extremities: a new concept. *Plast Reconstr Surg;* 87(6):1009–1018.

[9]   **Markman B, Barton FE Jr** (1987) Anatomy of the subcutaneous tissue of the trunk and lower extremity. *Plast Reconstr Surg;* 80(2):248–254.

[10]   **Pearce AI, Richards RG, Milz S, et al** (2007) Animal models for implant biomaterial research in bone: a review. *Eur Cell Mater;* 13:1–10.

[11]   **Rhinelander FW** (1968) The normal microcirculation of diaphyseal cortex and its response to fracture. *J Bone Joint Surg Am;* 50(4):784–800.

[12]   **Trueta J, Morgan JD** (1960) The vascular contribution to osteogenesis. I. Studies by the injection method. *J Bone Joint Surg Br;* 42:97–109.

[13]   **Chanavaz M** (1995) Anatomy and histophysiology of the periosteum: quantification of the periosteal blood supply to the adjacent bone with 85Sr and gamma spectrometry. *J Oral Implantol;* 21(3):214–219.

[14]   **Chen B, Pei GX, Jin D, et al** (2007) Distribution and property of nerve fibers in human long bone tissue. *Chin J Traumatol;* 10(1):3–9.

[15]   **Bjurholm A, Kreicbergs A, Brodin E, et al** (1988) Substance P- and CGRP-immunoreactive nerves in bone. *Peptides;* 9(1):165–171.

[16]   **Lundgaard A, Aalkjaer C, Holm-Nielsen P, et al** (1996) Method for assessment of vascular reactivity in bone: in vitro studies on resistance arteries isolated from porcine cancellous bone. *J Orthop Res;* 14(6):962–971.

[17]   **Olerud S, Strömberg L** (1986) Intramedullary reaming and nailing: its early effects on cortical bone vascularization. *Orthopedics;* 9(9):1204–1208.

[18]   **Shapiro F** (2008) Bone development and its relation to fracture repair. The role of mesenchymal osteoblasts and surface osteoblasts. *Eur Cell Mater;* 15:53–76.

[19]   **Harms J, van de Berg PA** (1975) [The venous drainage of the long bone after reaming and intramedullary nailing. An experimental study of the dog tibia]. *Arch Orthop Unfallchir;* 82(2):93–99. German.

[20]   **Brookes M** (1971) Cortex and Periosteum. *The blood supply of bone. An approach to bone biology.* 1st ed. London: Butterworth, 115–122.

[21]   **Trueta J, Harrison MH** (1953) The normal vascular anatomy of the femoral head in adult man. *J Bone Joint Surg Br;* 35:442–461.

[22]   **Chung SM** (1976) The arterial supply of the developing proximal end of the human femur. *J Bone Joint Surg Am;* 58(7):961–970.

[23]   **Klümper A** (1976) [Intra-osseous angiography of human tubular bone]. *Röfo;* 125(2):129–136. German.

[24]   **Jiang CC, Shih TT** (1994) Epiphyseal scar of the femoral head: risk factor of osteonecrosis. *Radiology;* 191(2):409–12.

[25]   **Ogden JA** (1979) Pediatric osteomyelitis and septic arthritis: the pathology of neonatal disease. *Yale J Biol Med;* 52(5):423–448.

[26]   **Inoue Y, Taylor GI** (1996) The angiosomes of the forearm: anatomic study and clinical implications. *Plast Reconstr Surg;* 98(2):195–210.

[27]   **Taylor GI, Pan WR** (1998) Angiosomes of the leg: anatomic study and clinical implications. *Plast Reconstr Surg;* 102(3):599–618.

[28]   **Attinger CE, Evans KK, Bulan E, et al** (2006) Angiosomes of the foot and ankle and clinical implications for limb salvage: reconstruction, incisions, and revascularization. *Plast Reconstr Surg;* 117(Suppl 7):261–293.

3 Mechanisms of soft-tissue injury

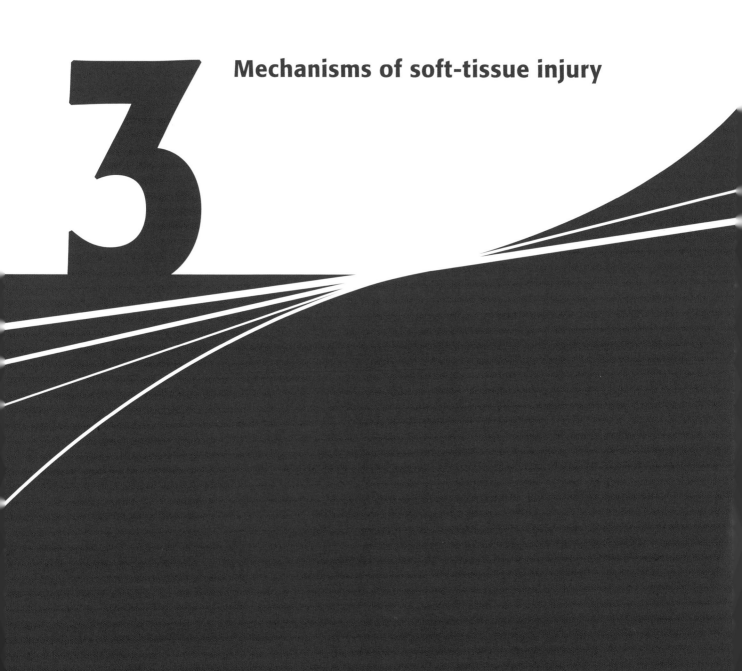

3.1 Blunt trauma

Author James R Ficke

3.1.1 Introduction

Blunt—usually direct—trauma may result in soft-tissue injury, which initially is often underestimated because it presents with a less dramatic clinical appearance than penetrating trauma. The extent of the injury may increase as pathophysiological processes continue for days after injury (chapter 10.3.3). Understanding the susceptibility of skin, muscle, nerves, and vascular structures to blunt or crushing occurrences enables the surgeon to thoroughly assess the condition of the injured area in order to formulate a treatment plan. This chapter describes such mechanisms, with emphasis on direct impact and crush injuries. As with any other type of injury, there is a substantial range of severity, from simple contusion to closed lacerations to devastating crush injuries. While closed injuries may not carry the same risk of infection as their penetrating or open crushing counterparts, they may have equally poor outcomes due to vascular injury or massive muscle necrosis.

3.1.2 Direct trauma

The most frequent cause of blunt trauma leading to significant soft-tissue damage is a direct blow, most often covering a larger area of impact than seen in penetrating injuries and with variable disruption of the integument. If the injury results from a more focal point of impact, disruption of the skin occurs, with possible concomitant vascular or neurologic injury. In a larger impact area, the energy is dissipated. Thus, open injuries are less frequent. However, this impact can still cause significant damage.

In a validated rat model, Crisco et al [1] found that the degree of damage incurred depended upon both the mass and velocity of the impacting object as well as the radius of curvature or dimensions of this object. They discovered a predictable time course of pathology, which follows initial injury. Immediately after impact, the gross appearance of the damaged muscle demonstrated marked hemorrhage and edema near the surface, which extended radially from the point of impact (**Fig 3.1-1**). Microscopically, this area showed intracellular formation of vacuoles within intact myofibrils and clear myofibril disruption of varying extent. There was no immediate change in quantities of collagen, and no early markers of fibroblast migration.

There appear to be three distinct zones of injury (**Fig 3.1-2**): the central or gap zone, directly beneath the point of impact; the regenerative zone, where edema develops over the initial few days, and the uninjured, surviving zone. These zones depend upon the amount of energy imparted to the soft tissue as well as its relationship to the surrounding hard tissues. A relationship also exists between muscle mass and the possibility for muscle displacement. Studies have demonstrated that a muscle, which is contracted at the time of injury, sustains less severe damage than muscle in a relaxed state. In the latter case, the zone of direct injury tends to be

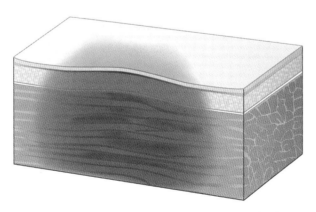

Fig 3.1-1 Intramuscular contusion. Note that the muscle fibers are more or less intact despite hemorrhage and edema extending radially from the point of impact.

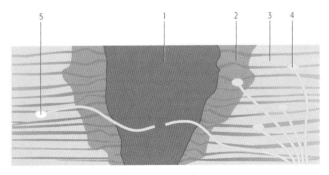

Fig 3.1-2 Three zones of injury in muscle.
1   Central gap zone.
2   Intermediate regenerative zone.
3   Peripheral zone of intact muscle.
4   Uninjured nerves.
5   Transected nerve.

displaced and deeper. The degree of damage initially present may clinically be difficult to determine. In severe injury, clear disruption can lead to hematoma, whereas lesser damage will rather create intramuscular hemorrhage.

A blunt impact creates damage that is highly dependent upon the material properties of the recipient tissue. When a considerable soft-tissue envelope is present, the impact creates shearing forces within adipose tissue, the underlying muscle, and neurovascular structures, which will dissipate some of the energy. However, when the soft-tissue envelope is minimal, skin and bone will typically be the first to fail. In case skin and bone remain intact even though the imparted energy is severe, a closed, complete laceration may occur. This is marked by failure and retraction of the muscle mass away from the zone of injury (chapter 10.3), resulting in an obvious defect. If linear structures are present, these are subjected to similar shear forces. Nerve tissue has very little tolerance in regard to stretching and prolonged compression.

Vascular injury has been described in conjunction with blunt trauma [2]. The degree of trauma inflicted in order to cause vascular injury is often severe enough to also cause associated limb loss, hemorrhage, and even life-threatening injury to the trunk, or a systemic inflammatory response. In these situations, careful clinical assessment, including peripheral neurovascular examination as well as an ankle-brachial index test, are mandatory. The nature of such an arterial injury is rather an avulsion (intimal tear) than a true crush and, therefore, loss of pulses is not consistently complete. Diagnosis requires awareness and detailed assessment. An ankle-brachial index (ABI) less than 0.9 has been found to be 100% correlated with occult lower-extremity vascular injury in healthy subjects [3].

3.1.3 Crush injury

Crush injury occurs when force is applied over an extended period of time to an immobilized portion of the body. Localized ischemia may occur as vessels are occluded by the external pressure. Crush injury of muscles is often associated with systemic effects of the ischemia, and may result in severe electrolyte imbalance, and myoglobinuria. The systemic effects have been described extensively, and are directly related to the severity and duration of tissue damage. They are manifested as an ischemic phase followed by reperfusion of the damaged area once the pressure is relieved (ischemia reperfusion injury) (**Fig 3.1-3**). Products of cellular death are then circulated, causing direct toxicity to end organs such as the brain, the lungs or the kidneys. Less frequently, a physical disruption of linear structures, such as vessels and nerves, is observed, precluding tissue reperfusion.

Crushing often exceeds the elasticity of the skin, causing it to burst (**Fig 3.1-4**). Tissues most sensitive to sustained pressure, such as vessels and nerves, fail early. Therefore, neu-

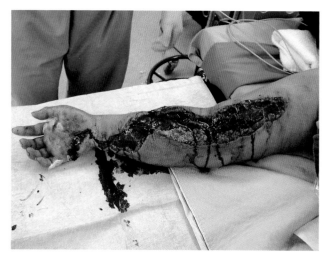

Fig 3.1-3 Arm with crush injury after fasciotomy, which extended from the elbow crease to the palm of the hand. Note the bloating of the arm and increased redness of the hand resulting from a profound interstitial edema and reperfusion, respectively.

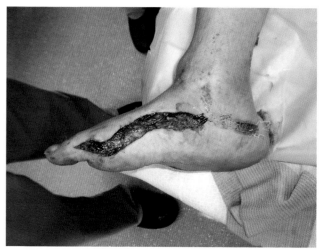

Fig 3.1-4 Severe "deck-slap" injury to the foot, causing overwhelming stretch forces when blunt impact exceeds the elastic capacity of the recipient soft tissue.

rologic deficits and perfusion failure are often observed and can be directly related to trauma or secondarily to ischemia (**Fig 3.1-5**). The clinical presentation of a prolonged crush injury is one of massive local soft-tissue damage, deformity, and associated fractures in the presence of a systemically unstable patient. In order to assess the involved damage correctly, the time interval between injury and rescue must be known, as it plays a large role in the development of subsequent reperfusion effects.

The pathophysiology at the site of injury is similar to blunt injury described above, however, with a substantially wider zone of injury. Actual muscle disruption occurs and hematomas will develop. In the setting of associated vascular injury, compartment syndrome may be imminent, but even without direct vascular injury, the reperfusion of ischemic muscle results in massive edema with delayed presentation of compartment syndrome. One study demonstrated the typical findings of severe blunt injury coupled with extreme capillary dilation beginning 2–4 days after crushing that was mediated by high nitric oxide levels [4]. Nitric oxide was shown to cause the characteristic hyperperfusion, and may have an additional destructive effect on compromised muscle due to increased blood flow, edema formation, and circulation of toxic mediators arising from areas of ischemia. The clinical impact is seen in a brisk response to bleeding when crushed muscle is debrided, and frequent difficulty in obtaining hemostasis.

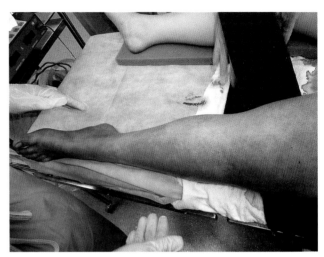

Fig 3.1-5   Severe crush injury to the lower extremity with concomitant vascular injury, which involved the entire femoral artery from the inguinal line to the mid thigh. Prolonged compression resulted in a limb, which was not salvageable. Note the mottled cyanosis present in the distal portion of the limb.

3.2   Penetrating trauma
Author   James R Ficke

3.2.1   Introduction

Penetrating injuries comprise a wide spectrum of soft-tissue injuries, from low-energy stab wounds to the systemic devastation of war-related blast injuries. Their severity is closely related to the affected structures and location, the degree of energy dissipation, and the behavior of the penetrating object within the tissue as well as the propensity for contamination. These determinants are critical for the amount of damage, lethality or long-term morbidity. While clinical treatment and evaluation of these injuries will be described subsequently, it is imperative to first understand the mechanisms leading to these injuries, and the associated pathology. This knowledge of the injury needs to include the degree to which these events impact the victim systemically as well as the associated injuries that are typically seen in

such contexts. This section will discuss such aspects, beginning with a basic overview of ballistic injuries, respectively the study of the impact of a projectile on the human body.

3.2.2   Ballistic injury

In order to fully understand the effect of ballistic trauma, one must know the meaning of several terms rarely used in clinical practice except in the field of penetrating injury. Ballistics encompasses three discrete aspects of the trajectory of a projectile during its flight. Internal ballistics relates to the behavior of a bullet within its firing tube or at the instant of explosion. External ballistics describes the flight path from tube to the object of impact, and terminal ballistics refers to the events upon impact. Terminal ballistics correlates to wound ballistics whenever it relates to living tissue upon impact. As the projectile passes through tissue, the area directly damaged is called the permanent cavity. The term temporary cavity has been used to describe the tissues that are stretched in response to a cavity being formed as the bullet becomes unstable and tumbles. Terminal or wound ballistics will be the focus of this section.

The ultimate damage that a projectile inflicts upon its target is directly related to the quantity of kinetic energy it transfers to that target, which is a function of the composition, configuration, and stability of the projectile at impact as well as the characteristics and location of the organs hit by the projectile. Kinetic energy follows the equation $KE = 1/2\,mv^2$, where m = the mass of the projectile and v = the velocity of the projectile [5]. Projectile mass can vary greatly from extremely small blast fragments to the 3.5 g round of the M16 military rifle to an artillery round weighing several kilograms. Throughout the history of studying ballistic injuries much emphasis has been placed upon velocity. In fact, while velocity is extremely important in laboratory settings, its significance to the study of human wounding patterns is much more ambiguous. In real life, velocity at the time of impact, is difficult to assess and depends upon the shape and composition of the projectile, the distance it has travelled as well as friction or drag from the surrounding air or material traversed. While arbitrarily defined, the most universally agreed upon terms for this subject define high muzzle velocity to be greater than 609.6 m/s (ie, 2000 ft/s). This velocity has previously been accepted as the point at which cavitation occurs within soft tissue. These factors are important in order to understand the behavior of a projectile immediately prior to impact. The most important consideration with respect to the damage caused by a projectile is the amount of kinetic energy imparted to the tissue rather than the velocity of the missile alone. This kinetic energy may not always be completely expended within the target. When a projectile has completely passed through a body, resulting in a perforated wound, it still retains part of its kinetic energy.

Upon impact with a human target, a projectile, whether it is a high-velocity bullet, a low-velocity shotgun pellet, arrow, or even a knife blade, will begin to transfer motion or kinetic energy to the target. The degree of damage is ultimately proportional to this transfer of energy, but is very much affected by additional forces acting upon the projectile. It becomes important to understand the behavior of the projectile within the tissue in order to understand the factors determining energy transfer. A nonspherical projectile with forward momentum meets a countering force acting to decelerate it—this is called friction or drag—which acts upon the leading surface. If the long axis of a nonspherical projectile is aligned with the direction of flight, this simply slows the projectile. However, if the bullet deviates from its track, the deceleration force turns into momentum and begins to tilt it out of the original direction of flight. This is defined as yaw. As yaw increases, the surface of the projectile imparting energy to the target is larger. This is known as the base-immersion phenomenon (**Fig 3.2-1**). A common mis-

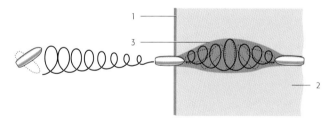

Fig 3.2-1 Idealized flight pattern of a rifle projectile. Yaw diminishes over distance traveled until the projectile enters another medium such as flesh. In a high-energy situation, the bullet becomes unstable and its yaw may increase up to the point when the bullet reverses by 180° and continuous moving end first, known as the base-immersion effect. When this occurs, there is an associated tremendous dissipation of energy into that part of the injured tissue.
1   Skin surface.
2   Deep tissues.
3   Permanent cavity.

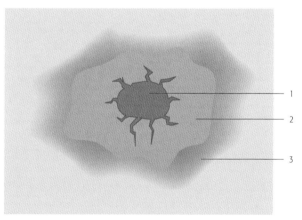

Fig 3.2-2 Idealized pathomorphology of a soft-tissue gunshot wound in skeletal muscle. Surface view. The wound consists of three zones:
1   Central zone of permanent cavity.
2   Intermediate zone of extravasation.
3   Peripheral zone of concussion.

conception is that yaw plays a significant role during flight prior to impact. If a projectile is spinning, such as occurs with the spiral grooves of a modern rifle, then yaw can be counteracted by gyroscopic forces that tend to minimize this deviation. For a variable distance after leaving the rifle tube, a bullet may have significant yaw, but this tends to decrease up to the time of impact. At impact, however, yaw can become more pronounced due to the marked difference in tissue density compared to air, and the bullet thus becomes unstable. In many situations the bullet completely rotates into a base-forward attitude within the second medium. Projectile studies in ballistic gelatin have demonstrated a consistent reversal at a penetration depth that is characteristic for each projectile [6]. The clinical significance of this effect lies in the explosive transfer of energy at the point when the bullet flips. This point can substantially be affected by previous impact with external objects—tree limbs, windows, clothing—or internally by contact with bone, fascial planes or tissues of different densities such as muscle and lung tissue. In such situations, the bullet may either impact with an enlarged surface and be deformed or else fragment into smaller missiles, each causing its own wound track. Occasionally, fragmentation of a primary projectile or impact with movable objects can propel multiple secondary projectiles. The path of destruction that the bullet leaves behind after it has passed is called the permanent cavity, and is divided into three zones (**Fig 3.2-2**): the central zone of permanent cavity, the intermediate zone of extravasation, and the peripheral zone of concussion [7].

The concept of cavitation pertains to a stretching of the soft tissue as the projectile travels through it. While cavitation, or stretching of soft tissues, has been demonstrated at all velocities, the marked expansion of this cavity consistently develops at velocities of over 609.6 m/s (ie, 2000 ft/s). This effect does not create the irreversible destruction that is seen from direct trauma within the permanent cavity, but certain tissues such as brain, nerves, and bone are less tolerant than more elastic tissues such as lung and liver. The cavity is very transient, but does create a vacuum, and it is this vacuum that can impel foreign debris and contamination into the cavity. Ballistic gelatin is a homogeneous material and readily demonstrates the phenomenon of cavitation (**Fig 3.2-3**, **3.2-4**). Cavitation is markedly reduced in living tissue due to the anisotropic properties of fascia and connective tissues. Therefore, cavitation does not have as profound an effect as previously theorized. It may still be implicated in the stretch injuries seen in nerve and vascular tissues in close proximity to the permanent cavity.

The notion that a projectile is sterile and wound contamination will not occur has been disproven [8]. In fact, in cavitation situations, the vacuum associated with the temporary cavity has been demonstrated to draw external material and even bacteria into that cavity. Sometimes this vacuum effect is also referred to as blowback.

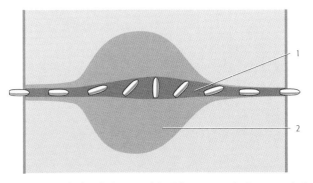

Fig 3.2-3 A high-velocity round (weight 150 g, velocity 863 m/s, ie, 2830 ft/s) that does not reverse within tissue creates a small permanent (1) and large temporary (2) cavity in a straight line. Cavitation in actual tissue depends on tissue planes, fascial compartments, and impact with hard structures.

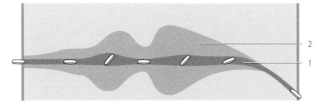

Fig 3.2-4 High-velocity round, which is slightly lighter and slower than that shown in **Fig 3.2-3**. It inverts to a base-forward attitude, creating explosion-type energy expenditure and fluctuating secondary missile cavities.
1   Permanent cavity.
2   Temporary cavity.

3.2.3 Pathophysiology

Perhaps the most important feature of penetrating ballistic wounds that needs to be understood is the mechanism by which a projectile disrupts the injured tissue. Tissue damage occurs by one or more of the following mechanisms [9]:

- **cutting**, due to direct contact
- **stretching**, due to transverse or shear waves created by the transfer of kinetic energy (cavitation)
- **compression**, due to longitudinal or shock waves in front of the projectile, and
- **heating**, due to the transfer of energy in the form of friction.

Much of the early work on wound ballistics was done in ballistic gelatin. This material is isotropic—ie, it behaves similarly in all directions and velocities and, therefore, fails to accurately model the human body. Skin, fat, fascial planes, and muscle layers can have a profound effect on the course of a projectile. It has been demonstrated that a round object requires ~76.2 m/s (ie, 250 ft/s) to penetrate human skin [10]. Notably, a sharp object such as a knife blade or arrow tip requires much less velocity and will penetrate skin with less local tissue damage. As demonstrated in the section regarding ballistics, the amount of kinetic energy at the time of impact and its subsequent transfer to the recipient tissue is of utmost importance. Additional factors include the stability of the projectile within the tissue; its size and construc-

tion; the tissue through which it travels within the body; the elasticity and density of the tissues traversed; the mechanism of tissue disruption; and finally the number of fragments involved [11].

Wounding studies on the effects of wounds caused in certain tissues have demonstrated that density of the tissue is less important than its effective elasticity. When a projectile enters muscle directly, the permanent cavity is linear but will be affected by fascial investments, proximity to bony attachments, and thickness. A projectile traversing the mid portion of a muscle will do less damage than a similar round at the point of a muscle insertion. Once a bullet becomes unstable, it will rotate and this creates more devastation than a linear permanent track. Similarly, impact with bone will often cause secondary fragmentation and multiple permanent tracks. Although less common, some projectiles may fragment even in soft tissues. Nerves and vessels are often spared direct transection, but the tension associated with cavitation can cause avulsion (tear of arterial intima), stretching (neurapraxia), or intraneural disruption (axonotmesis) [12]. These longitudinal structures are more frequently injured if bound tightly within tissue planes or in more distal injuries, where the smaller terminal branches are less elastic. Smaller-diameter structures are more at risk of direct injury and capillary damage rather than major vessels and largely contribute to the central zone of extravasation. There is an additional effect on the tissues that develops over time:

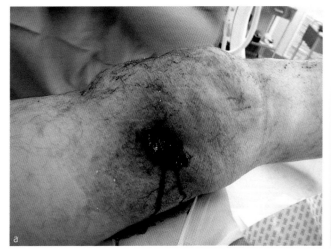 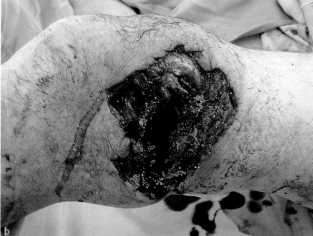

Fig 3.2-5a–b High-energy projectile which penetrated above the knee. Note the severe damage caused by bone fragments created when the bullet struck bone. Exit wounds are not always larger, depending on the bullet trajectory within the target tissue.
a Medial view: entry point.
b Lateral view: exit point.

immediately following the injury, the permanent track is visibly damaged, hemorrhagic, and physically disrupted, ie, the zone of extravasation redundancy. Within 24 hours the surrounding tissue shows signs of contusion, an apparent spread of the ischemia, severe inflammation and edema formation, and residual contamination. The microscopic examination of this intermediate zone of contusion appears similar to that of blunt injury. Finally, hollow organs are more sensitive to the pressure wave that accompanies the temporary cavity. Tissues of higher elasticity rebound from pressure while those associated with noncompressible fluid, such as intestines, bladder, or heart are subject to rupture. Therefore, these tissues can collapse or vessels attached to them are sheared off.

3.2.4 Weapon-specific effects

In general, the effectiveness of any specific weapon relies on its capacity to dissipate kinetic energy to the recipient tissue. When a low-velocity projectile penetrates tissue, it carries only a small amount of total kinetic energy to dissipate. While cavitation can occur with any projectile, the explosive effects are not often observed with low-energy rounds. Conversely, if a high-velocity round perforates, or passes completely through a soft-tissue target without disrupting or fragmenting bone, it imparts relatively little of its total kinetic energy (**Fig 3.2-5a–b**). Clear examples of the variability that can occur with the same type of projectile depending on its imparted energy are shotgun wounds. A shotgun can fire a large combination of pellet sizes and powder loads to propel the pellets, and is very dependent upon range to be effective. Specifically, the smaller caliber pellets seen in birdshot have very little mass individually, yet comprise a large amount of total energy. As these pellets are each subject to individual deceleration, their range is relatively short (**Fig 3.2-6**). The larger caliber pellets, such as buckshot or a single slug can mimic a similar caliber rifle bullet. In fact, the caliber of buckshot is very similar to a 22-caliber rifle round. The shotgun pellets, however, are subject to scatter, and within a few meters their energy begins to dissipate. Ordog et al described three grades of severity in relation to the distance of the target from the shotgun [13]. Type I wound patterns occur at distances > 6.4 m with individual pellets able to cause significant injury, but in general only create widely scattered skin perforations and multiple low-energy injuries. Type II wounds occur from 2.74–6.4 m and consist of multiple parallel tracks of destruction with a high degree of vascular injury of up to 35%. Type III wounds, inflicted at a distance < 2.74 m, are associated with total destruction in a straight path, regardless of shot size or powder load. These can often be recognized by a wound diameter of less than 15.24 cm. Type II and III injuries are associated with major fracture in up to 48%, and peripheral nerve injury up to 58% of patients (**Fig 3.2-7**). Nonetheless, shotgun wounds carry a disproportionately

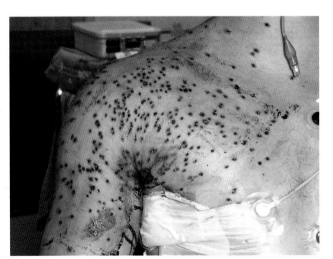

Fig 3.2-6 Shotgun wounds at extremely close range will have an appearance similar to a solid, high-energy round as the pellets have no time or distance to scatter. After a few meters, however, the pellets spread and create multiple penetrating wounds, frequently with complete energy dissipation, as in this shotgun blast to the shoulder.

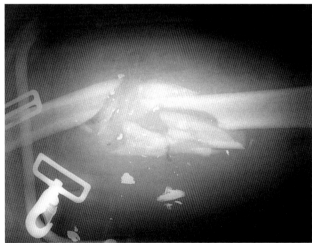

Fig 3.2-7 AP x-ray of a femoral fracture caused by a high-energy rifle shot. The round had first passed through a wooden door.

high rate of morbidity and even mortality in spite of this variability of projectile size and velocity.

On the other end of the spectrum, penetrating wounds caused by knife stabs impart a relatively low amount of kinetic energy, and consequently do not create the widespread local tissue damage seen with bullets or pellets. The damage of a knife-stab wound is most often directed via direct cutting, leading to the very limited permanent cavity of penetration. Injury to specific structures depends on the path of the knife, and unlike ballistic projectiles, this path typically follows a straight trajectory, independent of tissue elasticity or tissue planes. There is little stretching, compression, or heat injury with stab wounds [11]. Similarly, contamination is directly limited to that introduced by the utensil causing the skin penetration, and there is little to no contusion zone.

Much has been written regarding differences between handguns and high-energy weapons such as those used in military action. The basic principles described above apply to the entire spectrum of damage that can be seen. Handgun injuries must be assessed for associated neurovascular injury within the region injured, while nearly every rifle injury will cause extensive damage.

3.2.5 Blast injury

The final aspect of penetrating soft-tissue injury pertains to effects related to explosive blasts. Throughout the world, explosive blasts rank extremely high, both in regard to morbidity and mortality. In recent conflicts, injuries to the musculoskeletal system account for 54–70% of injuries and as high as 78% of these were related to explosions. Injury of the human occurs when the rapid expansion of gas surrounding the point of explosion propagates a supersonic shock wave in all directions from the blast. The spectrum of injuries related to blasts is categorized relative to the mechanism.

Primary blast injury results from the direct effect of the overpressure shock wave on the body, and occurs in very close proximity to the actual explosion. This affects hollow organs such as the lungs and digestive system. These injuries are thought to be related to the intense overpressure, and are rarely survived. In victims who do survive, scattered and rapidly confluent pulmonary hemorrhagic contusions occur, and can lead to progressive respiratory failure. In nearly all victims, a pneumothorax or hemothorax is encountered, but these victims usually do not survive unless

they are immediately rescued and receive treatment. Abdominal injury associated with primary blast affects gas-filled organs primarily, with colon rupture, bowel perforation, mesenteric shear injuries, and resultant hemorrhage. Tympanic membrane rupture is nearly universal and can be seen in all levels of blast injury. Soft-tissue injury is typically devastating, and, with this most severe subset, traumatic amputation is associated with very high rate of mortality.

Secondary blast injury results from flying debris that hits the body [14]. Within the scope of this chapter most penetrating injuries are due to secondary blast. Due to the initial propulsion, fragments can have extremely high initial velocities of as much as 1800 m/s (ie, 5,905 ft/s). All penetrating injuries from secondary debris should be considered high-energy wounds, associated with significant contamination and destruction.

Tertiary blast injury is most often a severe, blunt injury when the body itself is propelled into a stationary object. In these scenarios, the victim becomes the projectile and the injury is typically blunt trauma or impalement.

Quaternary blast injury finally comprises miscellaneous injuries such as burns, inhalation, crush, or radiation injuries, which may also be related to the explosion (**Fig 3.2-8**) [15].

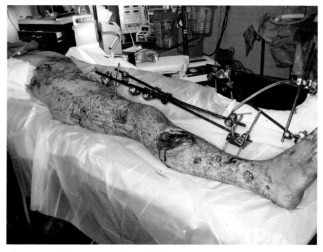

Fig 3.2-8 Blast injury with wide distribution of penetrating wounds. Debridement of larger wounds and stabilization of the limb. Variable size and depth of tissue injury is similar to shotgun injuries with rapid distribution of fragments, but near total dissipation of energy to target tissue. Irregular fragments cause more tearing, irregular wound patterns, and frequently more injury to nerves and vessels than those of bullets.

All these injury patterns are directly affected by the environment as well: enclosed spaces tend to compound effects from additional pressure waves, flying or collapsing material as well as the ability to evacuate the victims in time. Associated injuries such as skull fractures, burns, and penetrating abdominal injuries are common, and require immediate assessment. Penetrating material damages soft tissues either by cutting, tearing, crushing, or burning. This also applies to the pathophysiology of blasts. The projectiles from explosions can be anything from the weapon casing to household items to organic material. While bullets will often follow a predictable trajectory, the fragments from a blast, which are of extremely variable size and often irregular shape, will not. These missiles are aerodynamically unstable, and may even have extremely high velocity or mass at very close proximity to the explosion, but rapidly lose velocity [16]. Similar to shotgun injuries, the injury to soft tissue is directly related to the amount of kinetic energy imparted to the tissue. The variable, irregular and often jagged nature of the projectiles can compound the injury by accentuating the tearing or crushing of tissue. Additionally, these fragments more often injure longitudinal structures, which may resist stretching but are vulnerable to direct laceration. Due to the devastating effects of these mechanisms, the occurrence of compartment syndrome and crush injury is common due to massive tissue damage, prolonged extrication or delays due to mass casualty situations.

3.3 Shear injury

Author   James R Ficke

3.3.1   Introduction

Shear injury occurs when horizontal forces, especially friction, act between an adherent, immobile surface and the more elastic surface of the body. The skin, a durable protective cover, is the largest organ in the body. Moreover, in respect to evaluating injuries caused by shear or the application of a horizontal force to the soft tissues, a basic knowledge of this organ is important. Between the outer epidermis and the deeper dermis lies a strong basement membrane, beneath which small blood and lymphatic vessels run. The epidermis is resistant to shear, while the dermis is quite elastic. Deep within the subcutaneous layer, deposits of fat exist in varying amounts, depending on the region of the body and the individual body habitus. This underlying fat is resistant to impact, but less so to shear forces transmitted through the skin and all other tissue layers. The individual effect of shear force on these tissues depends on their adherence to the deeper skeletal structures. Regions with little adherence may tolerate shear at the superficial layers, yet lose their integrity within deeper layers. This section will first address the deepest layers affected by shear and conclude with the most superficial.

3.3.2   Closed degloving injury

The skin as a whole is relatively elastic, while the layer of microvasculature between the subcutaneous tissue and dermis can be affected by avulsive forces. In locations such as the lower lumbar region, the greater trochanter and the proximal thigh, and less commonly, the knee or the shoulder, the epidermal layer is relatively thick, and can withstand friction better than the deeper structures. A Morel-Lavallée lesion originally described an injury pattern commonly associated with detachment of the skin and subcutaneous layers from deeper fascia in pelvic fractures [17]. This type

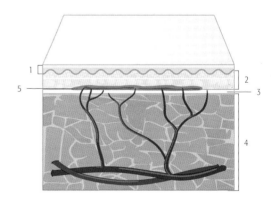

Fig 3.3-1   Pathology of a Morel-Lavallée lesion. A wide-spread, blood-filled space has formed on the muscle fascia as a result of shearing of skin and subcutaneous tissue against the underlying muscle fascia. Occasionally, a bulge forms and fluctuation may be present.
1   Epidermis and dermis.
2   Subcutis.
3   Muscle fascia.
4   Muscle.
5   Extensive hematoma.

of lesion is caused by compression and shear stress at the transition zones of subcutaneous tissue and muscle fascia or the periosteum of bone as seen in run-over accidents. It leads to shearing of skin and subcutaneous tissue from the underlying muscle, respectively bone, followed by the development of a blood-filled hollow space and fat liquefaction at predestined regions of the body (**Fig 3.3-1**). If the skin remains intact this closed degloving injury can persist for weeks or even months, and carries a risk of infection generally thought to be caused by hematogenous seeding. Up to 46% of closed degloving lesions may have culture positive aspirates prior to incision and debridement. The clinical appearance usually is a fluctuant mass with mobile skin, and bruising, but may also present as a solid tumor that could be confused with neoplasm. Once opened, these cases carry similar prognoses as full-thickness burns with severe infection and skin necrosis (**Fig 3.3-2**) [18].

3.3.3   Open degloving injury

In most areas of the body, shear forces cause disruption of the skin. Unlike the Morel-Lavallée lesion, these injuries are due to a higher level of energy. As a consequence of the energetic impact, these injuries are frequently associated with injuries to the deeper tissues, including fractures, disruption of muscle attachments, tearing of nerves and avulsion of vessels. Due to their more impressive nature, they are diagnosed much earlier (**Fig 3.3-3**) [19].

3.3.4   Fracture blisters

When the shearing forces to the skin arise from within, usually due to extensive edema, the lesion seems to occur superficially. Such superficial shearing injuries are called fracture blisters (chapter 12.1) and can appear as clear or blood-filled blisters. Clear blisters lie completely within the epidermis, but the hemorrhagic type often extends deeper into the dermis, compromising the crossing microcirculation (**Fig 3.3-4**). Giordano and Koval found that 7 of 53 patients with blood-filled fracture blisters developed complications after surgery, which were either caused by or located in the vicinity of these blisters, but no complications occurred with clear blisters [20]. Additional prospective evidence for standardized management of fracture blisters noted an incidence of 7.2% of blisters in all lower-extremity fractures, with 47% blood-filled, 43% clear, and 10% a combination of both. This study also validated a treatment protocol for unroofing the blister surface and applying silver sulfadiazine until the swelling of the skin permitted surgery and the blister appeared reepithelialized, on average after 7.7 days [21].

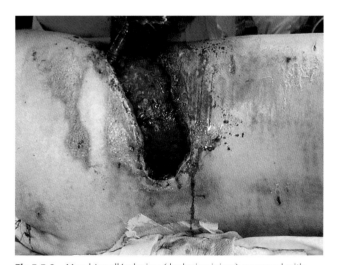

Fig 3.3-2   Morel-Lavallée lesion (degloving injury) managed with open debridement. There is a large cavity over the greater trochanter in a patient with an acetabular fracture. A small open wound reaches into this lesion. The cavity extends almost to the knee and across the mid line posteriorly.

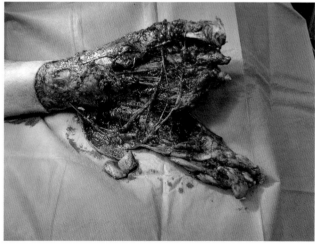

Fig 3.3-3   Open degloving injury of the foot, which occurred when the patient was run over by a car tire.

Finally, the most superficial type of shear injury is that of abrasion, where there is no chance for the skin to retain its elastic properties against the immobile surface. Here skin is literally torn off in layers, depending on the duration of the force applied and the thickness of the skin affected. Depending on the depth, shearing of microvessels within the superficial dermal layer occurs as well as subsequent contamination. With the superficial protective skin layer absent, the underlying structures are also at risk as the rate of exposure accelerates and progressively deeper layers are destroyed by continuing shear.

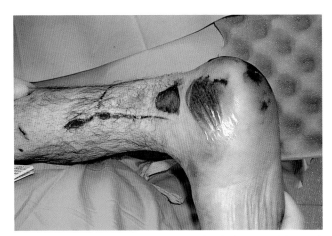

Fig 3.3-4 Fracture blisters in a patient with a high-energy injury and a closed calcaneal fracture.

References and further reading

[1] **Crisco JJ, Jokl P, Heinen GT, et al** (1994) A muscle contusion injury model. Biomechanics, physiology, and histology. *Am J Sports Med;* 22(5): 702–710.

[2] **Prêtre R, Bruschweiler I, Rossier J, et al** (1996) Lower limb trauma with injury to the popliteal vessels. *J Trauma;* 40(4):595–601.

[3] **Peck MA, Rasmussen TE** (2006) Management of blunt peripheral arterial injury. *Perspect Vasc Surg Endovasc Ther;* 18(2):159–173.

[4] **Rubinstein I, Abassi Z, Coleman R, et al** (1998) Involvement of nitric oxide system in experimental muscle crush injury. *J Clin Invest;* 101(6):1325–1333.

[5] *Wound Ballistics: an Introduction for Health, Legal, Forensic, Military and Law Enforcement People.* Film produced by the ICRC in cooperation with Robin M Coupland and Beat P Kneubuehl. International Red Cross, Geneva, Switzerland, 2008.

[6] **Jenkins D, Dougherty P** (2005) The effects of bullets. *Mahoney PF, Ryan J, Brooks AJ, Schwab CW (eds), Ballistic Trauma: a practical guide.* 2nd ed. London: Springer-Verlag, 40–44.

[7] **Wang ZG, Tang CG, Chen XY, et al** (1988) Early pathomorphologic characteristics of the wound track caused by fragments. *J Trauma;* 28(Suppl 1):89–95.

[8] **Tian HM, Deng GG, Huang MJ, et al** (1988) Quantitative bacteriological study of the wound track. *J Trauma;* 28(Suppl 1):215–216.

[9] **Bellamy RF, Zajtchuk R** (1991) The physics and biophysics of wound ballistics. *Jenkins DP, Zajtchuk R (eds) Conventional warfare: Ballistic, blast, and burn injuries.* Washington, DC: US Government Printing Office, 107–118.

[10] **DiMaio VJ, Copeland AR, Besant-Matthews PE, et al** (1982) Minimal velocities necessary for perforation of skin by air gun pellets and bullets. *J Forensic Sci;* 27(4): 894–898.

[11] **Bartlett CS** (2003) Clinical update: gunshot wound ballistics. *Clin Orthop Relat Res;* 408:28–57.

[12] **Lai X, Liu Y, Chen L** (1996) The effect of indirect injury to peripheral nerves on wound healing after firearm wounds. *J Trauma;* 40(Suppl 3):56–59.

[13] **Ordog GJ, Wasserberger J, Balasubramaniam S** (1988) Shotgun wound ballistics. *J Trauma;* 28(5):624–631.

[14] **Baskin TW, Holcomb JB** (2005) Bombs, mines, blast, fragmentation, and thermobaric mechanisms of injury. *Mahoney PF, Ryan J, Brooks AJ, Schwab CW (eds), Ballistic Trauma: a practical guide.* 2nd ed. London: Springer-Verlag, 45–66.

[15] **Stuhmiller JH** (1997) Biological response to blast overpressure: a summary of modeling. *Toxicology;* 121(1):91–103.

[16] **Covey DC** (2002) Blast and Fragment Injuries of the Musculoskeletal System. *J Bone Joint Surg Am;* 84-A(7):1221–1234.

[17] **Morel-Lavallée M** (1863) [Degloving of skin and underlying tissues]. *Arch Gen Med;* 1:20–38, 172–200, 300–332. French.

[18] **Sarlak AY, Buluç L, Alc T, et al** (2006) Degloving injury of pelvis treated by internal fixation and omental flap reconstruction. *J Trauma;* 61(3): 749–751.

[19] **Gwinn DE, Morgan RA, Kumar AR** (2007) Gluteus maximus avulsion and closed degloving lesion associated with a thoracolumbar burst fracture. A case report. *J Bone Joint Surg Am;* 89(2):408–412.

[20] **Giordano CP, Koval KJ** (1995) Treatment of fracture blisters: a prospective study of 53 cases. *J Orthop Trauma;* 9(2):171–176.

[21] **Strauss EJ, Petrucelli G, Bong M, et al** (2006) Blisters associated with lower-extremity fracture: results of a prospective treatment protocol. *J Orthop Trauma;* 20(9):618–622.

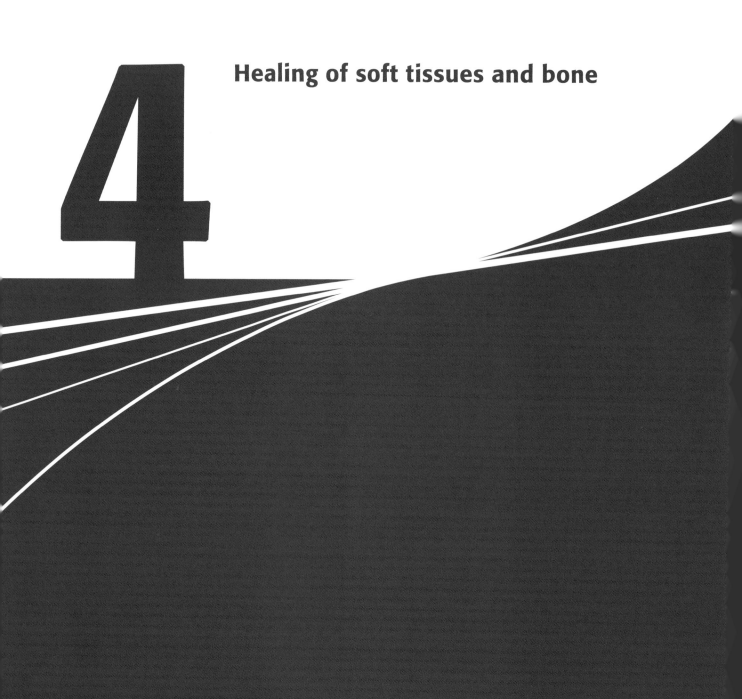

4 Healing of soft tissues and bone

4.1 Skin and subcutaneous tissue

Author   Jian Farhadi

4.1.1 General aspects of initial tissue response to injury

The normal response to tissue injury is a timely and orderly healing process resulting in restoration of anatomical and functional integrity [1]. Wound healing, however, is not a simple, linear process but rather a complex interaction of dynamic processes involving cell-to-cell and cell-to-matrix activities mediated by humoral messengers (**Fig 4.1-1a**) [2, 3]. Knowledge of the normal physiological process of tissue healing and repair helps to appreciate pathophysiological responses. Wound healing is characterized by three classic phases that, however, do not follow sequentially, but rather partially overlap in time (**Fig 4.1-1b**). The three phases are:

- **inflammatory or substrate phase** (hemostasis and inflammation)
- **proliferative or fibroblastic phase** (cellular migration and proliferation, protein synthesis)
- **remodeling and maturation phase** (wound contraction).

The goal of these well-orchestrated biological processes is the repair of the injured skin and subcutaneous tissue with fibroblast-mediated scar tissue. Various categories of wound healing have been described. However, a distinction must be made between primary and secondary healing. Primary wound healing or healing by first intention (**Fig 4.1-2a–c**) occurs within hours after closing of a surgical incision where wound edges are directly approximated without significant tissue loss (this generally signifies full-thickness) (chapter 10.1). Wound closure is performed with sutures, staples, or adhesive. A surgical incision only destroys a limited number of cellular constituents and scarring is minimal. In contrast, secondary wound healing or healing by secondary intention (**Fig 4.1-3a–c**) is characterized by the formation of granulation tissue, which contracts and finally reepithelializes (chapter 10.1). In such cases the wound may be superficial, intermediate, or full thickness. The different phases of wound healing are more distinct than in primary wound healing. Furthermore, granulation tissue only develops because there is a need for final wound closure. This may result in pronounced contraction of wounds.

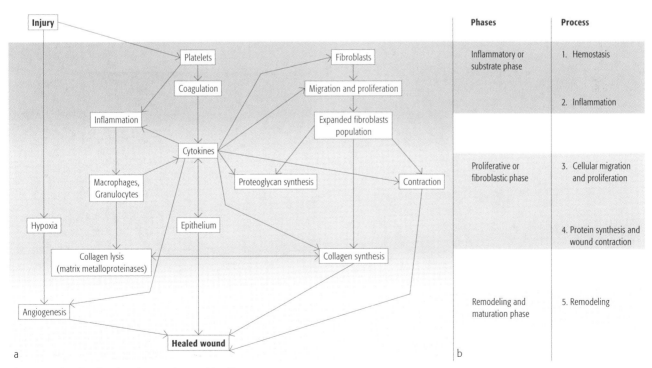

Fig 4.1-1a–b   Overlapping phases of wound healing.
a   Complex cell-to-cell and cell-to-matrix interactions mediated by humoral messengers.
b   The five distinct processes.

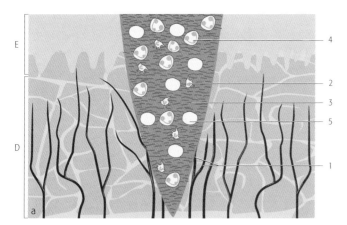

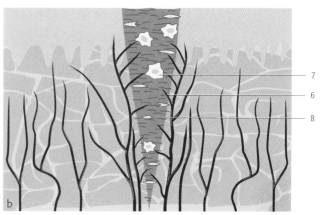

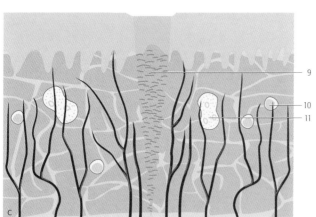

Fig 4.1-2a–c Three overlapping phases of primary wound healing. Epidermis (E) and dermis (D).

a Inflammatory phase (first hours): Vascular dilation (1), thrombocytes (2), activation and release of fibrin (3), transmigration of leukocytes (4) and erythrocytes (5) into the wound.

b Proliferative phase (days): Ingrowth of newly formed microvessels (6) originating from buds and sprouts. High density of macrophages (7) and fibroblasts (8) within the wound.

c Remodeling and maturation phase (weeks): Avascular collagenous fibers (9) replace woundmatrix. Presence of histiocytes (10) and giant cells (11) near sutures or staples (foreign bodies). The epidermal layer has been reestablished.

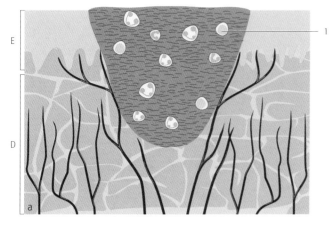

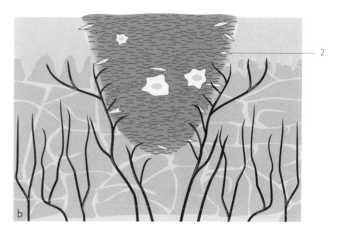

Fig 4.1-3a–c The three overlapping phases of secondary wound healing. Epidermis (E) and dermis (D).

a Inflammatory phase (several days): The wound defect is filled with granulation tissue (1) originating from inflammatory cells.

b Proliferative phase (weeks): Fibroblasts differentiate into myofibroblasts (2), resulting in wound contraction (arrows).

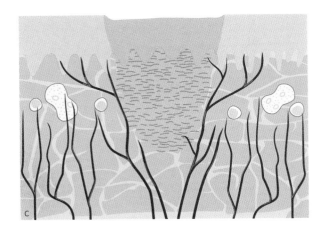

Fig 4.1-3a–c (cont)   The three overlapping phases of secondary wound healing. Epidermis (E) and dermis (D).
c   Remodeling and maturation phase (months).

4.1.2   Phases of wound healing

Inflammatory or substrate phase

Trauma to living tissue creates a vascular injury and bleeding, which in turn triggers the cellular and molecular responses to initiate hemostasis. The healing process cannot start before hemostasis has been accomplished. Any disturbance at this stage will lead to an impairment of wound healing. Key players in hemostasis are vasoconstriction, platelet aggregation, and fibrin deposition resulting in clot formation, which is primarily composed of embedded blood cells, aggregated platelets and a fibrin mesh [4]. Vasoactive amines are responsible for vasoconstriction, which starts as soon as the epidermis and dermis are penetrated. This process also triggers the secretion of prostaglandins, such as thromboxane. Platelet aggregation is stimulated by tissue factors released by damaged cells. Platelets adhere to the vascular endothelium and to each other in a process involving fibrinogen and von Willebrand factor [5]. Fibrin deposition in the clot seals the wound, preventing further fluid and electrolyte loss, and limiting the risk of contamination from outside. Fibrin is also the endogenous mesh material within the provisional wound matrix into which fibroblasts and other cells migrate as the healing process continues.

Inflammation was first described by John Hunter in 1794 as erythema, edema, heat, and pain (rubor, tumor, calor, and dolor). One of its main functions is to attract inflammatory cells to the injured area in order to repair the damaged tissue. Increased vascular permeability allows leucocytes and macrophages to migrate into the extravascular space starting phagocytosis, destroying bacteria, and eliminating debris in order to allow the repair processes to take over [6].

More explicitly, vasoconstriction is followed within 10–15 minutes after injury by vasodilation. Simultaneously, the endothelial cells lining the capillaries adjacent to the wound form intercellular gaps allowing leakage of plasma and cells into the extravascular space. The inflammatory phase is initiated and regulated by the release of numerous cytokines: α-granules liberate platelet-derived growth factor (PDGF), platelet factor IV, and transforming growth factor β (TGF-β), while vasoactive amines such as histamine and serotonin are released from dense bodies found in platelets. Platelet-derived growth factor acts as a chemotactic agent for fibroblasts and, along with transforming growth factor β, is a potent modulator of fibroblastic mitosis, leading to prolific collagen fibril construction in later phases. Fibrinogen is converted to fibrin and the framework for completion of the coagulation process is formed. Fibrin provides the structural support for the cellular constituents of inflammation. This process starts immediately after the insult and may continue for a few days.

Within the first 6–8 hours, the next phase of proliferation sets in, with polymorphonuclear leukocytes (PMN) engorging the wound. Transforming growth factor β facilitates migration of polymorphonuclear leukocytes from surrounding blood vessels into the extracellular space. The highest concentration of polymorphonuclear leukocytes is reached 24–48 hours after tissue injury. The start of their activity correlates with the termination of the inflammatory phase [7]. An imbalance of bacteria against polymorphonuclear leukocytes may lead to an acute infection, which becomes clinically visible after ~72 hours.

Proliferative or fibroblastic phase

Even before the inflammatory phase has come to an end, ie, 2–3 days after injury, fibroblasts begin to enter the wound, marking the onset of the proliferative phase that will last up to 14 days [2]. The process of angiogenesis starts concurrently with fibroblast proliferation when endothelial cells migrate to the area of the wound in order to supply the tissue with oxygen and other nutrients. The tissue in which angiogenesis has set in typically looks red due to the presence of numerous newly developed microvessels. Key factors in the angiogenic process include high lactate levels, acidic pH, and, in particular, decreased oxygen tension [8]. Angiogenesis is initiated by endothelial buds or sprouts deriving from preexisting, intact capillaries at the wound periphery and possibly from the wound ground [9]. These buds or sprouts grow by cellular migration and proliferation and may eventually come into contact with a bud or a sprout stemming from another nearby capillary. They interconnect and generate a new functional capillary network, ie, offering passage for cellular components such as erythrocytes and leukocytes. The two most important cytokines that contribute to angiogenesis are fibroblast growth factor 2 (FGF-2) and vascular endothelial growth factor (VEGF).

The resulting granulation tissue, which is typical for secondary wound healing, functions as rudimentary tissue. It first appears in the wound as early as the inflammatory phase, 2–5 days postinjury, and continues to grow until the wound bed is covered. Beside fibroblasts, inflammatory cells, endothelial cells, and myofibroblasts, granulation tissue consists of a new, provisional extracellular matrix as well as newly formed, patent blood vessels. Granulation tissue approximately contains 30% type III collagen.

Finally, reepithelialization of the wound is crucial for the reestablishment of the barrier function of the skin. Incisional skin injuries, with a minimal epithelial gap are typically reepithelialized within 24–48 hours. During the first 24 hours after injury, basal cells appear at the wound edge and begin to migrate across the denuded wound surface. If the initial injury does not destroy epithelial appendages such as hair follicles, sebaceous and sweat glands, these structures also contribute migratory epithelial cells to the healing process. The migration of epithelial cells continues until there is an overlap with other epithelial cells migrating from different directions. When two epithelial cells meet, "contact inhibition" stops their movement [10].

Remodeling and maturation phase

The quality and quantity of matrix deposited during this phase of healing significantly influences the strength of a scar [11]. Collagen constitutes more than 50% of the protein in scar tissue, and its production is essential to the healing process. Fibroblasts are responsible for the synthesis of collagen and other regenerative proteins during the repair process. Collagen synthesis is stimulated by transforming growth factor β, platelet-derived growth factors, and epidermal growth factors [12, 13]. Collagen synthesis also depends on the wound and the characteristic constitution of the patient's body including age, tension and pressure (chapter 4.4). Collagen synthesis continues at a maximum rate for 2–4 weeks and subsequently begins to slow down. Disturbed healing resulting in chronic wounds often is the result of aberrations in collagen deposition, for example, as observed in diabetic patients or smokers (chapter 4.4). Conversely, hypertrophic scar or keloid formations result from excessive collagen synthesis.

Initially the wound matrix is primarily composed of fibrin and fibronectin, which are gradually replaced by collagen and other proteins such as proteoglycans, the key components of a mature matrix. Additional proteins such as thrombospondin I and secreted protein acidic rich in cysteine (SPARC), which support cellular recruitment and stimulate wound remodeling, are also produced and found in the mature wound matrix [14]. The concentration of collagen subtypes varies among tissues. Type I collagen predominates and makes up 80–90% of the collagen seen in intact dermis. The remaining 10–20% consist of type III collagen.

Remodeling of the scar begins to dominate the wound-healing activities ~3 weeks after injury and can continue for up to 2 years. The rate of collagen synthesis reaches a peak by the third week, then starts to decrease and levels off at a balance with the rate of collagen breakdown. The downregulation of collagen synthesis is mediated by γ-interferon [15], tumor necrosis factor α (TNF-α) [16] and the collagen matrix itself [17]. Contraction of the wound is an ongoing process resulting in part from the proliferation of the specialized fibroblasts termed myofibroblasts, which resemble contractile, smooth muscle cells. Wound contraction occurs to a greater extent with secondary healing than with primary healing and greatly depends on the rate of fibroblasts differentiating into myofibroblasts (Fig 4.1-3b). Maximal tensile strength of the wound is achieved by the twelfth week. The ultimate resultant scar only has 80% of the tensile strength of the original skin, which has been replaced [18, 19].

4.2 Muscle and tendon

Author   Douglas W Lundy

4.2.1   Healing of muscle

The forces involved in producing a fracture almost always cause some degree of injury to the surrounding soft-tissue envelope. This injury can range from very minimal to a severe lesion with cavitation and loss of entire motor units (chapter 3).

The repair process is characterized by three phases, which run concurrently, respectively overlap in time (chapter 4.1). Immediately after injury, the damaged muscle enters the inflammatory phase. Proteases begin to degrade the necrotic portions of the muscle. As the surrounding vascular system has also been damaged, inflammatory cells invade the zone of injury from the lacerated vessels. These cells include macrophages, polymorphonuclear leukocytes and lymphocytes that release chemotactic factors and continue to enhance the inflammatory response (**Fig 4.2-1**). Interestingly, the local area affected by the injury is topographically contained by contraction bands that limit the repair process to the injured area. This intensifies the inflammatory effect within the zone of injury and protects normal tissue from the inflammatory cascade (chapter 10.3.3) [20, 21].

The proliferative phase starts at the earliest 7–10 days after the insult. The cytokine stimulus from the inflammatory cells triggers satellite cells that are dormant in the basal lamina. These muscle progenitor cells are activated and join the damaged muscle cells to promote healing and reconstitution of the muscle unit. This process of regeneration is at its climax ~2 weeks following the injury (**Fig 4.2-2**) and concludes ~2 weeks later [20, 21].

The formation of scar tissue within the damaged muscle is the hallmark of the final phase of remodeling and maturation (**Fig 4.2-3**). Granulation tissue is formed very early in the repair process under the influence of fibronectin and fibrin released from the hematoma. Fibroblasts migrate to the injured area and predominantly secrete fibronectin that subsequently increases the strength and elasticity of the repair tissue. As the proliferative phase draws to an end, the fibroblasts begin to produce type I collagen. Transforming growth factor β (TGF-β) and other growth factors stimulate this response, and collagen type I strengthens the fibrotic scar. The remodeling of the muscle is complete once the fibrotic scar has matured. However, the muscle never returns to its preinjury state as it will always be bridged by scar tissue [20, 21].

Healing of muscle is improved by a brief period of immobilization after injury. This helps to minimize contraction of the muscle edges as well as to decrease the size of the hematoma, which subsequently results in a smaller fibrotic scar [22].

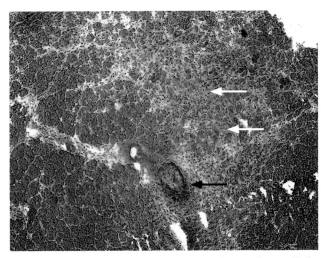

Fig 4.2-1   Blunt injury in a rat muscle at 1 week. Note the myofibril necrosis (white arrows) and the perivascular inflammation (black arrow).

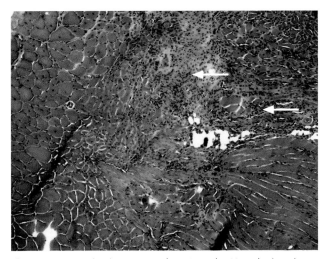

Fig 4.2-2   Contusion in a rat muscle at 2 weeks. Note the invasion of polymorphonuclear leukocytes (arrows) and early fibroblast ingrowth with widespread inflammation throughout the zone of injury.

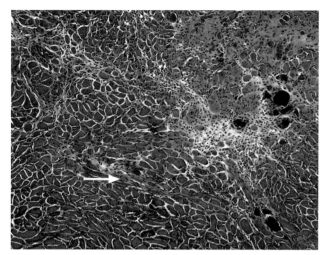

Fig 4.2-3 Contusion in a rat muscle at 4 weeks. Note the extensive ingrowth of fibroblasts (arrow) and persistent inflammatory reaction.

Extensive muscle loss will obviously hamper the function of a particular muscle unit. If there are other muscles remaining, the injured muscle unit may still be able to contribute to the overall function. However, the joint affected by the muscle loss may subsequently suffer from an imbalance of forces since formerly antagonistic muscle groups are now relatively unopposed.

4.2.2 Healing of tendon

Despite the fact that tendons basically are nonvascularized structures, they follow a similar healing pattern to that of traumatized skin or muscle, ie, vascularized tissue. The following process describes the healing mechanism of tendons covered by paratenon. After an injury to a tendon, the inflammatory phase begins with the migration of inflammatory cells into the area. Tenocytes are activated, developing into tenoblasts under the influence of fibronectin. Fibronectin also attracts fibroblasts to the damaged edges of the tendon. The paratenon and surrounding connective tissues combined constitute the source of the initial cellular response. Macrophages help to prepare the torn tendon edges for the repair process [20].

The next phase is the proliferative phase. During this phase, there is an increase in fluid content and of proteoglycan, hyaluronate, chondroitin sulfate and dermatan sulfate in the zone of injury. The gap in the injured tendon is filled by scar tissue comprised of collagen and fibroblasts. In this phase, collagen formation actually can be found as early as 3 days after injury. The initial collagen fibrils are rather disorganized but they become more longitudinally oriented within 4 weeks postinjury [1].

During the remodeling and maturation phase, the scar begins to mature. As the healing process proceeds, there is a decrease in cellular activity in the zone of injury, with an increase in the state of organization of the matrix and a conversion from type III collagen to type I collagen. Tendon remodeling is complete once type I collagen and proteins have formed the definitive scar in the tendon, and cellular activity has again returned to its preinjury level [20].

There are some differences in the way paratenon-covered tendons and sheathed tendons heal. The origin of the reparative cells is still unclear in sheathed tendons, while both an intrinsic and an extrinsic healing mechanism have been postulated. The formation of granulation tissue is postulated as the hallmark of the extrinsic response. The tendon sheath contributes the cells that form the granulation tissue while tenocytes are not involved in the healing process. The intrinsic mechanism is a newer theory, which assigns the source of healing cells to the epitenon and the actual tendon itself. Both mechanisms are likely to contribute to tendon healing with the extrinsic mechanism dominating the process early on and the intrinsic mechanism taking over in the later stages [23].

Smooth gliding of tendons within the tendon sheath is essential for effective function. If the tendon heals with exuberant tissue formation, resulting in a tendon that is too thick or bound to the sheath, the muscle-tendon unit will be ineffective in its performance. Tendon healing requires initial immobilization, followed by early protected motion in order to avoid adhesions. Healing tendons must be protected from excessive force that will endanger their repair. Adhesions may cause pain and swelling as well as loss of active joint motion due to decreased tendon excursion. About 20 weeks after tendon injury, the tendon histologically appears very similar to normal tendon, but in terms of biochemical and biomechanical characteristics the repaired tendon remains inferior to an uninjured one. Although the tendon may not return to its preinjury state, the final outcome is usually functionally acceptable [20, 23].

Tendon healing differs from muscle healing in several ways. The role of type III collagen in the initial stages of tendon repair and the eventual conversion from type III collagen to type I collagen is unique to tendon healing. Both tissues heal with a fibrotic scar, but, in contrast to muscle, tendons cannot tolerate thick scaring if a functional end result is to be achieved [20].

4.3 Bone

Author Douglas W Lundy

4.3.1 Phases of normal bone healing

After a fracture or osteotomy an immediate reduction of the blood flow within the bone of up to 50% can be observed [24]. This is the result of physiological vasoconstriction or disruption of periosteal and medullary vessels [25]. With the onset of bone healing—as an inflammatory reaction—hyperemia of intra- and extraosseous vessels sets in, with a peak at ~2 weeks, which slowly levels off again. Parallel to these vascular phenomena, bone healing itself begins with inflammation, followed by the phases: formation of soft callus, formation of hard callus, and remodeling. While each of the four phases has its own characteristics, they gradually merge, showing clear periods of overlapping as in skin and subcutaneous tissue (chapter 4.1).

The inflammatory phase is initiated by the forces causing the fracture as such and formation of hematoma and lasts from 1–7 days until a fibrous network has been formed (**Fig 4.3-1**). The effect of the hematoma is augmented by a localized increase in permeability of the adjacent blood vessels, while cytokines and inflammatory mediators are re-leased. The hematoma is invaded by polymorphonuclear leukocytes, macrophages, and mesenchymal stem cells followed by the development of new capillaries infiltrating the injured area and forming a network of fibrin, reticular and collagen fibrils. Subsequently the hematoma is replaced by granulation tissue. At the same time osteoclasts start to erode the necrotic cortical bone ends [21, 26, 27].

Formation of soft callus is part of the next phase, which corresponds to the proliferative phase of wound healing. It consists of intramembranous ossification, which starts at same distance from the fracture gap to form a cuff of immature, woven bone, while within the gap fibrous and cartilage tissue is invaded by new vessels as the callus slowly calcifies (**Fig 4.3-2**). This process starts in the periphery and moves towards the center, lasting for 2–3 weeks. Clinically, the pain subsides at this point as the callus becomes "sticky" and axial stability increases.

In the vicinity of the fracture gap, mesenchymal precursor cells proliferate and migrate through the callus, differentiating into fibroblasts and chondrocytes. Thereby the third

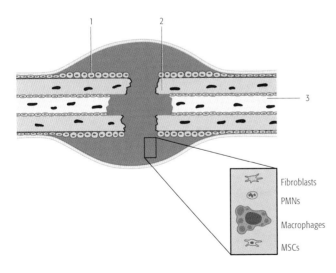

Fig 4.3-1 Inflammatory phase of bone healing: hematoma and inflammation. Note the presence of acute inflammatory cells: fibroblasts, polymorphonuclear leukocytes (PMNs), macrophages, and mesenchymal stem cells (MSCs).
1 Periosteum.
2 Necrosis.
3 Endosteum.

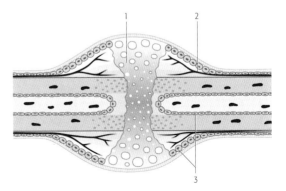

Fig 4.3-2 Repair phase in secondary bone healing. Note ingrowth of new blood vessels from periosteal vessels and the formation of a cartilage anlage, similar to endochondral ossification.
1 Cartilage anlage.
2 Capillary ingrowth.
3 Osteoblasts.

phase is initiated, which amongst others includes endochondral ossification. This process eventually converts the soft into hard, calcified callus.

The fracture callus continues to grow stiffer with time as the fracture progresses toward healing, as the width of the callus typically is wider than native cortical bone and the bending strength of bone correlates to the diameter cubed. This process lasts for about 3–4 months. Therefore, even though bone in the hard callus stage is woven bone, it is strong. In a canine model, torsional stiffness increases until the eighth week and then levels off [28]. If a fracture is exposed to increased strain for a prolonged period of time, the production of fibrous tissue and cartilage in the fracture gap will continue and, in the absence of calcification, a delay of bridging of the soft callus may result rather than bone healing, and the fracture can even result in a nonunion [21, 26, 27].

The remodeling phase is the final and longest period, lasting for up to 2 years until the bone has been completely restructured and has regained its original strength and form (**Fig 4.3-3**). The initial restoration that occurs during the remodeling phase is often disorganized; the order of the new bone is subsequently refined. Osteoclasts resorb the woven bone, and osteoblasts convert the immature bone into mature lamellar bone [24–26].

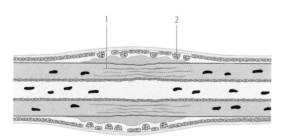

Fig 4.3-3 Remodeling phase of secondary fracture healing. Note that woven bone has been replaced by lamellar bone within the cortex.
1   Lamellar bone.
2   Osteoblasts.

The repair cells that modulate fracture healing originate from a variety of sources (**Fig 4.3-4**). Osteoclasts arise from either monoclastic bone marrow cells or circulating monocytes, while osteoblasts derive from undifferentiated mesenchymal cells that are in close proximity to the bone (periosteum, endosteum, etc) or the bone marrow. Osteoblasts eventually transform into osteocytes, and they are integrated within the new bone as the surrounding osteoblasts continue to synthesize osteoid. The fracture hematoma that develops due to trauma to the bone and soft tissues provides an accumulation point for fibroblasts and inflammatory cells [24–26].

4.3.2   Primary versus secondary bone healing

Primary bone healing, which should better be called direct bone healing, occurs if the fracture is rigidly fixed by interfragmentary compression (plate and screws), resulting in absolute mechanical stability. Under this condition, which is defined by the absence of micromotion at the fracture site under physiological loading, direct healing will take place with new osteons growing directly across the fracture line, interdigitating within the opposing cortices. There is no or only minimal periosteal or endosteal callus formation (**Fig 4.3-5a–b**). So-called gap healing occurs in areas where a small gap (150–200 μm) still exists between the bone ends, and which is first filled with lamellar bone. Thereafter osteons will be able to grow across it into the opposite fragment: Haversian remodeling occurs as the cortical bone is transformed. The induction of blood vessels and progenitor cells is influenced by the local oxygen tension. Areas with a higher oxygenation and decreased fracture strain tend to encourage the proliferation of osteoprogenitor cells that form lamellar bone. This requires fracture fixation that is sufficiently rigid in order to produce an environment of low fracture strain [21, 26, 27].

Secondary bone healing is also known as indirect or intramembranous ossification. This type of bone healing occurs if the cartilaginous callus is substituted into bone by the process of endochondral ossification (**Fig 4.3-2**). Fixation providing relative stability (intramedullary nailing, bridge plating and external fixation) results in fracture areas with an intermediate or rather high level of strain and lower oxygenation, which usually heals by secondary fracture healing similar to the "normal", biological healing pattern by callus formation as already described above [21, 26, 27].

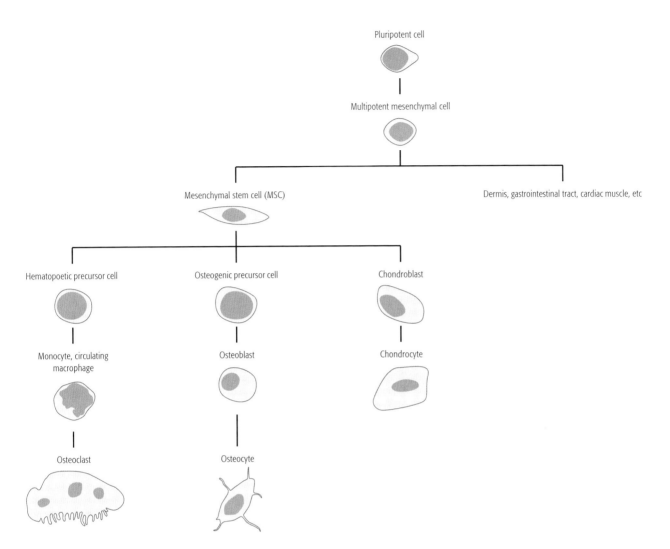

Fig 4.3-4   Origin of bone cells.

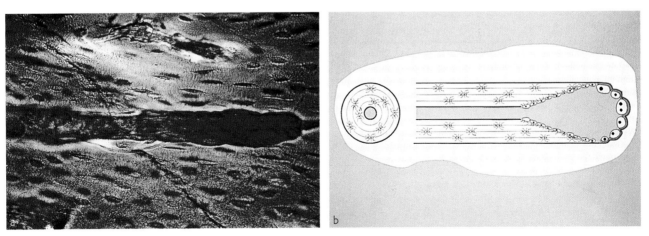

Fig 4.3-5a–b   Haversian remodeling.
a   Photomicrograph of bone after healing by direct (primary) bone healing.
b   Remodeling of cortical bone by cutting cones. Osteoclasts dissolve old or necrotic bone, creating a cutting cone, which is then filled in by osteoblasts.

4.4 Factors that affect healing

Author   Jian Farhadi

4.4.1   Overview

If undisturbed, wound healing generally progresses in a predictable sequence as described previously (chapter 4.1). There are, however, a number of factors which can affect the orchestrated wound healing process, and impairment can occur on different levels. These factors include gender, age, systemic diseases, immune response, iatrogenic factors, drugs, nutritional state, smoking, local and mechanical factors, which may affect any phase of the healing process (**Table 4.4–1**). A clear understanding of these mechanisms of disturbed wound healing is necessary when treating acute or chronic wounds.

Systemic factors	Gender	–
	Age	–
	Diseases affecting the vascular system	Atherosclerosis, vasculitis, diabetes, etc
	Drugs	Cytostatic drugs, steroids, nonsteroidal antiinflammatory agents, etc
	Nutrition	–
	Smoking	–
Local factors	Mechanism of injury	–
	Radiation	–
	Preexisting scars	–
	Hematoma and seroma	–
	Infection	–
	Necrotic tissue	–
	Surgical handling of tissues	–

Table 4.4-1   Factors that interfere with wound healing. Table modified according to: **Monaco JL, Lawrence WT** (2003) Acute wound healing: an overview. *Clinics in Plastic Surgery;* 30(1):1–12, Elsevier Science (USA).

4.4.2   Systemic factors

Introduction

Many common causes such as the patient's predisposition to atherosclerosis, vasculitis, renal failure causing uremia, impaired liver function resulting in hypoproteinemia, vitamin deficiencies, hormonal imbalance, neuropathy associated with disturbed sensation, and diabetes mellitus may often be treated, respectively taken into consideration prior

to a surgical procedure. The treatment of fresh wounds, of course, differs from that of chronic wounds (eg, in diabetic patients) in two respects:

1. Early decision on correct wound treatment, depending on wound extent and the exposure of vital structures (chapter 6).
2. Wound care as such, ie, irrigation and debridement to reduce further damage to the surrounding tissue (chapter 7.1, 7.2). Failure to do so can lead to more extensive loss of tissue as closure of the wound becomes a major challenge.

In chronic wounds it is more important to control the causes of disturbed healing than the treatment of the wound itself.

Gender

Androgenic and estrogenic steroids can affect normal healing of acute wounds. Testosterone and its metabolite 5α-dihydrotestosterone have been implicated in the inhibition of wound healing and repair [29, 30]. Factors such as the transforming-growth-factor-β-activated transcription factor Smad3 are said to act as inhibitors of androgens [29], whereas the proinflammatory and pleiotropic cytokine macrophage migration inhibitory factor (MIF) is responsible for delaying repair in ovariectomized female mice [30]. Interestingly, the male gender seems to be associated with decreased tissue necrosis and improved wound-healing capacity resulting from an increased tolerance to ischemic stress as compared to the female gender undergoing the same ischemic injury [31].

Age

Evidence for age-related effects on wound healing has mainly been derived from empirical observations without adjustment for confounding factors other than age. Age-related changes in the structure and function of the skin do occur. But some of these changes most probably result from chronic solar radiation and its consequences on the skin rather than aging as such. The tensile strength of wounds, the accumulation of wound-healing factors, and the rate of wound closure have all been examined in relation to chronological aging [32]. However, the clinical impact of such changes in acute wound healing appears to be small. Poor healing in chronic wounds, however, is more often related to comorbidities rather than age alone. Since the majority of these chronic wounds occur in the elderly, this has contributed to the conclusion that aging itself may influence healing. To date, the influence of aging as such has only been established in regard to a decreased survival of tissue, reduced formation of new collagen fibrils, and an impaired healing potential in senescent subjects, which is associated with an increased susceptibility to microvascular perfusion failure [33].

Drugs

A number of drugs are known to impair wound healing, but may be overlooked due to the patient's comorbidities [34]. Next to anticoagulants, immunosuppressive agents, ie, cytostatic drugs, steroids and nonsteroidal antiinflammatory agents are the most important drugs. Often, the medication cannot be discontinued, eg, in case of cytostatic drugs or some anticoagulants. The effects of coumarin derivatives and steroids can be reversed by the administration of vitamin K, respectively vitamin A. Yet, the effect of steroids on the tensile strength of wounds is dose and time dependent [35]. Low doses of steroids administered for short periods of time will not interfere with wound healing, nor will it impair tissue morphology, ie, lead to muscular and dermal atrophy or bleeding. With long-term administration of steroids, however, wound healing will be impaired for up to 1 year after cessation of drug intake.

As a general rule, minor surgical procedures at the skin level do not need any discontinuation of aspirin or any other nonsteroidal antiinflammatory agents [36]. In order to decide upon the operability of a patient, administration of coumarin derivatives need monitoring of the international normalized ratio (INR), [37]. If large dissections are performed as, for example, for a flap (eg, latissimus dorsi flap, gracilis muscle flap, etc.), abundant postoperative oozing is to be expected, possibly resulting in an increased risk of hematoma and seroma formation and hence impaired wound healing. These patients might benefit from discontinuation of any drug interfering with coagulation.

Nutritional state

Delayed wound healing is inevitable in a patient with a deficient nutritional state. Regardless of the nature of the wound, a careful initial assessment of the nutritional state is important as it may have a major impact for the further treatment plan. This includes:

- a history including questions about weight loss, appetite, vomiting, diarrhea, eating habits, and current medication.
- a physical exam including search for muscle wasting, subcutaneous fat loss, or edema associated with hypoproteinemia.

- a basic laboratory work-up including protein and albumin levels. Amino acids, in particular arginine and methionine, play a central role in wound healing through the production of collagen [38]. Amino-acid depletion can be caused by loss (nephrotic syndrome), consumption (trauma, burns, sepsis, chronic wounds), underproduction (liver disease), or inadequate intake (malnutrition). The consequences of protein depletion for wound healing comprise decreases in angiogenesis and fibroblast proliferation, which results in decreased synthesis, accumulation and remodeling of collagen [39].
- micronutrients such as vitamins and minerals that are critically important in wound healing and immune function. Many trace metals, including zinc, magnesium, copper, iron, and calcium are cofactors in collagen production, and deficiencies impair collagen synthesis [38].

Smoking

Cigarette smoking has long been known to have a detrimental effect on wound healing. Although the association between cigarette smoking and delayed wound healing is accepted in clinical practice, there are no controlled clinical studies to prove this relationship. Most studies are based on animal models that examined the individual components of cigarette smoke and tobacco, including nicotine, carbon monoxide, and hydrogen cyanide. Nicotine has significant vasoconstrictive properties that can last for up to 50 minutes after smoking [40]. Nicotine has also been shown to enhance platelet adhesion, whereby increasing the risk of thrombus formation in small vessels, challenging microcirculation. Finally, nicotine has been associated with an inhibitory effect on the proliferation of red blood cells, macrophages, and fibroblasts, which reduces the production of collagen and impairs wound healing [41, 42].

Active smokers have increased levels of carbon monoxide in their serum that will reduce tissue oxygenation due to carbon monoxide competing with oxygen in hemoglobin transportation. The result is a decreased delivery of oxygen to the tissues. Similarly high levels of hydrogen cyanide, a common by-product in tobacco smoke, are seen in smoking individuals. The enzyme system selectively inhibits the oxidative metabolism in oxygen transport on the cellular level, thus interfering with cellular respiration. Commonly, patients are asked to completely stop smoking 2–3 weeks before a planned surgical procedure. However, presently the evidence shows that only a 4-week abstinence from smoking significantly reduces smoking-associated complications to a level of nonsmokers [43, 44].

4.4.3 Local factors

Mechanism of injury

In every trauma, with or without association of the skeleton, the soft-tissue cover is involved. A small penetration of the skin may hide a complex injury of the skeletal system, and an extended degloving injury can be missed, if there are no apparent skin lesions or fractures (chapter 3). The history and assessment of the mechanism of injury is therefore paramount in the treatment of a fracture and the evaluation must include a careful examination of the soft-tissue envelope (chapter 5.1). A variety of classifications for the soft tissues and bones have been developed in order to establish a grading and severity score of the injury (chapter 5.2).

Wound conditions

Local factors that can influence wound healing include hematoma, seroma, infection, and necrotic tissue. The latter two are enhanced by foreign bodies such as sutures, staples, and implant material, while preexisting scars or postoperative radiation may disturb the local vascularity. Considerable hematoma and seroma will increase tension on the skin and impair microcirculation and oxygenation of the tissue, which is detrimental to wound healing. Although hypoxia is the strongest stimulus for angiogenesis, the wound will not proceed through the later phases of wound healing [45].

Foreign bodies can either act as a physical obstacle to wound healing or as a host for bacteria.

Too tight surgeon's knots, too much tension on the wound edges, or too many stitches can impair wound healing due to local ischemia, inflammation or infection. Foreign bodies prolong the inflammatory phase of wound healing (chapter 4.1) and delay contraction, respectively epithelialization of a wound. Additional incisions placed in parallel or using an acute angle to the preexisting scars may jeopardize microcirculation and lead to local skin necrosis. Necrotic tissue also inhibits healing and must be excised in order to allow a wound to heal [46].

Radiation has both acute and chronic effects on the skin. Acute effects include erythema, dry desquamation at moderate dose levels, and moist desquamation at higher dose levels. Chronic effects include increased or decreased pigmentation, thickening and fibrosis of the skin and subcutaneous tissues, telangiectasias, and alterations in sebaceous and sweat-gland function.

References and further reading

[1] **Lazarus GS, Cooper DM, Knighton DR, et al** (1994) Definitions and guidelines for assessment of wounds and evaluation of healing. *Arch Dermatol;* 130(4):489–493.

[2] **Clark RA** (1993) Biology of dermal wound repair. *Dermatol Clin;* 11(4):647–666.

[3] **Robson MC** (1991) Growth factors as wound healing agents. *Curr Opin Biotechnol;* 2(6):863–867.

[4] **Lawrence WT** (1998) Physiology of the acute wound. *Clin Plast Surg;* 25(3):321–340.

[5] **Cines DB, Pollak ES, Buck CA, et al** (1998) Endothelial cells in physiology and in the pathophysiology of vascular disorders. *Blood;* 91(10):3527–3561.

[6] **Majno G, Shea SM, Leventhal M** (1969) Endothelial contraction induced by histamine-type mediators: an electron microscopic study. *J Cell Biol;* 42(3):647–672.

[7] **Monaco JL, Lawrence WT** (2003) Acute wound healing: an overview. *Clin Plast Surg;* 30(1):1–12.

[8] **Witte MB, Barbul A** ([1] Lazarus GS, Cooper DM, Knighton DR, et al (1994) Definitions and guidelines for assessment of wounds and evaluation of healing. *Arch Dermatol;* 130(4):489–493.

[9] **Folkman J, Klagsbrun M** (1987) Angiogenic factors. *Science;* 235(4787):442–447.

[10] **Pilcher BK, Gaither-Ganim J, Parks WC, et al** (1997) Cell type-specific inhibition of keratinocyte collagenase-1 expression by basic fibroblast growth factor and keratinocyte growth factor. A common receptor pathway. *J Biol Chem;* 272(29):18147–18154.

[11] **Pierce GF, Vande Berg J, Rudolph R, et al** (1991) Platelet-derived growth factor-BB and transforming growth factor beta 1 selectively modulate glycosaminoglycans, collagen, and myofibroblasts in excisional wounds. *Am J Pathol;* 138(3):629–646.

[12] **Tamariz-Domínguez E, Castro-Muñozledo F, Kuri-Harcuch W** (2002) Growth factors and extracellular matrix proteins during wound healing promoted with frozen cultured sheets of human epidermal keratinocytes. *Cell Tissue Res;* 307(1):79–89.

[13] **Ignotz RA, Massagué J** (1986) Transforming growth factor-beta stimulates the expression of fibronectin and collagen and their incorporation into the extracellular matrix. *J Biol Chem;* 261(9):4337–4345.

[14] **Reed MJ, Puolakkainen P, Lane TF, et al** (1993) Differential expression of SPARC and thrombospondin 1 in wound repair: immunolocalization and in situ hybridization. *J Histochem Cytochem;* 41(10):1467–1477.

[15] **Granstein RD, Murphy GF, Margolis RJ, et al** (1987) Gamma-interferon inhibits collagen synthesis in vivo in the mouse. *J Clin Invest;* 79(4):1254–1258.

[16] **Buck M, Houglum K, Chojkier M** (1996) Tumor necrosis factor-alpha inhibits collagen alpha1(I) gene expression and wound healing in a murine model of cachexia. *Am J Pathol;* 149(1):195–204.

[17] **Madden JW, Peacock EE Jr** (1968) Studies on the biology of collagen during wound healing. I. Rate of collagen synthesis and deposition in cutaneous wounds of the rat. *Surgery;* 64(1):288–294.

[18] **Stephens FO, Hunt TK, Dunphy JE** (1971) Study of traditional methods of care on the tensile strength of skin wounds in rats. *Am J Surg;* 122(1):78–80.

[19] **Ono I** (2002) The effects of basic fibroblast growth factor (bFGF) on the breaking strength of acute incisional wounds. *J Dermatol Sci;* 29(2):104–113.

[20] **Beason DP, Soslowsky LJ, Karthikeyan T, et al** (2008) Muscle, tendon and ligament. *Fischgrund JS (ed), Orthopaedic Knowledge Update 9.* Rosemont, IL: American Academy of Orthopaedic Surgeons, 35–48.

[21] **Buckwalter JA, Einhorn TA, Bolander ME, et al** (1996) Healing of the musculoskeletal tissues. *Rockwood CA, Green DP, Bucholz RW, et al (eds). Rockwood and Green's Fractures in Adults. 4th ed.* Philadelphia: Lippincott-Raven, 261–304.

[22] **Kirkendall DT, Garrett WE Jr** (2002) Clinical perspectives regarding eccentric muscle injury. *Clin Orthop Relat Res;* 403 Suppl; S81–S89.

[23] **Frank CB, Shrive NG, Lo IKY, et al** (2007) Form and function of tendon and ligament. *Einhorn TA, Buckwalter JA, O'Keefe RJ (eds) Orthopaedic Basic Science: Foundations of Clinical Practice.* 3rd ed. Rosemont, IL: American Academy of Orthopaedic Surgeons, 191–222.

[24] **Grundnes O, Reikerås O** (1992) Blood flow and mechanical properties of healing bone. Femoral osteotomies studied in rats. *Acta Orthop Scand;* 63(5):487–491.

[25] **Kelly PJ, Montgomery RJ, Bronk JT** (1990) Reaction of the circulatory system to injury and regeneration. *Clin Orthop Relat Res;* (254):275–288.

[26] **Brown CR, Boden SD** (2008) Fracture Repair and Bone Grafting. *Fischgrund JS (ed), Orthopaedic Knowledge Update 9.* Rosemont, IL: American Academy of Orthopaedic Surgeons, 13–22.

[27] **Miclau T III, Bozic KJ, Tay B, et al** (2007) Bone Injury, Regeneration and Repair. *Einhorn TA, Buckwalter JA, O'Keefe RJ (eds) Orthopaedic Basic Science: Foundations of Clinical Practice.* 3rd ed. Rosemont, IL: American Academy of Orthopaedic Surgeons, 331–348.

[28] **Markel MD, Wikenheiser MA, Chao EY** (1991) Formation of bone in tibial defects in a canine model. Histomorphometric and biomechanical studies. *J Bone Joint Surg Am;* 73(6):914–923.

[29] **Gilliver SC, Ashworth JJ, Mills SJ, et al** (2006) Androgens modulate the inflammatory response during acute wound healing. *J Cell Sci;* 119(Pt 4):722–732.

[30] **Ashcroft GS, Mills SJ, Lei K, et al** (2003) Estrogen modulates cutaneous wound healing by downregulating macrophage migration inhibitory factor. *J Clin Invest;* 111(9):1309–1318.

[31] **Harder Y, Amon M, Wettstein R, et al** (2010) Gender-specific ischemic tissue tolerance in critically perfused skin. *Langenbecks Arch Surg;* 395(1):33–40.

[32] **Thomas DR** (2001) Age-related changes in wound healing. *Drugs Aging;* 18(8):607–620.

[33] **Harder Y, Amon M, Georgi M, et al** (2007) Aging is associated with an increased susceptibility to ischaemic necrosis due to microvascular perfusion failure but not a reduction in ischaemic tolerance. *Clin Sci (Lond);* 112(8):429–440.

[34] **Burns JL, Mancoll JS, Phillips LG** (2003) Impairments to wound healing. *Clin Plast Surg;* 30(1):47–56.

[35] **Ehrlich HP, Hunt TK** (1969) The effects of cortisone and anabolic steroids on the tensile strength of healing wounds. *Ann Surg;* 170(2):203–206.

[36] **Billingsley EM, Maloney ME** (1997) Intraoperative and postoperative bleeding problems in patients taking warfarin, aspirin, and nonsteroidal antiinflammatory agents. A prospective study. *Dermatol Surg;* 23(5):381-383; discussion 384–385.

[37] **Dixon AJ, Dixon MP, Dixon JB** (2007) Bleeding complications in skin cancer surgery are associated with warfarin but not aspirin therapy. *Br J Surg;* 94(11):1356–1360.

[38] **Ruberg RL** (1984) Role of nutrition in wound healing. *Surg Clin North Am;* 64(4):705–714.

[39] **Brown KL, Phillips TJ** (2010) Nutrition and Wound healing. *Clin Dermatol;* 28(4):432–439.

[40] **Jensen JA, Goodson WH, Hopf HW, et al** (1991) Cigarette smoking decreases tissue oxygen. *Arch Surg;* 126(9):1131–1134.

[41] **Kwiatkowski TC, Hanley EN Jr, Ramp WK** (1996) Cigarette smoking and its orthopedic consequences. *Am J Orthop (Belle Mead NJ);* 25(9):590–597.

[42] **Jorgensen LN, Kallehave F, Christensen E, et al** (1998) Less collagen production in smokers. *Surgery;* 123(4):450–455.

[43] **Hoogendoorn JM, Simmermacher RK, Schellekens PP, et al** (2002) [Adverse effects if smoking on healing of bones and soft tissues]. *Unfallchirurg;* 105(1):76–81. German.

[44] **Knobloch K, Gohritz A, Reuss E, et al** (2008) [Nicotine in plastic surgery: a review]. *Chirurg;* 79(10):956–962. German.

[45] **Knighton DR, Hunt TK, Scheuenstuhl H, et al** (1983) Oxygen tension regulates the expression of angiogenesis factor by macrophages. *Science;* 221(4617):1283–1285.

[46] **Steed DL** (2004) Debridement. *Am J Surg;* 187(5A):71S–74S.

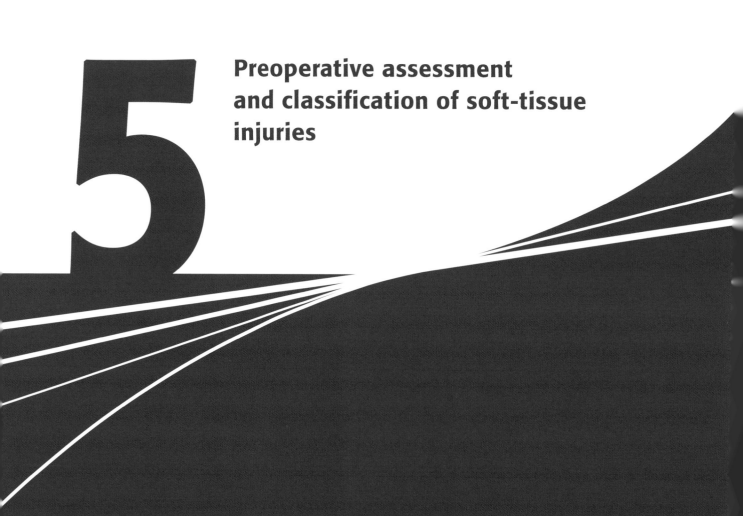

5

Preoperative assessment and classification of soft-tissue injuries

5.1 Preoperative assessment of soft-tissue injuries

Authors   Farid Rezaeian, Reto Wettstein, Dominique Erni, Yves Harder

5.1.1 Basic principles of assessment

Examination of wounds, soft-tissue defects, and concomitant injuries in orthopaedic trauma is based on a systematic survey that must be performed in a standardized manner in order to assess the injury correctly (chapter 6.1). A detailed case history goes hand in hand with clinical, laboratory, and radiographic evaluation—everything aimed at rapidly obtaining a diagnosis that is as accurate as possible. History and assessment must be surveyed and recorded immediately. However, emergency measures that are not directly related to the soft-tissue injury may sometimes delay assessment, for example, in a polytraumatized patient. Furthermore, the evaluation of an unconscious patient requires laboratory and radiographic support, or even deferral of the examination. The value of the assessment of injured soft tissues and the classification of their severity greatly depends on the examiner's experience (chapter 5.2). The most experienced surgeon in house should, therefore, be the one to assess the patient. If the diagnostic procedure is delegated or performed by a junior physician on call, he or she must be in close contact with the consulting specialist. A systematic examination of the patient in general and of the injury in particular will allow the surgeon to be thorough and efficient. This is a prerequisite for appropriate subsequent decision making and preoperative planning. Moreover, initial and definitive treatment options, including reconstructive needs, as well as the coordination with all the team members involved, must be taken into consideration (chapter 6.2). Regardless of their extent, th e assessment of soft-tissue injuries must address the medical history as well as the following clinical issues:

- factors affecting the general condition of the patient (eg, age, gender, vascular diseases, diabetes, drugs, nicotine, alcohol, tetanus immunization, or infection with HIV, hepatitis B or C)
- mechanism and energy of injury
- agent that caused the wound
- time of injury
- localization, size, extent, and character of the wound (eg, crush, abrasion, defect, degloving)
- wound contamination or presence of foreign bodies
- involvement of surrounding structures (eg, nerves, vessels, muscles, tendons, bone, cartilage, or any combination of these).

Several systems for the classification of traumatized soft tissues are in clinical use such as the Gustilo-Anderson classification [1, 2], the AO soft-tissue classification [3], and the Hanover fracture scale [4, 5] (chapter 5.2). The following description will explain in detail some of the already mentioned general statements on the history of the injury as well as the clinical and nonclinical (ie, laboratory and radiographic) assessment.

5.1.2 Assessment of trauma history

Knowledge about the mechanism and the involved energy of an injury will help to judge the severity of the resulting lesions. It will also influence the therapeutic approach and subsequent decisions (**Fig 5.1-1a–b**). This information may roughly indicate the extent of the zone of injury (chapter 10.3.3), the potential capacity for wound healing and the possible extent of contamination. In addition, it will also supply an estimate of the risk of complications and functional damage [6]. Superficial abrasions, simple cuts, and low-energy injuries that heal by secondary intention or simple primary wound closure will be classified and approached differently compared to high-energy crush injuries, deep, multistructural soft-tissue defects, or extensive degloving as well as severely contaminated wounds or farming injuries (chapter 5.2).

Furthermore, it is of utmost importance to include the patient's age and associated comorbidities in the assessment, because senescence [7], diabetes [8], or smoking [9, 10] may not only affect wound-healing capacity, but may even be associated with decreased survival rates in polytraumatized patients.

Treatment of infected wounds and soft-tissue defects with associated injuries to tendons, muscles, blood vessels, nerves, or bone should be addressed rather aggressively. Definite assessment of the local soft-tissue injury can sometimes only be performed during emergency irrigation and debridement, or even after repeated debridement (chapter 6.1, 7.1, 7.2). Once an assessment has been carried out, closure of the defect not only depends on the condition of the adjacent tissues, but also on the general status of the patient, the availability, experience, and skills of the surgeon in charge and the whole team in the operating room.

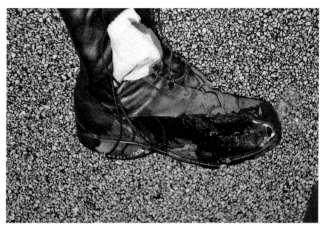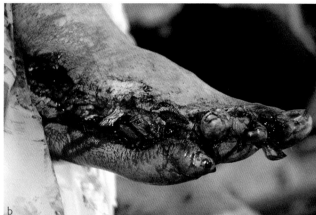

Fig 5.1-1a–b Injury of the right lateral foot after being struck by a lawn edger.
a Heavy boot lacerated by the edger.
b Injury with extensive skin laceration, torn tendons, exposed and fractured bone, as well as partial degloving of the sole.

5.1.3 Clinical assessment of injury and tissue viability

Clinical examination must be performed on the undressed patient under sterile conditions both of the injured area (sterile drapes) and the examiner (sterile gloves, face mask, etc) using an adequate light source. Often, full assessment of the extent of soft-tissue injury can only be carried out in the operating room. Room temperature is indicated for the assessment of the soft-tissue injuries in order to minimize temperature-induced changes of the skin's perfusion that could influence the assessment. Exact localization, type (ie, clean, dirty, contaminated, infected), and extension of the injury as well as involved neighboring structures must be recorded, documented, and photographed (chapter 5.1.5). Traumatized soft tissues must be compared with adjacent healthy tissues. General anesthesia is recommended for more extensive injuries, especially if they are associated with single or multiple fractures.

Severe soft-tissue injury not only involves skin and subcutaneous tissue, but also muscles, tendons, nerves, vessels and/or bone (**Fig 5.1-2a–b**). In practice, soft-tissue assessment is performed from superficial to deep layers, starting out with the skin. With some experience, examination of the skin allows a relatively good appraisal of perfusion that can be obtained by examination of color, capillary refill, turgescence, and surface temperature. It is recommended to always use a reference area for comparison. Differences in skin temperature of as little as 1°C can be perceived from the dorsum of the hand. Assessing perfusion by skin color may not be practical in the absence of an adequate light source, or in heavily pigmented or very pale skin. In addition, venous stasis may be mimicked by bruising due to trauma and/or intradermal hemorrhage. Capillary refill is examined by applying light pressure on the skin with a finger or instrument, which is then quickly released (**Fig 5.1-3a–c**). Scarification of the skin with a sharp needle or a scalpel may sometimes be helpful in order to judge capillary bleeding. Adequate perfusion is then validated by judging color (eg, light or dark red) and flow of the capillary bleeding. Absent capillary bleeding is suggestive of nonviable tissue. Nevertheless, skin may reperfuse after trauma. Accordingly, the assessment must not only include the time interval since and mechanism of the trauma, but also skin color. Bluish discoloration will indicate some injury to the skin, which it may survive, whereas greyish discoloration of the skin will indicate changes beyond the skin's ischemic tolerance. All these clinical signs should be used in order to assess perfusion of normal skin or of a flap (**Table 5.1-1**). In contrast, muscle viability may be determined by assessing the four "C"s: color, contractility by mechanical or electrical stimulation, consistency, and the capacity of the muscle to bleed. Absent pulses may suggest a severely injured artery proximal to the region of interest. The presence of a pulse more distally does not guarantee intact vascularity, because retrograde perfusion of the injured vessel may maintain a palpable pulse through collateral vessels. Therefore, clinical examination must include palpation of the respective vessel, using the finger to occlude flow proximal to the supposedly injured vessel.

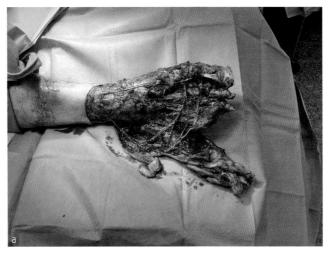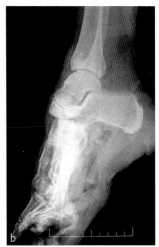

Fig 5.1-2a–b Severe trauma to the right foot and distal tibia. Considerable skin loss and degloving including skin, subcutaneous tissue, muscle, and bone.
a Dorsal view of the foot.
b Mediolateral x-ray.

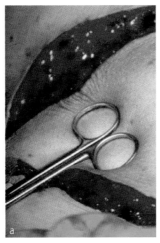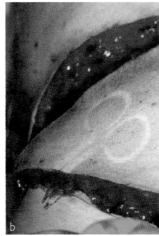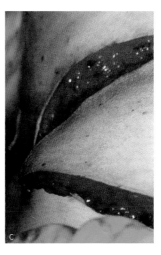

Fig 5.1-3a–c Capillary refill.
a By gently pressing scissors onto the region of interest, capillary refill can be tested.
b Observation of the imprint of the scissors.
c Fading of the imprint. A fading within ~3 seconds is normal. Rapid or slowed fading may indicate venous occlusion or arterial inflow obstruction, respectively.

	Bruise	Inflammation / infection	Arterial insufficiency	Venous congestion
Color	Purple	Red	Pale	Dark red, purple
Capillary refill	Normal	Accelerated	Slow to absent	Accelerated
Turgescence	Increased	Increased	Decreased	Increased
Surface temperature	Normal	Increased	Decreased	Normal to increased

Table 5.1-1 Clinical signs indicating compromised skin perfusion.

In case a wound is situated over a tendon, the examination should include testing the tendon's function actively and passively. If in doubt, wound exploration must be carried out in the operating room and the surgeon must be prepared to repair the tendon at that time. The viability of a tendon cannot be judged in a freshly injured patient. Necrotic tendons, however, that were exposed over a period of days, will macerate and develop a greenish discoloration.

Axial malalignment of the limb and crepitation are typical for a fractured bone, which must be verified by radiography (see below).
The following clinical signs may indicate significant injury to nerves and must be assessed immediately:

- severe pain and dysesthesia resulting from acute swelling of a limb, respectively compression of a nerve (eg, compartment syndrome)
- massive contusion or transection of a nerve resulting in paralysis and functional deficit of a limb, foot, or hand, eg, drop foot (deep fibular nerve), wrist drop (radial nerve), claw hand (ulnar nerve), monkey hand (median nerve), or traumatic paresis of the brachial plexus
- absence of two-point discrimination (ie, ability to discern that two nearby sharp objects touching the skin are felt as two distinct points)
- lack of response to strong and painful stimuli and absence of peripheral reflexes.

5.1.4 Nonclinical assessment of injury and tissue viability

Full assessment of a soft-tissue injury often requires further investigations using various devices. Several techniques are available to assess the viability of skin (**Tab 5.1-2**).

Indirect variables

Temperature measurement

Temperature measurement for the assessment of tissue perfusion of soft tissues, including flaps, depends on several factors that must be fulfilled:

- exposure of the patient to room temperature in order to avoid errors caused by external heating or cooling by convection
- reference measurement of normal skin in the vicinity of the tissue under investigation
- continuous registration of temperature for comparison
- repeated measurements at exactly the same spot
- suitable and reliable instruments such as a temperature probe that can be fixed to the skin, an ear thermometer, or an adhesive thermometer.

If the above prerequisites are fulfilled, temperature measurement is easy to handle and a reliable method in order to monitor skin or flap perfusion. However, such options may not always be available as in cases of buried flaps or in very small flaps surrounded by well-vascularized tissue. Note that the surrounding temperature of the tissue is able to maintain an adequate temperature of the flap even despite inadequate perfusion, which can be misleading.

Tissue oxygenation

Tissue oxygenation can either be assessed by measuring partial oxygen tension or oxygen saturation of the tissues. Both are determined by the difference between oxygen delivery and consumption, the former being defined as the product of blood flow and arterial oxygen content. The value obtained with partial oxygen tension measurement reflects the oxygenation value in the surrounding intercellular space. The value for oxygen saturation, however, is mainly

	Invasiveness	Reliability	Quantification	Ease of handling
Temperature	No	Some	Some	Yes
Tissue oxygenation	Yes	Yes	Yes	Some
Acoustic Doppler	No	Some	No	Yes
Laser Doppler flowmetry	No	Some	Some	Some
Duplex, color Doppler	No	Yes	Yes	No
CT imaging	Yes	Yes	No	No
Fluorescent dyes	Yes	Yes	Some	No

Table 5.1-2 Advantages and disdvantages of nonclinical techniques to assess skin blood flow.

determined by the venous blood pool in the area under investigation, which is the major contributor to the total number of hemoglobin molecules present in this tissue volume. Partial oxygen tension may easily be assessed on the tissue's surface or within the tissue using Clark type microprobes (polarographic electrodes inside of an oxygen-sensitive microcell) or fiber-optic microprobes measuring partial oxygen pressure (pO_2) by fluorescence quenching of a dye. Oxygen saturation is usually measured with white-light spectrometry or near-infrared spectrometry [11]. Provided that arterial oxygen content and oxygen consumption are constant, partial oxygen tension and oxygen saturation can be used to assess blood flow, especially in areas of the body that are difficult to reach (eg, buried flaps). However, malpositioning of the probe or temperature-dependent changes in blood flow may bias the true values of tissue oxygenation.

Fluorescent dyes

The perfusion of a skin area may be visualized by injecting a fluorescent dye, ie, indocyanine green. The light emission induced by excitation with a laser light can be recorded by a video camera equipped with a filter corresponding to the wavelength of the emitted light. The fluorescence intensity is quantified in terms of assessing the increase of intensity after dye injection [12]. The technique may reflect the perfusion of large skin surfaces. However, injection of fluorescent dyes in order to detect the extent to which skin or muscle is perfused is an invasive technique. Moreover, it may lead to false results in acute settings due to reactive vasoconstriction or centralization of the blood flow as experienced in severely injured patients suffering from significant blood loss or hypothermia.

Direct variables

Radiological imaging

Whereas conventional angiography is still the method of choice to visualize patency and particularly intraluminal characteristics of peripheral arteries, new technologies based on magnetic resonance (MR) or computed tomography (CT) have evolved. They allow for detailed imaging with accurate 3-D reconstruction of the arborization, the diameter, and the putative interruption of arteries and/or veins of less than 1 mm in diameter, including their course through the surrounding tissues [13]. In many institutions, conventional angiography has been substituted by CT angiography, generally using up to 64-slice scanning, made possible by the introduction of multidetector row scanners. In case of trauma involving an extremity, CT may also represent an excellent tool in order to assess the geometry of complex fractures,

usually involving joints. Multi-slice CT—used conventionally or as a CT angiography—offers high accuracy, low cost and low inter-observer variability, particularly, if the recorded images undergo 3-D reconstruction of the designated anatomical region. In some cases, contraindications include claustrophobia, intolerance to the contrast medium and, to some extent, radiation load. The latter may be overcome with high-resolution MR angiography in the near future. MR tomography, and particularly MR angiography, provides very precise images of the soft tissues (ie, muscles, tendons, menisci, nerves, and vessels) without radiation, especially if 3-D reconstruction is involved. However, data acquisition is still very time consuming, expensive, and cumbersome for a traumatized patient. It cannot provide the essential information for soft-tissue damage in orthopaedic trauma, particularly in emergency situations.

Conventional angiography, although it is by far the most invasive radiological tool for vascular mapping, still represents a good backup tool whenever intraoperative assessment of a putative vascular lesion is required.

Plain x-rays of the injured area still constitute the gold standard for the radiological examination of orthopaedic trauma and, therefore, are mandatory. These x-rays should be obtained in two different planes during initial patient evaluation. Exceptionally, one x-ray plane may give sufficient information for primary diagnostics in cases of severely comminuted fractures or total or subtotal amputations. The x-ray is primarily intended to exclude or confirm, a fracture, as well as to define its type and complexity. Sometimes, the x-ray may even indicate the presence and severity of any associated damage to be expected. Beside the bone structures, special attention should be given to inclusion of air, radio-opaque shadows, or foreign bodies within the soft tissues.

Methods based on the Doppler effect

This effect, named after Christian Andreas Doppler, who first described it in 1842, is defined as the change in wavelength that occurs if the source of the wave and the recipient move in relation to each other. In medicine, this effect is applied by measuring the shift of the wavelength of an optical or acoustic signal caused by moving particles, eg, blood cells.

Acoustic Doppler velocimetry

An ultrasonic acoustic burst is emitted towards a vessel, where the particles moving within its lumen cause a shift in frequency and phase of the emitted sound, which is proportional to the velocity of the particles. These phase and frequency shifts are recorded and transduced either into an acoustic or a visual signal that reflect the flow velocity of the red blood cells. If diameter measurement is included, volumetric blood flow can be calculated and visualized (color Doppler or Duplex Doppler), whereas the acoustic Doppler is usually used to localize a vessel or to prove its patency, allowing for the discrimination between an artery and a vein. The method allows assessing vessels as small as 1 mm in diameter (**Fig 5.1-4a–b**).

In addition to vascular mapping, ultrasound may easily detect soft-tissue swelling caused by hematoma or seroma formation as well as significant lesions to tendons (eg, rupture of the rotator cuff or the patellar tendon, or the Stener lesion of the thumb). Muscles and foreign bodies that are not radio-opaque may also be visualized.

Laser Doppler flowmetry (LDF)

Laser Doppler flowmetry uses laser light, which is emitted towards a tissue surface [14]. The light penetrates the tissue to a depth of about 1 mm, where its wavelength is shifted by all particles moving within the sampled tissue volume. The extent of the shift correlates with the speed of the particles, and the sum of shifted laser light corresponds to the amount of moving particles, which allows calculation of volumetric blood flow within the sampled tissue area. The data are expressed in virtual perfusion units (PU), which only allow the assessment of relative, time-dependent changes. In addition, the interpretation of the values is complicated due to the phenomenon that an LDF signal may still be obtained by movement of artifacts, even in case of total ischemia (biological zero). Furthermore, the conventional application of LDF is restricted to an area of 1 mm², whereas new scanning technologies allow blood-flow mapping of larger surface areas (**Fig 5.1-5a–c**).

Which method to use?

Multi-slice CT angiography has become the most reliable tool for vascular mapping. Acoustic Doppler is the cheapest, most easily applicable method in order to spot upstream and downstream vascular structures and to assess their patency. For their further characterization and blood-flow quantification, Duplex Doppler or color Doppler is required. Clinical evaluation by an experienced examiner provides a good estimate of tissue perfusion even in the operating room, except for muscle tissue or pigmented skin. The techniques based on ultrasonic waves are noninvasive and easy to apply. However, they are often very time consuming and investigator dependent.

Temperature and laser Doppler flowmetry monitoring are easy to handle and can therefore be used to monitor time-dependent changes. Yet, the validity of both methods may be jeopardized by external factors (ambient temperature, light) that may lead to artifacts and misinterpretation of the data. The same holds true for the measurement of tissue oxygen saturation, whereas partial oxygen tension provides the most useful information on tissue oxygenation. The drawback of this method as well as the fluorescent dye method is their invasiveness. The pros and cons of each method are summarized in **Table 5.1-2**. All in all, some of the above mentioned techniques are not used on a regular basis in the acute setting, because they will not provide vital information for the therapeutical decision making right after trauma. However, they may be very useful in the follow-up surveillance of selected cases with damaged skin and muscle or with flaps.

5.1.5 Documentation of the injury

All findings and diagnoses identified during the primary survey in the emergency department (ED) should be recorded in detail and documented on the patient's chart. For fractures and especially for soft-tissue injuries, a simple drawing of the injury, its location and extent is very helpful. Photographic documentation of the soft-tissue injury is a necessity for the consulting specialists, further planning and decision making as well as for follow-up, scientific, or legal reasons. Sometimes photographs may also keep too many people from wanting to inspect the injured area, which would otherwise greatly increase the risk of infection. Unfortunately, photographic documentation is often forgotten or not performed in sufficient quality. For a good documentation, a digital pocket camera with sufficient resolution is recommended. Overviews of the injury are important, but close-ups are needed to supplement the overview with details. The injured area is best presented on a clean, sterile cloth. Gross contamination and blood clots should first be removed. Direct flashlight is preferred to room light or operating room light. Photographs must carry the date of exposure and always be assignable to the patient. They are best stored with the operating room report, with copies for the surgeon in charge. For common understanding, the injury then has to be documented, using an appropriate classification system with acceptable reliability, and consequences for the treatment as well as for the prognosis, knowing that all fractures involve some degree of soft-tissue injury (chapter 5.2).

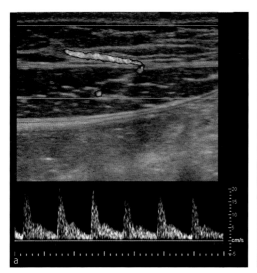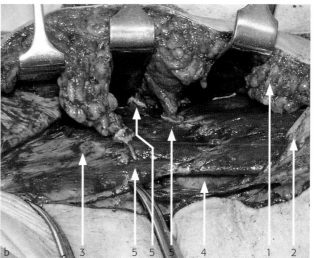

Fig 5.1-4a–b Vascular monitoring using Doppler.
a Visualization of an artery perforating the rectus abdominis muscle and its pulsatile flow velocity by ultrasound Doppler imaging (Siemens Acuson SC2000).
b Corresponding intraoperative visualization after dissection of various perforating vessels.
  1 Subcutaneous tissue.
  2 Anterior rectus sheath.
  3 Rectus abdominis muscle.
  4 Posterior rectus sheath and peritoneum.
  5 Perforating vessels.

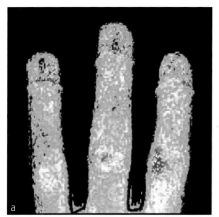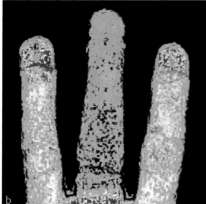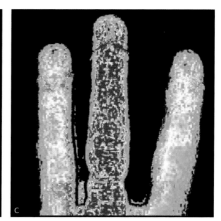

Fig 5.1-5a–c Semi-quantitative monitoring of blood-flow changes in the fingers II to IV of the left hand using laser Doppler when applying tourniquet-induced ischemia to the middle finger. Normal perfusion (yellow) is present throughout the index and ring finger, whereas total ischemia (green, blue) occurs during vascular occlusion, followed by hyperperfusion (red) after removal of the tourniquet (ie, restoring perfusion).
a Before tourniquet application.
b During tourniquet application.
c After tourniquet application.

5.2 Classification systems

Author   David A Volgas

5.2.1   Overview

All classification systems are designed to highlight similarities or differences between individual injuries. By grouping patients with comparable injuries, sufficient numbers of patients with such injuries may be studied in order to determine outcomes. This information may then be used to guide the treatment of individual patients with similar injuries. Unfortunately, soft-tissue injuries are even more diverse than fractures. While the x-rays of a fracture usually provide hard, reproducible, and objective facts, descriptions of soft-tissue injuries depend on rather subjective judgment, allowing different interpretations even in the presence of initial photographic documentation of the injury. Moreover, the extent of the injury may change dramatically following the development of necrosis and repeated debridement procedures. Therefore, numerous classification systems exist, which are based on anatomical and/or physiological observations. Some are limited to the injured part or even limited to specific types of injury, while others include systemic factors of the patient. All depend on the personal experience of the surgeon, and some may be appropriate in clinical settings while others in research.

5.2.2   Gustilo-Anderson classification

The Gustilo-Anderson classification is probably the most commonly used classification system for open fractures, as it is short, simple and easy to remember. However, it is not very detailed. This classification system was developed by examining 1,025 open fractures and the characteristics of the soft-tissue injury associated with them [1]. Note that the original description was of types, not grades, but in current usage, many surgeons use the term "grade" synonymously. Gustilo, Mendoza and Williams later further subdivided the type III injuries [2].

Type I: There is a small (< 1 cm) wound, typically felt to be caused by bone protruding through the skin from inside-out. By definition, these do not include contaminated wounds. The bone injury is of a simple type such as a spiral or short oblique fracture (**Fig 5.2-1a–b**).

Type II: There is a larger skin laceration of 1–10 cm, but little evidence of additional damage such as crushing or muscle contusion. The fracture pattern is more complex (**Fig 5.2-2a–b**).

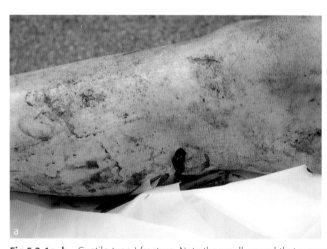 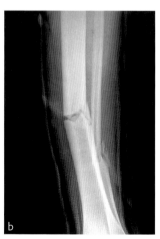

Fig 5.2-1a–b   Gustilo type I fracture. Note the small wound that appears to come from inside to outside.
a   Clinical photograph.
b   AP x-ray.

Type III: There is extensive soft-tissue injury, which may include:

- severely damaged or even necrotic skin and subcutaneous tissue
- large, single or even multiple lacerations
- contusion or crushing of muscle
- lesions of major vessels and/or nerves or gross contamination.

Certain injuries justify immediate classification and treatment as type III injuries such as farmyard injuries, shotgun wounds, high-energy gunshot wounds, or delayed initial treatment of open wounds, all of which are prone to infection.

Type III: These injuries are further subdivided into three subcategories:

- **Type IIIA:** These wounds meet criteria for inclusion as type III injuries, but generally do not require flap or vascular repair and there is no periosteal stripping of the bone (**Fig 5.2-3a–b**).
- **Type IIIB:** These injuries are associated with extensive soft-tissue injury or loss, usually heavily contaminated. There is periosteal stripping and exposure of bare bone, requiring soft-tissue coverage (**Fig 5.2-4a–b**).
- **Type IIIC:** These injuries are associated with a vascular injury, which requires repair irrespective of the degree of soft-tissue lesion (**Fig 5.2-5a–b**). Note that fractures associated with a vascular injury, but which do not require repair, such as a radial artery injury with an intact and dominant ulnar artery, are classified according to the soft-tissue injury.

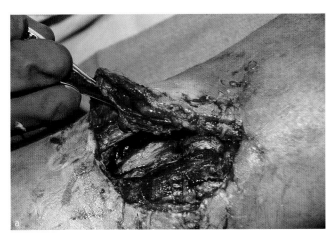
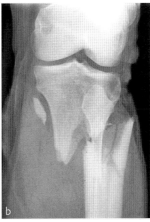

Fig 5.2-2a–b Gustilo type II fracture. Note that the wound is small, ~5 cm, and there appears to be minimal periosteal stripping.
a Clinical photograph.
b AP x-ray.

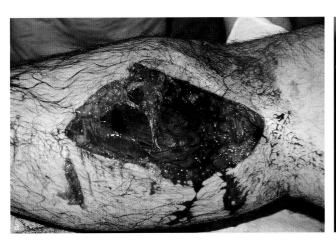
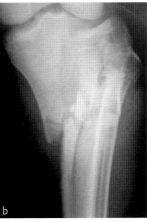

Fig 5.2-3a–b Patient who was bitten by an alligator. He sustained a crush injury to the muscle and deep contamination, which classifies this as a Gustilo type IIIA fracture.
a Clinical photograph.
b AP x-ray.

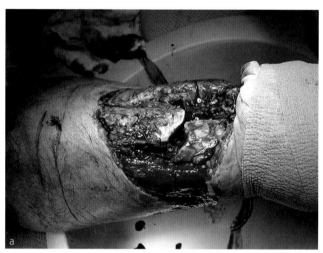

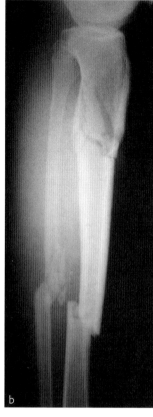

Fig 5.2-4a–b Patient involved in a motor-vehicle collision. This wound requires vascularized tissue (eg, muscle flap) for coverage and represents a Gustilo type IIIB fracture.
a   Clinical photograph.
b   AP x-ray.

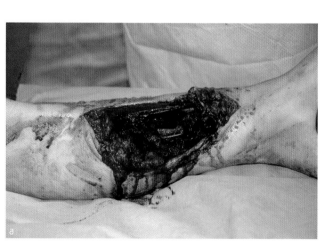

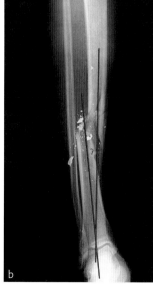

Fig 5.2-5a–b Gunshot wound to the leg that requires vascular repair of the posterior tibial artery. This is a Gustilo type IIIC fracture. The red lines indicate the axial malalignment.
a   Clinical photograph.
b   AP x-ray.

5.2.3 Hanover fracture scale (HFS)

The Hanover fracture scale (**Table 5.2-1**) was developed in 1982 [4] and revised in 1998 [5]. It was first designed as an extension of the Tscherne soft-tissue classification, which was the first system to not only describe open fractures, but to also include soft-tissue injuries in closed fractures [15]. The Hanover fracture scale was initially derived from a retrospective study of 948 open fractures and attempted to predict the risk of osteomyelitis from these cases, but later was used to predict limb salvage.

The Hanover fracture scale has been revised to become a very comprehensive assessment tool for every important facet of fracture pathology, including soft-tissue damage, fracture pattern, time to initial treatment, contamination, and bacteriological data. Its main drawback is that it is time consuming and cumbersome to use until the evaluator has become familiar with the system. The criteria for assessing each variable, however, are precise. Nonetheless, many centers do not take cultures from the wound until the first debridement. Therefore, this important component is often missing. At present, the Hanover fracture scale is most useful in a research setting, as it is not particularly helpful in determining limb salvage, especially in light of the lower extremity assessment project (LEAP) study and recent advances in prosthetic care [15, 16].

5.2.4 AO soft-tissue classification

The AO developed an anatomical classification system, which includes assessment of the skin (integument), the muscle-tendon system, and the neurovascular system [3]. Fractures are assessed using the Müller AO classification of fractures—long bones.

For the classification of the skin (integument) component, injuries are subdivided into closed (**Table 5.2-2**) and open (**Table 5.2-3**). This classification system uses the prefix IC (integument closed) or IO (integument open) in addition to a scale from 1 (ie, minimal injury) to 5 (ie, most severe injury). Unfortunately, the condition of the subcutaneous fat was not included and, furthermore, classification of an injury may change during the assessment period as swelling, fracture blisters, and wound erythema change, which of course may also affect classifications by other systems.

The muscle-tendon assessment (**Table 5.2-4**) is conceptually easy, but much more difficult to apply in clinical practice, especially in closed injuries. As with many classification systems, the extremes of no injury versus compartment syndrome are fairly easy to distinguish, but there is a great deal of variability in the assessment of intermediate grades. The assessment of this component may also need to be changed with time, though usually, the initial assessment is most commonly used, especially in research.

Perhaps the most reproducible aspect of the AO soft-tissue classification is the neurovascular assessment (**Table 5.2-5**). However, careful examination of small peripheral nerves (eg, deep fibular nerve) is essential in order to correctly classify the wound. Often, either due to sedation, brain injury, or relative lack of time during emergency department management, these examinations may not be performed adequately, or this component may not be recorded, again limiting the usefulness of this classification (chapter 5.1).

5.2.5 International Red Cross war wound classification

Coupland developed a simple classification system designed to provide a rapid, easily learned system to stratify war wounds, especially projectile wounds [17]. It is widely used in International Red Cross hospitals. Major features of the classification system include assessment of the entrance and exit wounds, presence of metal objects in the wound, assessment of the wound cavity, consideration of the fracture, and presence of any injuries to vital organs (**Table 5.2-6**). Wounds are scored after initial assessment or surgery. However, only the two most serious injuries are scored. Entries, which cannot be assessed or which do not apply are coded with a "?" after the entry, eg, E2 X0 C? F2 V0 M2 (**Table 5.2-6**). While useful as an epidemiologic tool, this does not have any direct impact on the management of wounds.

A Fracture type	Points
Type A	1
Type B	2
Type C	4
Bone loss	
< 2 cm	1
> 2 cm	2

C Ischemia/compartment syndrome	Points
No	0
Incomplete	10
Complete	
< 4 hours	15
4–8 hours	20
> 8 hours	25

B Soft tissues	Points
Skin (wound, contusion)	
No	0
< 1/4 circumference	1
1/4–1/2	2
1/2–3/4	3
> 3/4	4
Skin defect (loss)	
No	0
< 1/4 circumference	1
1/4–1/2	2
1/2–3/4	3
> 3/4	4
Deep soft tissues (muscle, tendon, ligaments, joint capsule)	
No	0
< 1/4 circumference	1
1/4–1/2	2
1/2–3/4	3
> 3/4	6
Amputation	
No	0
Subtotal/total guillotine	20
Subtotal/total crush	30

D Nerves	Points
Palmar/plantar sensations	
Yes	0
No	8
Finger/toe motion	
Yes	0
No	8

E Contamination	Points
Foreign bodies	
None	0
Single	1
Multiple	2
Massive	10

F Bacteriological smear	Points
Aerobe 1 germ	2
Aerobe > 1 germ	3
Anaerobe	2
Aerobe/anaerobe	4

G Onset of treatment	Points
(Only if soft-tissue score > 2)	
6–12 hours	1
> 12 hours	3

Classification	Total A–B	
Fr. O 1	2–3	points
Fr. O 2	4–19	points
Fr. O 3	20–69	points
Fr. O 4	> 70	points

Classification	Total C–G	
Fr. C 0	1–3	points
Fr. C 1	4–6	points
Fr. C 2	7–12	points
Fr. C 3	> 12	points

Table 5.2-1 Hanover fracture scale with correlation of the fracture scale score to the Tscherne classification of open and closed fractures [5].

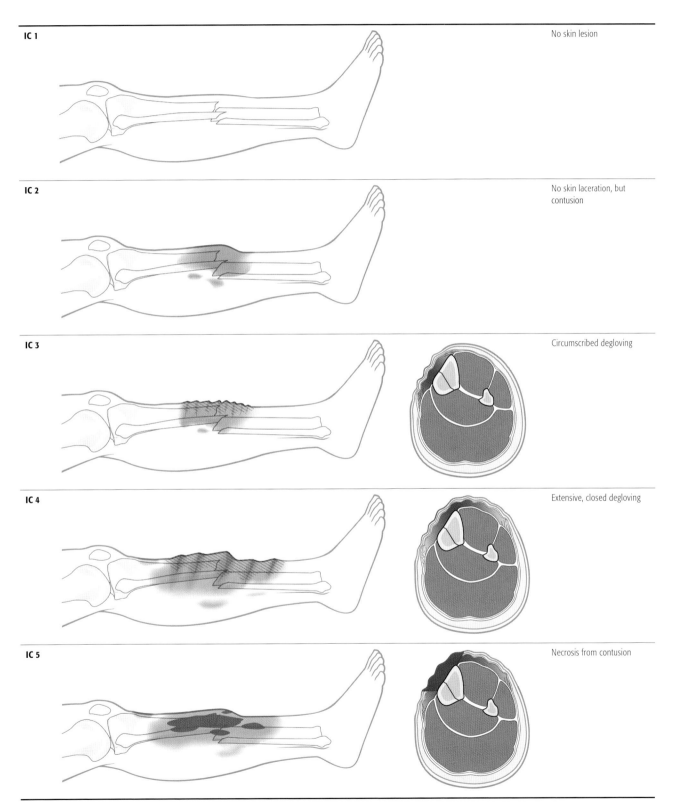

IC 1 — No skin lesion

IC 2 — No skin laceration, but contusion

IC 3 — Circumscribed degloving

IC 4 — Extensive, closed degloving

IC 5 — Necrosis from contusion

Table 5.2-2 AO soft-tissue classification: closed skin lesions (IC) [3].

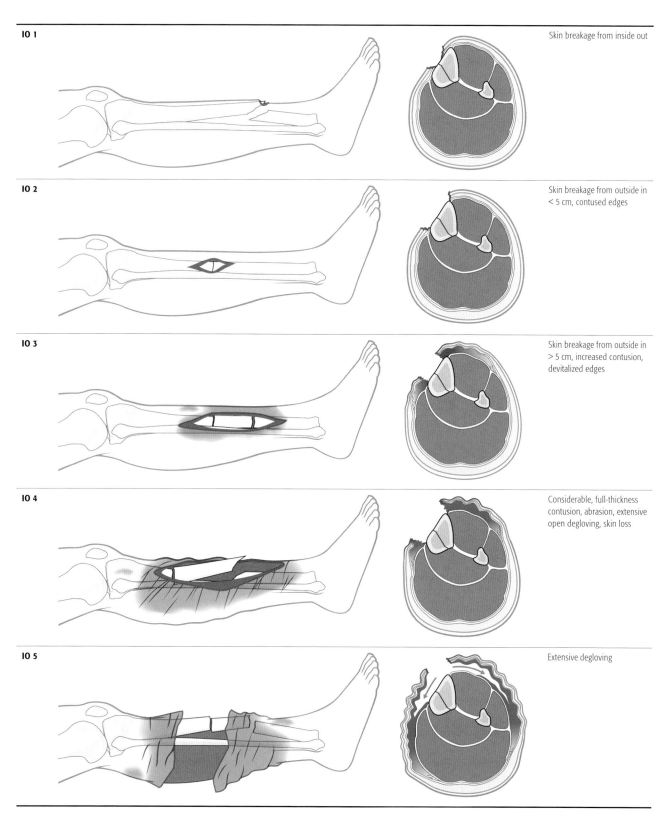

IO 1   Skin breakage from inside out

IO 2   Skin breakage from outside in < 5 cm, contused edges

IO 3   Skin breakage from outside in > 5 cm, increased contusion, devitalized edges

IO 4   Considerable, full-thickness contusion, abrasion, extensive open degloving, skin loss

IO 5   Extensive degloving

Table 5.2-3   AO soft-tissue classification: open skin lesions (IO) [3].

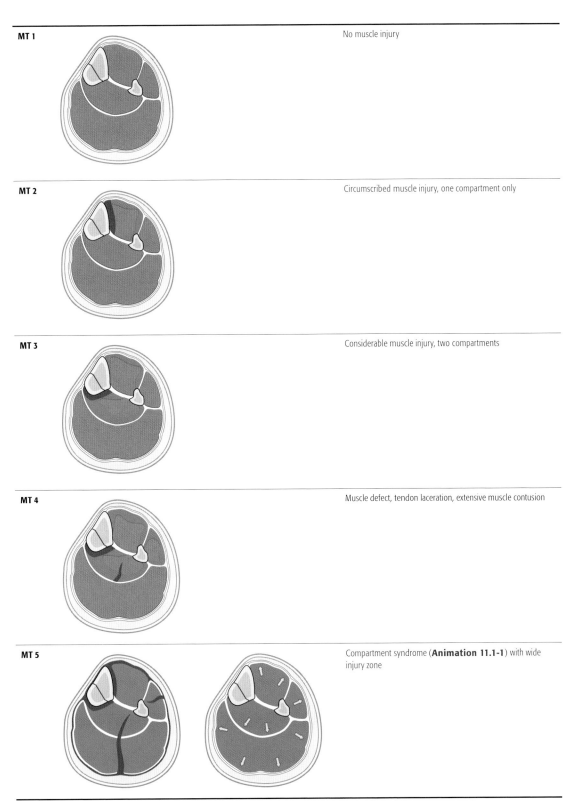

MT 1	No muscle injury
MT 2	Circumscribed muscle injury, one compartment only
MT 3	Considerable muscle injury, two compartments
MT 4	Muscle defect, tendon laceration, extensive muscle contusion
MT 5	Compartment syndrome (**Animation 11.1-1**) with wide injury zone

Table 5.2-4 AO soft-tissue classification: muscle and tendon lesions (MT) [3].

NV 1 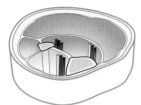 No neurovascular injury

NV 2 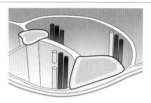 Isolated nerve injury

NV 3 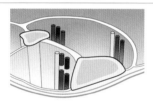 Localized vascular injury

NV 4 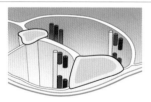 Extensive segmental vascular injury

NV 5 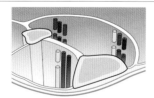 Neurovascular injury including subtotal or even total amputation

Table 5.2-5 AO soft-tissue classification: nerve and vessel lesions (NV) [3].

E = entry	Estimate the maximum diameter of the entry in centimeters.
X = exit	Estimate the maximum diameter of the exit (X = 0 if no exit) in centimeters.
C = cavity	Can the surgeon fit two fingers into the cavity before surgery? No: C = 0 Yes: C = 1 This may be obvious before surgery or only established after skin incision. For chest and abdominal wounds it refers to the wound of the chest or abdominal wall.
F = fracture	No fracture: F = 0 Simple fracture, clinically insignificant comminution: F = 1 Segmental bone loss or clinically significant comminution: F = 2
V = vital structure	Are brain, viscera (breach of dura, pleura, or peritoneum), or major vessels injured? No: V = 0 Yes: V = 1
M = metallic body	Bullet or fragments visible on x-ray. None: M = 0 One metallic body: M = 1 Multiple metallic bodies: M = 2

Table 5.2-6 International Red Cross war wound classification [17].

5.3 Limb salvage—pros and cons

Author David A Volgas

5.3.1 Overview

In recent years, as rescue times have decreased, neurovascular repair techniques have also improved. Therefore, attempts to salvage compromised extremities have been performed more frequently. The indication to perform this surgery is based upon classifications, which try to define

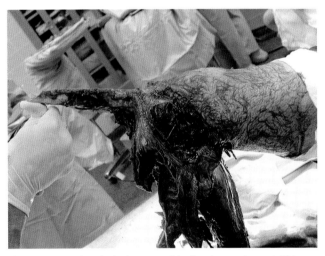

Fig 5.3-1 Massive degloving caused by farming equipment. This lower limb is not salvageable.

whether limbs are salvageable are not. Many of these early classification systems, such as the mangled extremity severity score (MESS), have tried to determine salvageability from a technical point of view. Recently, the more important question of which limbs should reasonably be salvaged from a functional point of view has received more attention.

While there are clear cases that cannot be salvaged (**Fig 5.3-1**), the trauma surgeon is more commonly confronted with severe limb injuries, which technically could be salvaged. However, limitations of skill, timing, or resources preclude this. When limb salvage is not possible, there is little decision making needed, except to plan the level of amputation in order to preserve as much function as possible. Fortunately, the majority of cases present with a technically salvageable extremity. The question confronting the surgeon is whether the patient will functionally be better off following reconstruction and limb salvage than following amputation.

The mangled extremity severity score is a score developed from a retrospective review of factors associated with amputation in 25 trauma patients, who had sustained severe injuries of the lower extremities [18]. In this scoring system, points are assigned based on skeletal and soft-tissue injury, time of limb ischemia, shock, and the patient's age (**Table 5.3-1**). In the first series, a mangled extremity severity score of 7

Type		Characteristics	Injuries	Points
Skeletal/soft-tissue	1	Low energy	Stab wounds, simple closed fractures, small-caliber gunshot wounds	1
	2	Medium energy	Open or multiple-level fractures, dislocations, moderate crush injuries	2
	3	High energy	Shotgun blast (close range), high-velocity gunshot wounds	3
	4	Massive crush	Logging, railroad, oil rig accidents	4
Shock	1	Normotensive hemodynamics	Blood pressure stable in field and operating room	0
	2	Transient hypotension	Blood pressure unstable in field, but responsive to intravenous fluids	1
	3	Prolonged hypotension	Systolic blood pressure < 90 mmHg and responsive to intravenous fluids only in the operating room	2
Ischemia	1	None	Pulsatile limb without signs of ischemia	0*
	2	Mild	Diminished pulses without signs of ischemia	1*
	3	Moderate	No pulse by Doppler, sluggish capillary refill, paresthesia, diminished motor activity	2*
	4	Advanced	Pulseless, cool, paralyzed and numb without capillary refill	3*
Age	1	< 30 years	–	0
	2	30–50 years	–	1
	3	> 50 years	–	2

Table 5.3-1 Mangled extremity severity score (MESS) [18]. Points are totaled after doubling ischemia scores if ischemic time is > 6 hours (*). Scores of 7 points or greater are associated with 100% predictive value for amputation.

or greater predicted amputation with a 100% accuracy. Later studies confirmed that scores lower than 7 are associated with higher salvage rates, however, high scores did not necessarily predict amputation [15, 19, 20].

The limb salvage index (LSI) similarly is based on a retrospective review of risk factors that showed that scores greater than or equal 6 were associated with amputation in 19 out

of 19 patients, whereas scores less than 6 were associated with limb salvage in 51 out of 51 cases (**Table 5.3-2**) [21]. Like other scores, later studies using the LSI prospectively did not confirm its absolute value in clinical decision making for individual patients [22, 23].

The nerve injury, ischemia, soft-tissue injury, skeletal injury, shock and age of the patient score (NISSSA) was

Location	Points	Extent of injury
Artery	0	Contusion, intimal tear, partial laceration or avulsion (pseudoaneurysm) with no distal thrombosis and palpable pedal pulses; complete occlusion of one of the three shank vessels or profunda
	1	Occlusion of two or more shank vessels, complete laceration, avulsion or thrombosis, or femoral or popliteal without pedal pulses
	2	Complete occlusion of femoral, popliteal or three of three shank vessels with no distal runoff
Nerve	0	Contusion or stretch injury, minimal clean lacertion of femoral, fibular or tibial nerve
	1	Partial transection or avulsion of sciatic nerve, complete or partial transection of femoral, fibular or tibial nerve
	2	Complete transection or avulsion of sciatic nerve, complete transection or avulsion of both tibial and fibular nerves
Bone	0	Closed fracture at one or two sites, open fracture without comminution or with minimal displacement; closed dislocation without fracture; open joint without foreign body; fibular fracture
	1	Closed fracture at three or more sites on same extremity; open fracture with comminution or moderate to large displacement; segmental fracture; fracture dislocation; open joint with foreign body; bone loss < 3 cm
	2	Bone loss > 3 cm; Gustilo type IIIB or IIIC fracture (open fracture with periosteal stripping), gross contamination, extensive soft-tissue injury-loss)
Skin	0	Clean laceration; single or multiple or small avulsion injuries, all with primary repair; first degree burn
	1	Delayed closure due to contamination; large avulsion requiring split-thickness skin graft or flap closure; second or third degree burns
Muscle	0	Laceration or avulsion involving a single compartment or single tendon
	1	Laceration or avulsion involving two or more compartments; complete laceration or avulsion, or two or more tendons
	2	Crush injury
Deep vein	0	Contusion, partial laceration or avulsion; complete laceration or avulsion if alternate route of venous return is intact; superficial vein injury
	1	Complete laceration, avulsion, or thrombosis with no alternate route of venous return
Warm ischemia time	0	< 6 hours
	1	6–9 hours
	2	9–12 hours
	3	12–15 hours
	4	> 15 hours

Table 5.3-2 Limb salvage index (LSI) [21]. Scores of 6 points or greater are associated with 100% amputation rate.

developed as a modification of the mangled extremity severity score (MESS) (**Table 5.3-3**) [24]. By adding nerve injury and splitting the soft tissue/fracture assessment into two separate scores, sensitivity and specificity of the system as well as its predictive value were improved.

The Hanover fracture scale was a further attempt to facilitate decision making as to whether a limb was salvageable or not [5] by incorporating detailed anatomical and physiological assessment of the injured extremity (**Table 5.2-1**). As it involves many more parameters than the mangled extremity severity score, it is of limited clinical use.

All of these different types of scores emphasize the technical capability of salvaging limbs in a major trauma center, which has the immediate availability of surgeons for plastic/

reconstructive surgery including vascular surgery, and offers total intensive care for the trauma patient. These prerequisites do not necessarily apply to less well-equipped trauma centers. Nor do they address outcomes after limb salvage or amputation.

The lower extremity assessment project (LEAP) studied functional outcomes after lower-extremity trauma and found that no functional difference could be detected between patients, who had undergone amputation and those whose limbs had been salvaged after severe lower-extremity trauma. Earlier, the LEAP study group published a report challenging the dogma that an insensate foot was an indication for amputation [16]. Against this background, this chapter will examine a comprehensive decision-making process for deciding whether to proceed with salvage or amputation.

Type of injury	Degree of injury	Points	Description
Nerve injury (N) Assessed in the emergency department	Sensate	0	No major nerve injury
	Dorsal	1	Deep or superficial nerve, femoral nerve injury
	Plantar partial	2	Tibial nerve injury
	Plantar complete	3	Sciatic nerve injury
Ischemia (I) Double scores if ischemia time > 6 hours	None	0	Good to fair pulses, no ischemia
	Mild	1	Reduced pulses, perfusion normal
	Moderate	2	No pulses, prolonged capillary refill, Doppler pulses present
	Severe	3	Pulseless, cool, ischemic, no Doppler pulses
Soft tissue/contamination (S)	Low	0	Minimal or no contusion, no contamination (Gustilo type I fracture)
	Medium	1	Moderate soft-tissue injury, low-velocity gunshot wound, moderate contamination (Gustilo type II fracture)
	High	2	Moderate crush, degloving, high-velocity gunshot wound, moderate soft-tissue injury, may require soft-tissue flap, considerable contamination (Gustilo type IIIA fracture)
	Severe	3	Massive crush, farmyard injury, severe degloving, severe contamination, requires soft-tissue flap (Gustilo type IIIB fracture)
Skeletal (S)	Low energy	0	Spiral fracture, oblique fracture, no or minimal displacement
	Medium energy	1	Transverse fracture, minimal comminution, small caliber gunshot wound
	High energy	2	Moderate displacement, moderate comminution, high velocity gunshot wound, butterfly fragments
	Severe energy	3	Segmental fracture, severe comminution, bone loss
Shock (S)	Normotensive	0	Blood pressure normal, always < 90 mmHg systolic
	Transient hypotension	1	Transient hypotension in field or emergency department
	Persistent hypotension	2	Persistent hypotension despite fluids
Age (A)	Young	0	< 30 years
	Middle	1	30–50 years
	Old	2	> 50 years

Table 5.3-3 Nerve, ischemia, soft-tissue, skeletal, shock, and age (NISSSA) score [24].

5.3.2 Upper extremity

There are few scores, which have been used to predict limb salvage outcomes of upper extremity injuries. The mangled extremity severity score has been tested and found not useable [15]. The prevailing opinion is that in the upper extremity every attempt should be made to salvage the limb (**Fig 5.3-2a–j**).

Unfortunately, there nevertheless are cases when amputation is still the best option (**Fig 5.3-3**). Some cases are clearly not salvageable, such as massive crush injuries with segmental bone and soft-tissue loss as well as extensive neurovascular injury. Other situations are more questionable, such as when there is traumatic loss of both the flexor and extensor compartments, or in case of compartment syndrome, but vascular supply is still present. Since most patients prefer a nonfunctional limb to a prosthesis in the upper extremity, reconstruction is more often attempted.

During the initial assessment of an injured upper extremity, the surgeon should make a thorough inventory of the intact muscles, vessels, and nerves in order to facilitate the decision-making process. Until a large-series study demonstrates more clear-cut outcome differences between salvage and amputation, the trauma surgeon should attempt to salvage the limb as long as this is technically feasible.

In contrast, there has been tremendous progress in regard to technically advanced prostheses in recent years. A poorly functioning or nonfunctional hand, or a hand that causes chronic pain and has no sensation is often not as good as a good stump, especially if it is on the nondominant side. Such conditions, most often in young men, hinder reintegration into the working process. These patients, therefore, not only suffer a lot, but cost society more than an initial, respectively delayed, amputation. Currently, hand or arm allotransplantation gets quite a lot of attention in the media, and is vigorously discussed in professional circles. Such

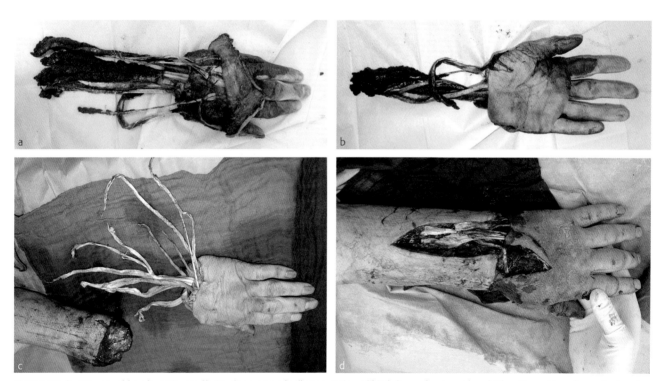

Fig 5.3-2a–j 50-year-old male patient suffering from a treadmill amputation of his left nondominant hand. The attempt to salvage the hand was successful.
a Dorsal view of the amputate 45 minutes after amputation. Note the extensive dirt, particularly at the tendon level.
b Palmar view.
c Dorsal view of the amputate and the stump after thorough surgical debridement.
d Dorsal view after replantation of the hand including internal fixation, anastomosis of two arteries (radial and ulnar artery), three veins (the radial and an ulnar concomitant vein (deep draining system), and the cephalic vein (superficial draining system). Note the bluish skin flap at the hand's dorsum.

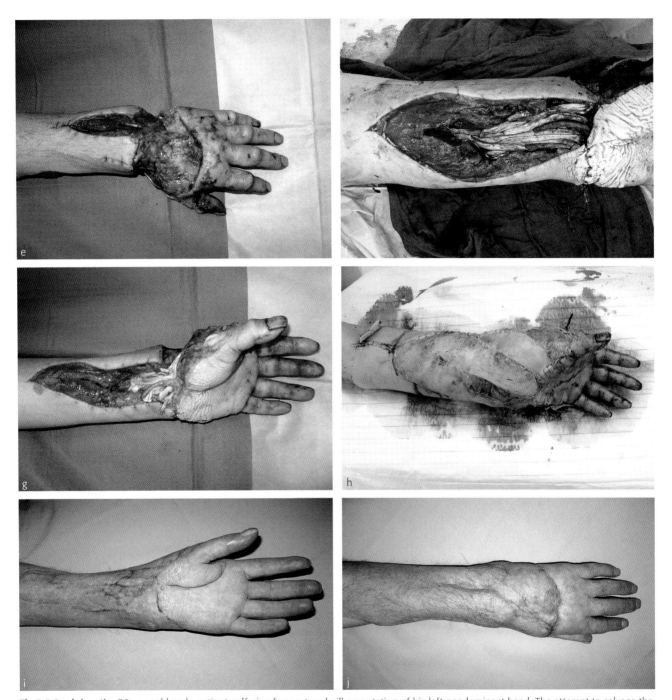

Fig 5.3-2a–j (cont) 50-year-old male patient suffering from a treadmill amputation of his left nondominant hand. The attempt to salvage the hand was successful.

e Dorsal view 2 weeks after replantation. Part of the skin flap has developed necrosis and has been debrided.

f Palmar view after replantation. Note the extensive cutaneous skin defect.

g Palmar view with exposed flexor tendons.

h Palmar view 3 days after coverage of the defect using a chimeric free muscle flap (latissimus dorsi and serratus anterior muscles) and split-thickness skin graft.

i Dorsal view: Follow-up at 12 months. Note the good color and texture match of the skin-grafted flap that has significantly atrophied.

j Palmar view: Follow-up at 12 months. Note the good color and texture match of the skin-grafted flap, the slight bulkiness of the flap dorsally, and the well-perfused hand with normal trophicity. Functional adduction of the fingers (intrinsic muscles).

interventions are thought to overcome the disability of these amputated patients. Since this treatment is still associated with life-long immunosuppression and all its drawbacks, limb transplantation of composite tissue will only become an option in very selected cases, performed by specialized teams.

If surgery or allotransplantation is not an option for the patient, a myoelectric prosthesis could be a valuable alternative in the future. The myoelectric prosthesis is an "intelligent" replacement of the arm of hand that can be controlled by muscle contraction.

5.3.3 Lower extremity

The surgeon should approach severe trauma to the lower extremity with a different set of criteria than for the upper extremity, because of the differences in perception of body image and the functionality of the available reconstructive options. In the upper extremity, a variety of tendon or muscle transfers are possible, which may restore the function of the hand. In contrast, in the lower extremity, there are much fewer options, because the impairment caused by losing motion of a toe is far less than that of a finger. Moreover, many very good foot or ankle prosthetic replacements are available, which can replicate different functions of the foot.

In the lower extremity, more factors should be assessed before deciding on limb salvage or amputation, in large part because the function of well-planned stumps at the level of

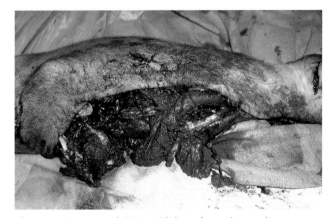

Fig 5.3-3 Severe crush injury with loss of vascular supply, gross contamination, loss of all muscles in the forearm, and a comminuted fracture of both bones, which was sustained in a mining accident. Amputation is the method of choice.

the mid foot, lower leg, or thigh fitted by effective and well-tolerated prostheses are usually very good. As in the upper extremity, absolute indications for amputation are:
- nonreconstructible vascular injury (eg, segmental and/or very distal vascular injury)
- crush injury comprising a wide zone of the extremity, such as after hydraulic press injury
- insensate foot
- the patient's age, comorbidities, and general state of health at the time of the injury
- overwhelming infection or necrotizing fasciitis.

If a lower extremity is considered to be technically salvageable, then a decision must be reached whether salvage should be attempted or not. In most situations, the functional outcome should be the primary determinant of salvage or amputation. In some cultures, the integrity of the body and especially of the limbs may be even more important than function and this fact should not be ignored.

While an easy concept, function should be considered from a broad perspective. Prosthetic function must be compared with the potential functional outcome of a salvaged limb. The lower extremity assessment project demonstrated that more than half of all patients with an insensate foot recover plantar sensation within 2 years [16]. There is little data concerning the functional recovery of injured or denervated muscle, however, lacerated or crushed muscle is not likely to regain significant function and may lead to contractures.

Surgeons should carefully assess the entire environment and circumstances in which the patient lives. They must, whenever possible, present the likely outcome of salvage versus amputation to the patient and his or her relatives and allow them to participate in the decision-making process, unless the limb is truly unsalvageable. Surgeons should consider the following when explaining options to the patient and/or family:
- occupation and activity of the patient
- availability of suitable prosthetics
- general health, compliance, and expectations of the patient, who may have to undergo multiple procedures in order to reconstruct the limb (eg, age, smoking, medication, diabetes, nutritional state, profession)
- risks associated with limb salvage procedure(s): anesthetic risks, bleeding, vascular occlusion, infection, wound breakdown, malunion, nonunion, persistent pain, multiple surgeries, long rehabilitation time, possibility of secondary amputation, long process of professional and/or social reintegration, etc

- risks associated with amputation: wound breakdown, phantom sensation, phantom pain, replacement costs of prosthetics, etc
- time it may take to reconstruct a limb versus recovery time from an amputation
- function of the limb if all reconstructive efforts (fracture healing, soft-tissue coverage, etc) are successful
- function of the prosthesis in the context of the patient's occupation and activities

- social and cultural environment of the patient (in some cultures, amputees are ostracized from society).

Patients must be made to feel that there is no right or wrong choice, only alternative ways of restoring function. Some patients and physicians will view amputation as a failure. This should be discouraged. Restoration of preinjury activities is the goal. By carefully considering the path to this goal, both patient and physician can reach the best decision.

References and further reading

[1] **Gustilo RB, Anderson JT** (1976) Prevention of infection in the treatment of one thousand and twenty-five open fractures of long bones: retrospective and prospective analyses. *J Bone Joint Surg Am;* 58(4):453–458.

[2] **Gustilo RB, Mendoza RM, Williams DN** (1984) Problems in the management of type III (severe) open fractures: a new classification of type III open fractures. *J Trauma;* 24(8):742–746.

[3] **Rüedi TP, Buckley RE, Moran CG** (2007) *AO Principles of Fracture Management.* 2nd ed. Stuttgart New York: Georg Thieme Verlag.

[4] **Tscherne H, Oestern HJ** (1982) [A new classification of soft-tissue damage in open and closed fractures]. *Unfallheilkunde;* 85(3):111–115. German.

[5] **Krettek C, Seekamp A, Köntopp H, et al** (2001) Hannover Fracture Scale '98—re-evaluation and new perspectives of an established extremity salvage score. *Injury;* 32(4):317–328, Elsevier.

[6] **Berk WA, Osbourne DD, Taylor DD** (1988) Evaluation of the 'golden period' for wound repair: 204 cases from a Third World emergency department. *Ann Emerg Med;* 17(5):496–500.

[7] **Clement ND, Tennant C, Muwanga C** (2010) Polytrauma in the elderly: predictors of the cause and time of death. *Scand J Trauma Resusc Emerg Med;* 13:18–26.

[8] **Kline AJ, Gruen GS, Pape HC, et al** (2009) Early complications following the operative treatment of pilon fractures with and without diabetes. *Foot Ankle Int;* 30(11):1042–1047.

[9] **Castillo RC, Bosse MJ, MacKenzie EJ, et al** (2005) Impact of smoking on fracture healing and risk of complications in limb-threatening open tibia fractures. *J Orthop Trauma;* 19(3):151–157.

[10] **Nåsell H, Adami J, Samnegård E, et al** (2010) Effect of smoking cessation intervention on results of acute fracture surgery: a randomized controlled trial. *J Bone Joint Surg Am;* 92(6):1335–1342.

[11] **Ferrari M, Mottola L, Quaresima V** (2004) Principles, techniques, and limitations of near infrared spectroscopy. *Can J Appl Physiol;* 29(4):463–487.

[12] **Mothes H, Dönicke T, Friedel R, et al** (2004) Indocyanine-green fluorescence video angiography used clinically to evaluate tissue perfusion in microsurgery. *J Trauma;* 57(5):1018–1024.

[13] **Inaba K, Potzman J, Munera F, et al** (2006) Multi-slice CT angiography for arterial evaluation in the injured lower extremity. *J Trauma;* 60(3):502–507.

[14] **Rajan V, Varghese B, van Leeuwen TG, et al** (2009) Review of methodological developments in laser Doppler flowmetry. *Lasers Med Sci;* 24(2):269–283.

[15] **Bosse MJ, McCarthy ML, Jones AL, et al** (2005) The insensate foot following severe lower extremity trauma: an indication for amputation? *J Bone Joint Surg Am;* 87(12):2601–2608.

[16] **Mackenzie EJ, Bosse MJ** (2006) Factors influencing outcome following limb-threatening lower limb trauma: lessons learned from the lower extremity assessment project (LEAP). *J Am Acad Orthop Surg;* 4(10):205–210.

[17] **Coupland RM** (1992) The Red Cross classification of war wounds: the E.X.C.F.V.M. scoring system. *World J Surg;* 16(5):910–917, Springer.

[18] **Johansen K, Daines M, Howey T, et al** (1990) Objective criteria accurately predict amputation following lower extremity trauma. *J Trauma;* 30(5):568–573, Lippincott Williams & Wilkins, Wolters Kluwer Health.

[19] **Bosse MJ, MacKenzie EJ, Kellam JF, et al** (2001) A prospective evaluation of the clinical utility of the lower-extremity injury-severity scores. *J Bone Joint Surg Am;* 83-A(1):3–14.

[20] **O'Sullivan ST, O'Sullivan M, Pasha N, et al** (1997) Is it possible to predict limb viability in complex Gustilo IIIB and IIIC tibial fractures? A comparison of two predictive indices. *Injury;* 28(9–10):639–642.

[21] **Russell WL, Sailors DM, Whittle TB, et al** (1991) Limb salvage versus traumatic amputation. A decision based on a seven-part predictive index. *Ann Surg;* 213(5):473–480; discussion 480–481, Lippincott Williams & Wilkins, Wolters Kluwer Health.

[22] **Dagum AB, Best AK, Schemitsch EH, et al** (1999) Salvage after severe lower-extremity trauma: are the outcomes worth the means? *Plast Reconstr Surg;* 103(4):1212–1220.

[23] **Durham RM, Mistry BM, Mazuski JE, et al** (1996) Outcome and utility of scoring systems in the management of the mangled extremity. *Am J Surg;* 172(5):569–573; discussion 573–574.

[24] **McNamara MG, Heckman JD, Corley FG** (1994) Severe open fractures of the lower extremity: a retrospective evaluation of the Mangled Extremity Severity Score (MESS). *J Orthop Trauma;* 8(2):81–87, Lippincott Williams & Wilkins, Wolters Kluwer Health.

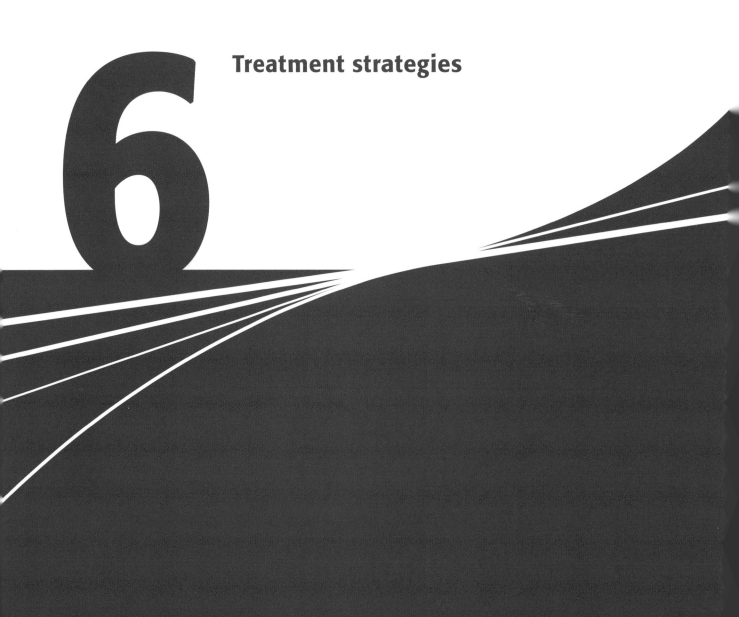

6 Treatment strategies

6.1 Emergency department management

Authors   Ulrich Stöckle, Hans-Günther Machens

6.1.1 Introduction

Soft-tissue trauma—including thermal injury—embraces a wide range of lesions from minor to life-threatening, which necessitate immediate and coordinated action by all surgical specialties involved. Prehospital assessment and decision for or against referral to the trauma center can sometimes be subject to an over- or underestimation of the severity of a trauma, which needs to be corrected within the treatment algorithm.

The situation in a trauma bay is often filled with action, adrenaline, and agitation when trauma patients arrive. There is often a flurry of activity, which, if uncoordinated, can waste valuable time and resources. Crucial to the care of severely injured or critically-ill patients is a well-rehearsed plan of action, which begins even before the patient arrives at the hospital.

6.1.2 Organizational aspects of the emergency department

Communication with emergency department personnel should begin prior to the patient's arrival at the hospital. Skilled first responders should have radio contact with the receiving hospital and should provide an accurate field assessment of the extent of injuries, or at least the mechanism of injury. The mechanism of injury (eg, high-energy trauma versus low-energy, blunt trauma versus penetrating trauma) (chapter 3) may determine the destination of the patient, eg, patients with high-energy injuries should preferably be diverted to specialized (level I) trauma centers. This early triage can help avoid unnecessary delays in definitive treatment, which occur when patients are first taken to a lower-level care facility, where they are evaluated, and then have to be transferred to a higher-level care facility [1]. While the mechanism of injury itself is not diagnostic, it may heighten awareness of the trauma team regarding unrecognized injury [2], and eventually reduce the economic costs resulting from complex injuries of the extremities that affect bone and soft tissues [3].

Upon arrival at the trauma center, every patient admitted to the emergency department should be seen and managed primarily by an experienced general or trauma surgeon, who is in charge of the evaluation, resuscitation, and coor-

dination efforts [4]. As a matter of course, the evaluation of the patient and the injuries varies, based on the available resources and the extent of suspected injury.

In emergency management, it is the duty of the team leader to involve the consulting experts from other specialties according to the different injuries (**Fig 6.1-1**). In case of severe soft-tissue injury—either as an isolated trauma or polytrauma—it is essential to include a soft-tissue specialist, preferably the plastic surgeon as early as possible [5, 6]. Even though such organizational structures are not always available in every trauma center, there is evidence that an early interdisciplinary approach will help to correctly diagnose and classify the severity of soft-tissue lesions, thus preventing a delay in the appropriate treatment [7, 8].

Depending on the infrastructure of the hospital and the availability of qualified personnel, the trauma leader must decide whether the hospital is capable of taking care of certain types of injuries or whether a referral to a specialized

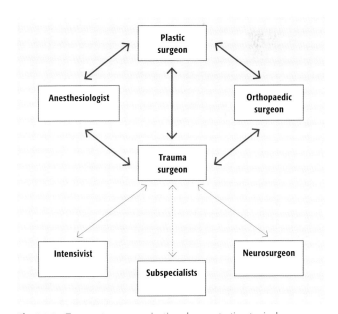

Fig 6.1-1 Trauma team organization demonstrating typical communication pathways between team members. The role of the trauma surgeon may be filled by orthopaedic or general surgeons or by emergency physicians, depending on local practice. Subspecialists often involved in trauma care: burn specialist, gynecologist, hand surgeon, oral and maxillofacial surgeon, ophthalmologist, oto-rhino-laryngologist, urologist, vascular surgeon.

trauma center should be arranged. Clear and individualized decision trees should be implemented for every hospital with an emergency department admitting trauma patients.

6.1.3 General management of trauma patients

Isolated extremity trauma

The focus of an isolated extremity trauma in an otherwise healthy patient should be on the assessment of the severity of the injury. Good communication with the prehospital care team and collection of all available information about the mechanism of injury is of highest priority [5]. The type of injury to be expected varies, depending on whether the patient sustained a car or a skiing accident, a gunshot wound, or, as a pedestrian, was hit by a car. The mechanism of injury provides important clues as to the location (eg, fracture of the proximal third of the tibia in a pedestrian struck by a car) and the potential severity of the lesions. The rescue team transporting the patient to the emergency department should further supply information about the initial condition of the patient as well as the time interval since the accident.

In patients with closed and benign-appearing soft tissues, the condition and real extent of the injury must be assessed carefully (chapter 5.1). In alert patients, the clinical evaluation with respect to pain, perfusion, and peripheral movement, eg, the ability to flex and extend the toes, most often is sufficient in order to detect or exclude compartment syndrome. In case of doubt, the additional measurement of compartment pressure can be helpful, especially if the measurements are repeated during the clinical course or performed on an unconscious patient (chapter 5.1, 11.1).

In open injuries, a primary inspection must be performed in the trauma bay. However, everybody involved must respect the local guidelines regarding sterility (ie, face masks as well as sterile gloves, cloth, bandages, and instruments). The size of the wound and the involvement of bone, muscles and/or neurovascular structures must be assessed, recorded, and adequately documented during the primary survey. Thereafter, a sterile wound dressing is mandatory, which should not be removed again until further treatment in the operating room is initiated. Inspection and evaluation of the structures peripheral to the injury is the next step.

Pallor of the skin and/or unequal palpation of the peripheral pulses when compared to the uninjured side are suspicious signs of vascular compromise. This condition mandates immediate assessment of the peripheral circulation, which means checking temperature, capillary refill, making use of Doppler sonography or angiography in order to confirm any vascular lesion, as well as to determine its extent and location. Furthermore, asymmetrical pulses after reduction of an articulation (eg, knee dislocation) as well as bluish discoloration and swelling of the extremity, which may indicate impaired venous drainage, are conditions that warrant a vascular study. If not already involved, the vascular or plastic surgeon needs to be informed and included in the decision-making process.

X-rays of the injured area are mandatory and can be obtained during the initial evaluation. Exceptionally, one x-ray plane may give sufficient information in case of total or subtotal amputations for primary diagnostics, whereas CT scans are sometimes necessary to adequately evaluate comminuted fractures with involvement of a joint. Beside the bone structures, special attention should be given to shadows and foreign bodies within the soft tissue, while the extent of the injury may often be judged on plain x-rays indicating the severity of the injury.

The information obtained at this point of the evaluation is sufficient to begin the multidisciplinary planning process, which will determine the time and nature of treatment.

Polytrauma

The basic approach to the evaluation of extremity injuries in a polytrauma patient is the same when compared to isolated injuries of the extremity, including the soft tissues. The soft-tissue injury should be incorporated into the polytrauma algorithm, and assessed and managed according to the priorities set by the overall patient condition. Soft-tissue trauma due to high-velocity/severe deceleration events are often associated with abdominal or cerebral injuries, which necessitate immediate surgical intervention after clinical and radiological diagnostics and stabilization of the vital parameters. An organized trauma team with well-defined roles and protocols for every single member of the trauma team or the emergency department staff will allow efficient assessment and rapid treatment of critically-injured patients, leading to a reduction in the rate of morbidity and mortality. In busy trauma centers, individual team members have preassigned roles and the initial resuscitation and evaluation proceeds automatically, with little direction from the team leader. It is important to have a person assigned to record vital signs and interventions as they occur, who does not have to participate directly in the starting of intravenous medication or any other tasks.

Together, the anesthesiologist, the intensivist and all consulting specialists who will be involved according to the type of injury, will follow the polytrauma algorithm for primary evaluation as defined by the advanced trauma life support (ATLS) criteria [5]. Initially, the goal is to resuscitate and stabilize the patient, which requires that primary evaluation and decision making must be fast and precise. This includes a check and record of all vital signs, such as airway and circulation. Problems are addressed as they are identified. Simultaneously, the primary clinical survey from head to toe is directed to find obvious instabilities that might include the pelvic ring, fractures of the long bones, and injuries of the soft tissues. Initial diagnostics such as x-ray (chest, pelvis, lateral cervical spine), blood tests including hematocrit, blood type and cross-match, and electrolytes, abdominal ultrasound or rapid-sequence CT scans are carried out in parallel in order to detect or exclude sources of major bleeding and potentially life-threatening injuries. The degree of consciousness is documented using the Glasgow coma scale (GCS), if the patient has not yet been intubated.

At this point, obvious diagnoses are summarized and recorded, while treatment priorities are set. With a successfully resuscitated and stabilized patient, further diagnostic steps may now be performed as clinically indicated. Severe soft-tissue injuries need to be included in the decision-making process as well.

6.1.4 Debridement and irrigation in the trauma bay

Radical debridement and irrigation of the wound usually are procedures to be performed in the operating room under anesthesia and sterile conditions (chapter 7.1)(eg, chapter 12.2). In the trauma bay only emergency procedures may be carried out. In open injuries with severe contamination an initial irrigation (chapter 7.2) and disinfection as well as a careful removal of foreign bodies and obviously devitalized or contaminated tissue can be performed during the initial wound inspection before sterile wound coverage (eg, chapter 12.2). This will not cause any additional pain, since only devitalized tissue is removed. In open wounds with significant blood loss, obvious sources of bleeding such as lacerated small vessels can be cauterized or ligated, while major vessels can even be tamponaded temporarily or closed definitively using microclamps, thereby stabilizing the general condition of the patient. As a general rule, thorough irrigation and debridement of the wound should only be performed in the trauma bay in exceptional situations. Definitive irrigation and debridement requires adequate sterility, anesthesia, lighting and instruments—conditions only rarely given in the trauma bay.

6.1.5 Role of microbiological cultures, antibiotics, and tetanus

In open injuries, swabs of the wounds can be taken during wound assessment. However, they need to be taken under strictly sterile conditions. Instead of swabs, it is recommended to take several bits of representative wound tissue in order to obtain a suitable microbiological work-up. Many surgeons therefore postpone the initial bacteriological wound assessment until the patient is in the operating room.

Short-term antibiotic prophylaxis is to be initiated as early as possible and according to the specific protocol used in the hospital. Generally, first- or second-generation cephalosporins are considered adequate for simple wounds, while penicillin should be added for farmyard injuries, and an aminoglycoside for Gustilo type III fractures. Antibiotic prophylaxis should be limited to 24–48 hours. Thereafter, therapeutic coverage—if indicated—is best administered based on the results of cultures. In all patients with insufficient or questionable tetanus status, an immunization is to be initiated immediately.

6.1.6 Field coverage of the wound

If the rescue team reported an open wound or open fracture, and the wound was primarily covered with a sterile dressing, the dressing should be left in place in the trauma bay if the patient is expected to go to the operating room regardless of the findings. However, if there is any question about whether the wound requires operative management, wound inspection is allowed by an experienced senior surgeon under strictly sterile precautions. After inspection and photographic documentation, the wound is disinfected and covered with sterile dressings. In addition to wound coverage, the injured extremity should temporarily be immobilized with a splint and only removed for x-ray evaluation and further treatment.

6.2 Interdisciplinary decision making and staging of treatment

Authors   Hans-Günther Machens, Ulrich Stöckle

6.2.1 Introduction

Despite technological progress in the surgical management of fractures and reconstruction of soft-tissue injuries, patients with severe, traumatic soft-tissue defects still represent a major surgical challenge, requiring an interdisciplinary approach [9]. Due to the etiology of trauma (eg, high-velocity accidents) (chapter 3), the soft-tissue damage in many cases is more extensive than initially apparent and equals the zone of injury (chapter 10.3.3). Especially inexperienced colleagues or residents tend to underestimate soft-tissue injuries and direct patients on to an inadequate therapeutic path [10].

It has been demonstrated that decision making and treatment plans for an individual patient are often incorrect and that correction often comes too late, when the patient has already left the emergency department. Such mismanagement often delays the start of treatment, which may result in more complicated surgical and postoperative courses, prolonged hospitalization time, and ultimately higher costs [11]. The multidisciplinary treatment strategy—including timing for complex injuries of the extremities—is guided by the injury pattern, the ischemia time of the tissues, and the general condition of the patient (eg, additional injuries, polytrauma, shock).

6.2.2 Role of the trauma/orthopaedic surgeon

Depending on the educational background and national differences, it will either be an orthopaedic surgeon with special interest in extremity trauma or a trauma/general surgeon with an interest in fracture management, who will be taking care of the injured patient in the emergency department. Regardless of specialization—orthopaedic or trauma surgeon—it appears crucial that a single physician, preferably a senior colleague, is responsible for a specific patient—as a "trauma team leader". This person should be the first one to see and examine the patient in the trauma bay. During primary survey, the trauma team leader must assess the patient as a whole, recognizing the injury pattern and the severity of each injury, and will then decide which specialty consultants (burn specialist, gynecologist, hand surgeon, ophthalmologist, oral and maxillofacial surgeon, oto-rhino-laryngologist, urologist, vascular surgeon, etc

(Fig 6.1-1)) to call in. They will then establish the initial treatment plan and priorities based on the ATLS trauma protocol.

In patients with soft-tissue trauma, the severity and extent of the soft-tissue injury should ideally be assessed by the trauma surgeon in charge and a plastic surgeon. Special attention should be paid to muscles, fascia, tendons, and neurovascular structures. Injuries of the hand nearly always require primary consultation of a hand surgeon. In consultation with subspecialists and based on available resources, the trauma team leader will guide the timing and set the priorities for planned surgical interventions. The decision to include a specialist for the management of the soft tissues should be made liberally and as early as possible. Likely indications for an early interdisciplinary management of soft-tissue injuries are Gustilo type IIIC fractures, extended soft-tissue defects with or without segmental bone loss, and amputation injuries with the option of replantation (Fig 6.2-1) (chapter 5.2).

6.2.3 Role of the plastic surgeon

If available and in house, a plastic surgeon should immediately be included in the decision-making process while the patient is in the emergency department. Because of their expertise in the treatment of extended soft-tissue injuries, an early involvement to formulate a detailed treatment plan is of crucial importance and will improve outcome.

Today, technology-supported decision-making tools such as teleconsulting may help to fill such a gap if properly used. A telemedicine system using a mobile camera-phone as communication tool has been suggested as feasible and valuable alternative for early diagnosis and triaging of soft-tissue injury in emergency cases, with online verbal communication and review of the image transmitted [12]. Although such systems have the advantages of easy use, low cost, and high mobility, they cannot substitute the personal physical examination by the experienced clinician. Even with the appropriate clinical expertise and use of the relevant scores such as the mangled extremity severity score (MESS) (chapter 5.3), interdisciplinary decision making for amputation will be necessary in selected cases of severe soft-tissue injuries in order to preserve the patient's "life before limb".

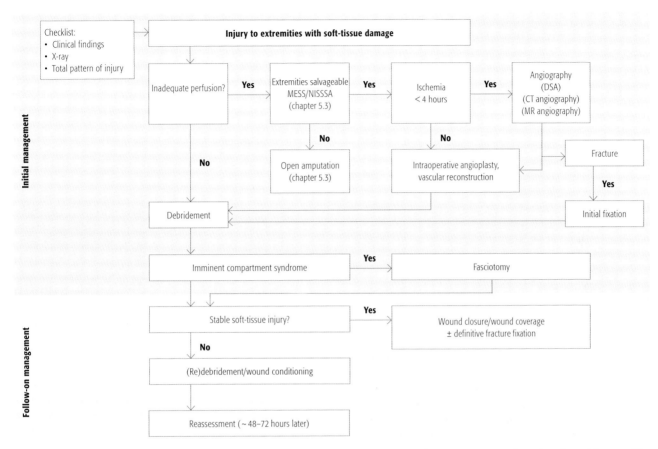

Fig 6.2-1 Algorithm for the management of complex soft-tissue injuries. Note that repeated reassessment is indicated until a stable wound is obtained.

6.2.4 Decision making for limbs at risk

Once a complex injury has been fully evaluated, including conventional x-ray, CT scan, Doppler, angiography, etc (chapter 5.1), and a surgical reconstruction appears feasible, the further steps will have to be established together with the plastic surgeon in a general treatment plan. Simultaneously, therapeutic priorities must be set (eg, fracture fixation before vascular repair or vice versa, temporary shunting, immediate soft-tissue coverage versus delayed soft-tissue coverage) in order not to lose valuable time.

Generally, the procedure will start with a meticulous inspection of the wound ("inventory") in the operating room, debridement of all necrotic tissue, dead bone fragments, and foreign bodies (chapter 7.1), and wound irrigation (chapter 7.2). Only then will it be possible to once more assess the extent of the injury in more detail, which might require an adaptation of the next therapeutic step(s).

Next, if necessary, the type of fracture fixation has to be decided upon—either by internal or external fixation. Today, in diaphyseal fractures, intramedullary nailing is clearly preferred. In articular fractures of major joints, temporary bridging with an external fixator will be the primary option. The same applies to fractures with complex vascular and/or soft-tissue defects. However, it is very important that the placement of the fixator pins is well planned as they should not impede secondary debridements, nor interfere with later reconstructive procedures (ie, pedicled or free flap surgery). In some cases, primary shortening of the bone may be chosen. Nevertheless, early stabilization of the fracture has to be performed (chapter 7.3).

In the presence of compartment syndrome or after a successful vascular reconstruction, it is mandatory to perform an adequate release of the different muscle compartments in order to avoid muscle damage. Nerve lesions will only exceptionally be approached at this early stage. However, the specialist should be consulted with regard to how the severed nerve ends should be tagged in order that they can be easily relocated during subsequent surgery. Their exact position must be recorded in the operating room report, preferably together with a drawing.

Although the different options of wound closure and coverage will be discussed in detail in the following chapters, this question must be addressed from the very beginning in the decision making and treatment plan (chapter 10.1 to 10.6).

6.2.5 Staging of therapeutic procedures

Several reasons may lead to a staged treatment of a complex injury of the extremity:

- The severity of the bone or joint injury and/or soft tissue is such that a primary definitive repair appears too extensive and risky.
- The patient's condition—usually due to multiple concomitant injuries—does not allow any prolonged surgical procedure, but, nevertheless, requires stabilization of the long bones and large joints according to the principle of damage-control surgery.
- The infrastructure is not suitable, eg, unavailability of an experienced surgical team, inadequte equipment in the operating room, lack of postoperative treatment capacity, ie, intensive care unit.

A well-defined treatment plan that may include a staged therapeutic approach is therefore a prerequisite. This plan should, whenever possible, be established together with all subspecialists that are needed. Basically, the approach is identical in comparison to one-stage surgery, including intraoperative survey of the injury, wound irrigation and de-

bridement. However, the stabilization of the fractured bone or bones that may include joints will often be achieved by external fixation–either within a long bone or by bridging a major joint. Again the placement of pins is crucial, as it should not interfere with any subsequent surgical procedure of the treatment plan. Depending on the general recovery of the patient and the local conditions (ie, swelling of the soft tissues), the second stage is usually planned for 3–5 days after the accident, while second-look debridement is usually performed earlier, after 24–72 hours [13].

The second stage may include definitive stabilization of the open fracture, including bone replacement with nonvascularized or vascularized bone. In such cases, consulting a plastic surgeon may be particularly helpful in order to decide upon the most adequate soft-tissue coverage (eg, local versus free flap) to be used so that bone healing and stable wound closure can be achieved. If the type of fixation has to be changed from an external to an internal fixator (eg, intramedullary nail or plate osteosynthesis), it should be done as early as possible—ideally within the first 10 days after the injury—as this will reduce the risk of osteitis. If the soft-tissue defect does not yet appear ready for closure, wound conditioning may be performed before the next stage (chapter 9.3), always taking into account that the true zone of injury extends beyond the visibly damaged tissue (chapter 10.3.3).

The third stage of reconstruction should be delayed until wound healing appears complete and the patient has recovered fully, including the completion of an early rehabilitation period. This stage will include secondary bone grafting, nerve reconstruction, or tendon/muscle transfers for the restoration of motor function as well as refinement surgery of the soft tissues in order for footwear to fit as well as to be aesthetically pleasing.

References and further reading

[1] **Sampalis JS, Denis R, Fréchette P, et al** (1997) Direct transport to tertiary trauma centers versus transfer from lower level facilities: impact on mortality and morbidity among patients with major trauma. *J Trauma;* 43(2):288–295; discussion 295–296.

[2] **Frink M, Zeckey C, Haasper C, et al** (2010) [Injury severity and pattern at the scene. What is the influence of the mechanism of injury?]. *Unfallchirurg;* 113(5):360–365. German.

[3] **Schwermann T, Grotz M, Blanke M, et al** (2004) [Evaluation of costs incurred for patients with multiple trauma particularly from the perspective of the hospital]. *Unfallchirurg;* 107(7):563–574.German.

[4] **Regel G, Bayeff-Filloff M** (2004) [Diagnosis and immediate therapeutic management of limb injuries. A systematic review of the literature]. *Unfallchirurg;* 107(10):919–926. German.

[5] **Vasconez HC, Nicholls PJ** (1991) Management of extremity injuries with external fixator or Ilizarov devices. Cooperative effort between orthopedic and plastic surgeons. *Clin Plast Surg;* 18(3):505–513.

[6] **Pape HC, Hildebrand F, Krettek C** (2004) [Decision making and priorities for surgical treatment during and after shock trauma room treatment]. *Unfallchirurg;* 107(10):927–36. German.

[7] **Wurmb T, Frühwald P, Roewer N, et al** (2009) [Clinical pathway, quality circle and standard operating procedures as tools for quality management in the trauma suite]. *Z Evid Fortbild Qual Gesundhwes;* 103(1):49–57. German.

[8] **Bernhard M, Becker TK, Nowe T, et al** (2007) Introduction of a treatment algorithm can improve the early management of emergency patients in the resuscitation room. *Resuscitation;* 73(3):362–373.

[9] **Schaser KD, Melcher I, Stöckle U, et al** (2004) [Interdisciplinarity in reconstructive surgery of the extremities]. *Unfallchirurg;* 107(9):732–743. German.

[10] **Tscherne H, Oestern HJ (**1982) [A new classification of soft-tissue damage in closed and open fractures]. *Unfallheilkunde;* 85(3):111–115.

[11] **Machens HG, Kaun M, Lange T, et al** (2006) [Clinical impact of operative multidisciplinarity for severe defect injuries of the lower extremity]. *Handchir Mikrochir Plast Chir;* 38(6):403–416. German.

[12] **Archbold HA, Guha AR, Shyamsundar S, et al** (2005) The use of multi-media messaging in the referral of musculoskeletal limb injuries to a tertiary trauma unit using: a 1-month evaluation. *Injury;* 36(4):560–566.

[13] **Karanas YL, Nigriny J, Chang J** (2008) The timing of microsurgical reconstruction in lower extremity trauma. *Microsurgery;* 28(8):632–634.

7 Stabilization of the wound

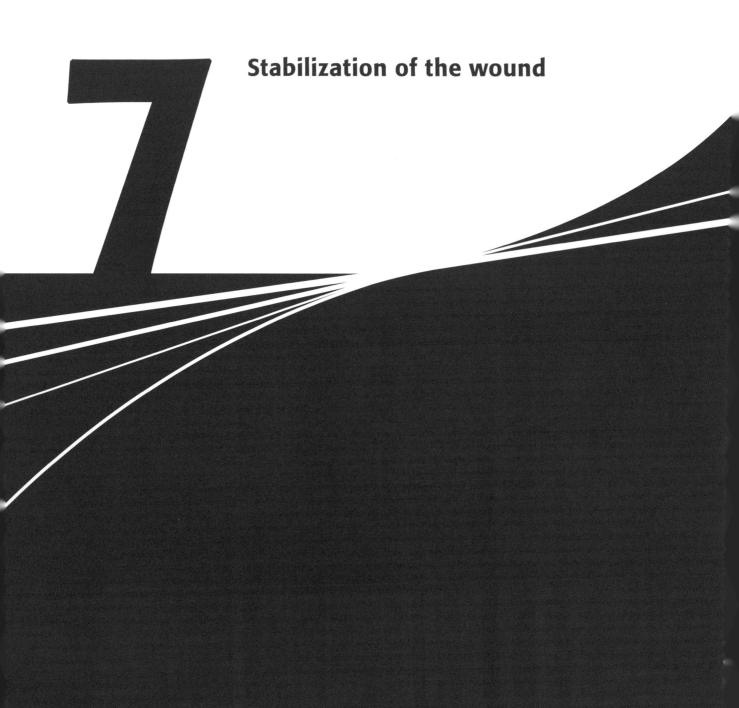

7.1 Principles of debridement

Author   Robert D Teasdall

7.1.1   Introduction

Debridement is the cornerstone of modern surgical treatment of open wounds. The term "debridement" originated with the French word "débrider", which literally meant to unbridle or release something that was confining. It was used to describe the release of tight tissues around a wound. Today, debridement has come to mean the systematic removal of all grossly contaminated or nonviable, necrotic tissue from a wound with the ultimate goal to create a clean or even sterile wound. Effective debridement has been attempted for many centuries, eg, through the use of changed dressing or the application of maggots (chapter 9.4) [1]. However, during the Napoleonic Wars, the French surgeons Larrey and Desault strongly advocated the use of incision of traumatic wounds to allow drainage, conversely, John Hunter, the English father of surgery, felt that covering the wound with salve and a dressing was the mainstay of treatment. Not until the dawn of the 20th century has debridement turned into mainstream thought. This concept was cemented in surgical practice after the positive experiences gathered during World War I [2].

Despite major advances in the understanding of wound pathophysiology and bacteriology, little has changed during the past two centuries with regard to the basic techniques and assessment of tissues.

7.1.2   Assessment of viability (Video 7.1-1)

General considerations

Ideally, the final examination of a wound involving a complex soft-tissue defect should be carried out with the patient under anesthesia in order to allow full assessment of the extent of the injury without causing further pain (**Fig 7.1-1**). A systematic approach to the wound should be used, beginning with an examination of the skin and subcutaneous tissue, followed by fascia, muscles, tendons, neurovascular structures, and, finally, bone and periosteum (chapter 5.1).

Skin

Viable skin has a healthy subcutaneous layer firmly attached to the dermis. Skin that shows significant ecchymosis within the subcutaneous fat is at risk (**Fig 7.1-2**). Skin that has been avulsed from the subcutaneous fat—as may be observed in elder patients—is likely to lose its viability and, thus, may be debrided at once. Heavily contaminated skin should be removed because contaminants cannot be thoroughly removed without compromising the skin's integrity significantly. Often, the subcutaneous layer may be avulsed from the underlying fascia (**Fig 7.1-3**) (chapter 3.3). If the subcutaneous fat does not show ecchymosis, it may be left, but larger areas of avulsed fat will often become necrotic. Harvesting of the skin in order to use it as a split-thickness skin graft to cover the defect may sometimes be an option.

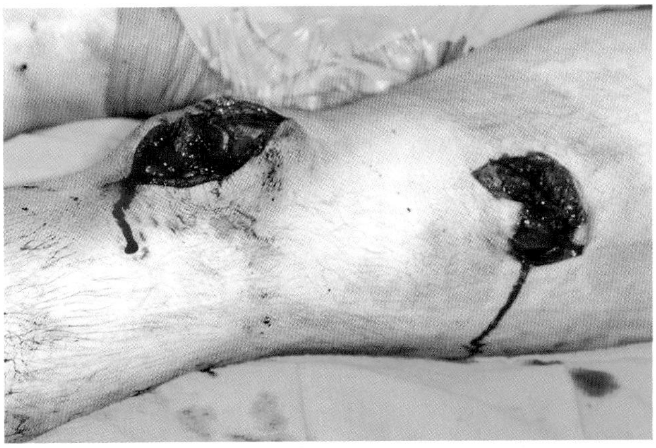

Fig 7.1-1   Assessment of the injury. The first examination of the wound occurs in the trauma bay, but the wound is not fully evaluated until the patient is properly anesthetized and the wound can be explored surgically.

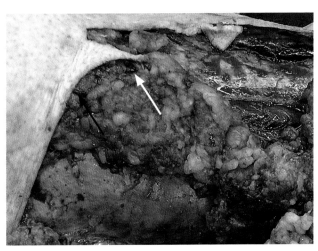

Fig 7.1-2   Degloving injury of a leg. Note the ecchymosis in the subcutaneous layer (white arrow). Also note the thrombosis in the subcutaneous veins (black arrow).

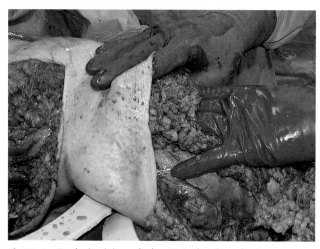

Fig 7.1-3 Degloving injury of a leg. Note that the subcutaneous tissue is neither attached to the skin nor to the underlying muscle fascia.

Muscle

Muscle viability can be assessed by checking the following four "C"s (**Fig 7.1-4a–c**) (**Video 7.1-1**):

- color
- consistency
- capacity to bleed
- contractility.

Although very subjective, this time-honored method of assessing muscle viability is still acceptable [3]. Muscles should appear bright red in color, as dark red muscle indicates rupture of muscle capillaries and intramuscular hematoma formation. In that case, the muscle must be searched for areas of bruising (**Fig 7.1-5**). Such a bruised muscle may survive, but there is a risk of future necrosis. Gray muscle tissue is already necrotic and must be removed, especially if there is continued risk of contamination, because such tissue provides the ideal conditions for infection to take hold.

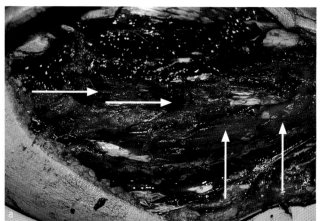

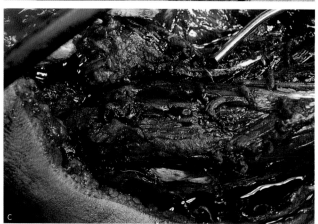

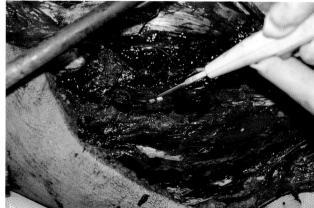

Fig 7.1-4a–c Assessment of muscle viability relies on the four "C"s: color, consistency, capacity to bleed, and contractility.
a Areas of dark red muscle (horizontal arrows) in comparison to healthy muscle, which is beefy red (vertical arrows).
b Muscle contractility can be demonstrated with electrocautery or by direct tapping.
c Healthy muscle will bleed when cut with a scalpel.

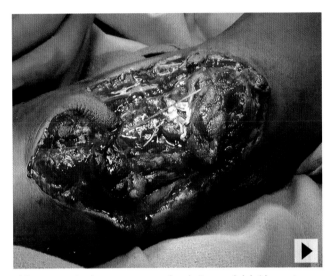

Video 7.1-1 Basic assessment and techniques of debridement: high-energy gunshot wound to the forearm and leg injury caused by a motor vehicle.

Surgeons should be familiar with the consistency of viable muscle. The muscle should exhibit good turgor and should not pull apart with gentle teasing. Consistency remains good until muscle is clearly necrotic and, therefore, its loss is a rather late sign. The capacity to bleed is less reliable, because muscle with extensive rupture of capillaries may bleed initially as a result of an intramuscular hematoma. Furthermore, cutting muscle back to bleeding may require excision of some viable tissue. Muscle contractility is judged most commonly by touching the muscle with the electrocautery pencil, but it will respond to tapping or pinching with a forceps. Viable muscle should contract with direct stimulation, even when a depolarizing anesthetic substance has been administered or spinal cord injury has denervated the muscle. As muscle contractility may be decreased initially following blunt trauma, great care should be taken when assessing it.

Bone and periosteum
The latter should be carefully assessed especially if stripped from bone. Ecchymosis within the periosteum indicates a rather severe injury, but does not necessarily require excision. If there is good continuity with the remainder of the periosteum, the damaged periosteum is likely to survive. However, periosteum that is separated both from its overlying muscle and from the rest of the periosteal sleeve is not likely to provide much supply for the bone and may be removed. Bone that has lost all its attachments to surrounding tissues is probably dead and should be removed. In relatively clean wounds, small fragments may be left, but all necrotic bone must be excised, especially if the risk of contamination is high.

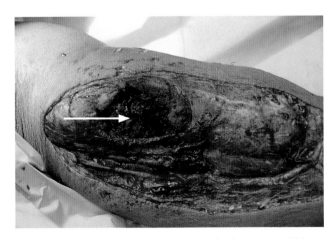

Fig 7.1-5 Gunshot wound to the arm. Note the hematoma within the muscle (arrow).

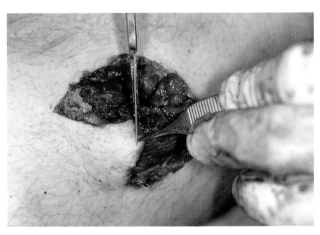

Fig 7.1-6 Debridement should be approached systematically, beginning with the skin and proceeding to the subcutaneous tissue, muscle, periosteum, and bone.

7.1.3 Techniques of debridement (Video 7.1-1)

There are many techniques for surgical and nonsurgical debridement of open wounds. Wounds that are not heavily contaminated and that do not have a great deal of necrotic tissue may be treated nonoperatively with changes of dressing. Chemical debridement is useful for very superficial, chronic wounds. High-pressure irrigation is not recommended in fresh wounds, but may be useful to clean infected and chronic environments (chapter 7.2). The most commonly used procedure for debridement of open wounds is sharp surgical debridement with a scalpel. Regardless of the methods used, the end result should be a macroscopically clean wound, which allows natural repair processes to proceed.

Many surgeons perform debridement procedures with a tourniquet, particularly if vessels and nerves are exposed. If after release of the tourniquet punctate bleeding of the exposed tissues is insufficient, additional debridement can be performed, even without tourniquet.

The surgeon must aggressively seek out and—by meticulous excision—remove all dead and devitalized tissues and foreign matter. This should be done in a thorough manner while avoiding additional trauma to the tissues as a result of excessively aggressive dissection (chapter 11.2). Surgical debridement ranks as the most important single activity influencing outcome in the management of the open fractures.

The cost of leaving dead, necrotic tissue in the wound is high. In case of doubt and if the first debridement was not extensive enough, a second or even third debridement must be performed within 48–72 hours. Any wound that received delayed initial care or that was grossly contaminated, should be considered for second debridement. Debridement should thus be regarded as a staged procedure. Surgical debridement of the contaminated wound is urgent before bacterial proliferation approaches the critical inoculum, above which infection becomes highly likely.

When using sharp debridement, care should be taken to prevent any further damage, especially to uninjured surrounding tissues. Excessive retraction or clamping must be avoided. A sharp scalpel with frequent changing of blades creates clean cuts and is most helpful, while the use of scissors should, whenever possible, be avoided as they cause local crushing of tissue (chapter 1).

Of course, debridement commences on the outside working inwards (**Fig 7.1-6**). Skin that is manifestly dead and macerated should be excised. Skin of dubious viability can safely be left for the second look, when its status will be obvious (eg, avulsion injury). Damaged subcutaneous fat should be thoroughly excised.

Leaving devitalized muscle in the wound may have catastrophic consequences, even within a short period of time. Careful attention must thus be paid to muscle in the initial

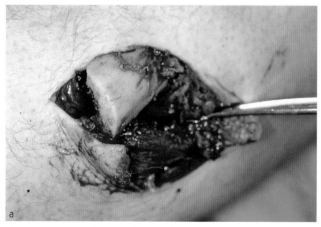
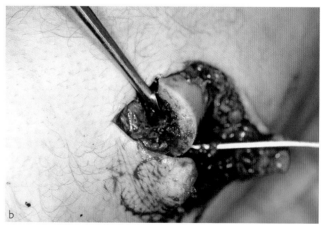

Fig 7.1-7a–b Debridement in open fractures.
a Care must be taken to preserve any viable periosteum, but to remove any nonviable tissue.
b The surgeon must also take care to debride the medullary canal.

debridement. All muscle of dubious viability must be resected to pink bleeding edges, which contract when gently pinched. This implies that debridement procedures are performed without tourniquet. The intact tendon can be cleaned and reexamined during the second look. Major neurovascular structures should be preserved and repaired, if necessary.

Bone ends should be scrupulously cleaned mechanically, and any foreign material must be removed from the medullary cavity (**Fig 7.1-7a–b**). Bone ends must be exposed and debrided. Any loose fragments of bone, or bone without soft-tissue attachments, are removed from the wound and discarded. In some exceptional situations a large segment of bone might be preserved in order to help axial alignment and/or as a spacer.

Surgeons should realize that any penetrating injury may involve far more extensive damage below the skin, and a larger incision is required to allow for adequate deep debridement (**Fig 7.1-8a–b**). Most small wounds should be extended in order to allow full assessment of the underlying tissue.

7.1.4 Summary

Debridement and irrigation of a wound needs good judgment and much experience and, therefore, should never be delegated to the junior resident or an inexperienced surgeon. Despite the simple concepts behind debridement, it is the task that is most often inadequately performed. Surgeons should treat debridement in the same manner an architect treats the foundation of a building. Its design is simple, compared to the elaborate designs of the rooms of the building, but unless it is well designed and well executed, the building will fall. A "laissez-faire" attitude toward this procedure may put the limb and the patient at risk.

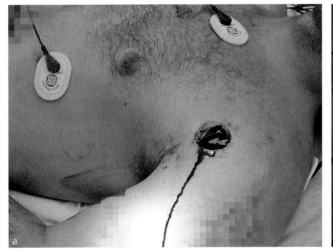 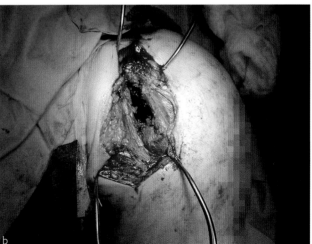

Fig 7.1-8a–b Patient, who sustained a shotgun wound to the left shoulder.
a   The injured shoulder prior to surgical intervention.
b   After extension of the wound, the true damage to underlying tissues can be assessed.

7.2 Techniques of irrigation

Author   Jeffrey Anglen

7.2.1   When and why to irrigate?

Irrigation of wounds is one of the most commonly performed procedures in the care of the injured patient, and one of the most ancient. The purpose is to prevent infection and promote wound healing by cleansing the wound of material that may inhibit the healing process or promote infection: foreign matter, microscopic pathogens, and toxic substances. In some cases wound irrigation has been used as a drug delivery method. It is usually performed in association with surgical debridement, which is the more important aspect of appropriate wound care (chapter 7.1). Relatively little scientific inquiry has been directed at the details of the wound irrigation procedure.

The parameters of wound irrigation include timing of the procedure, volume and pressure of the irrigating solution, type of solution, and method of administration. With regard to timing, it is believed that the sooner after the injury or contamination the irrigation procedure is performed, the more effective it will be in removing contaminants. Bacterial infection of a wound is a time-dependent process, which occurs in several stages, beginning with the attraction and attachment of bacteria to surfaces in the wound, their proliferation, and the production of an extracellular glycocalyx slime, or biofilm. The initial attraction of bacteria to a surface is mediated by electrostatic, van der Waals, or hydrophobic forces and occurs within minutes. Covalent bonding of bacterial cell walls to surface proteins then follows over a period of hours. Proliferation of bacteria and synthesis of complex molecules composing the extracellular matrix results in a biofilm. Very little is known about the rate of development of a full biofilm, and it is likely to be affected by many variables, including the specific genetic composition of the bacterial species, available nutrients and conditions as well as the size of the inoculum. Foreign material may be more difficult to remove with time due to desiccation of tissues and suppuration. In an in vitro study of contaminated bone surfaces, Bhandari et al [4] demonstrated a reduction in the ability of low pressure irrigation to remove surface bacteria after 6 hours. Using an animal model of goat wounds contaminated with bioluminescent bacteria and then irrigated at 3, 6, or 12 hours, Owens and Wenke [5] demonstrated improved bacterial removal with earlier irrigation. While it seems true that efficacy of irrigation is improved with an earlier onset of the procedure, this is only one and probably a minor factor in whether a wound ultimately develops infection (**Video 7.2-1**).

7.2.2   Role of volume irrigation

"The solution to pollution is dilution."

The volume of irrigation solution used for cleansing wounds is usually described as "copious" or "ample". Published volume recommendations for irrigation of wounds associated with open fractures have ranged from 7–15 l, but these are not evidence-based. Available in vitro and animal studies suggest that increasing the irrigation volume improves removal of foreign material and bacteria up to a point, but the relationship is not linear; there seems to be a plateau effect [6]. The highly variable nature of wounds, including size and 3-D geometry, requires considered judgment. One empiric protocol, based on the availability of 3-l bags of irrigation solution, recommends one bag (ie, 3 l) for Gustilo type I fractures, two bags (ie, 6 l) for type II, and three bags (ie, 9 l) for type III [7]. This is probably in excess of what is necessary for fresh and relatively clean wounds. The important thing is that an irrigant is used to actively wash all parts of the wound including cavities and recesses, and not to simply flood a particular area with water.

7.2.3   Role of antibiotic irrigation

A wide variety of irrigation solutions have been advocated. Thus, water, saline, antiseptics, antibiotics, chelating agents, and soaps have been proposed. For simple lacerations and fresh animal bites seen in the emergency department, tap water seems to be a safe and effective irrigant, and equal to

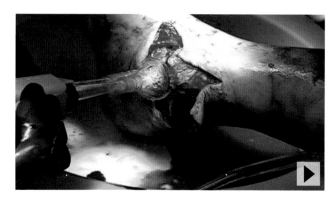

Video 7.2-1   Principles of active and passive irrigation in open fractures.

saline in efficacy. In combat or wilderness situations, field water can be rendered safe for wound irrigation by addition of sodium hypochlorite to form a 0.025% Dakin's solution (ie, 5 ml bleach per liter of water). However, the use of most antiseptics (eg, povidone-iodine, hydrogen peroxide, alcohol) in open wounds with or without fractures should be avoided due to their toxicity to host tissues, particularly immune cells and osteoblasts. The threshold host-toxic concentration of most antiseptics is exceeded before the bactericidal efficacy is reached.

In the orthopaedic setting, antibiotics have commonly been added to irrigation of open fractures, apparently based on literature derived from general surgical or gynecologic wound care practice [8–10]. No animal or clinical studies of musculoskeletal wounds or open fractures are available that support the use of antibiotics delivered via irrigation. Moreover, there is some concern with adding antibiotics:

- increased costs
- low but reported incidence of adverse drug effects including severe anaphylactic reactions
- potential promotion of antibiotic resistance.

The use of soaps or detergents to clean wounds was a common practice in the preantibiotic era. Soaps, which belong to the category of molecules called surfactants, function by disrupting the electrostatic or hydrophobic interactions that bind particles to surfaces, corresponding to the initial stage of bacterial attachment to the wound. Surfactants form micelles surrounding the bacterial particles, which allows them to be flushed from the wound. Some types of soap have bactericidal properties as well, through effects on the bacterial cell membrane. Animal studies of contaminated complex musculoskeletal wounds support the use of soap irrigation over antibiotics or saline alone [7, 11]. In vitro studies demonstrate that soap solution was the most effective at removing adherent bacteria from bone, and the least toxic to osteoblasts when used with low-pressure irrigation, compared to antiseptics and antibiotics [12].

A prospective, randomized, controlled trial compared irrigation of open lower-extremity fractures with a bacitracin solution to a solution of liquid Castile soap. No difference was found in the incidence of wound infection or delayed bone healing. However, the antibiotic solution group did have a significantly higher incidence of soft-tissue wound-healing problems [13]. The soap solution used was made by adding 80 ml of liquid Castile soap (not sterile) to a 3-l irrigation bag of normal saline.

7.2.4 Role of pressure irrigation

There are a wide variety of methods and equipment to deliver irrigation to a wound, from a simple squeeze bottle or bulb syringe to expensive power tools with a selection of different nozzles. There is no evidence to suggest that any particular type of tip or fluid stream geometry is superior, nor is there evidence that intermittent or pulsatile flow dynamics are more effective than constant flow. However, there do seem to be differences in irrigation effectiveness as well as potential tissue damage based on pressure. Although the terms "low" and "high" pressure are not well defined, in general they refer to fluid pressures at the irrigation nozzle of < 15 pounds per square inch (psi) (775 mmHg) or > 25 psi (1293 mmHg) [6]. High pressures are provided by power lavage systems (**Fig 7.2-1a–h**), and low pressures are provided by bulb syringe (~1–3 psi) or gravity flow systems. Impact pressure at the wound or bone surface may vary substantially from the nozzle pressure.

Animal studies from the 1970s demonstrated that high-pressure lavage (HPL) removed inorganic, particular debris from soft-tissue wounds better than low-pressure lavage (LPL). The current literature about the ideal pressure to be used is inconclusive. Nevertheless, the advantage of high-pressure lavage was recently demonstrated, using the previously mentioned model of goat wounds contaminated with bioluminescent bacteria [6]. Although a recent study using muscle cubes reinvigorated older concerns about damaging tissue, increasing dispersal of bacteria into the tissues, and impairment of the resistance of the tissue to infection, clinical experience has not been negative, and high-pressure lavage of soft-tissue wounds has become a well-accepted tool in the management of soft-tissue wounds that are or are not associated with fractures. However, studies of high-pressure lavage on bone have also suggested some potential problems. Using a rabbit model with a fresh intra-articular distal femoral fracture, Dirschl et al [14] demonstrated that high-pressure lavage has a detrimental effect on early bone healing compared to low-pressure. Animals, whose fractures were subjected to pulsatile irrigation with a commercially available jet lavage system, produced significantly less new bone in the first 2 weeks than those, whose fractures were irrigated with a bulb syringe. Similarly, an in vitro study using human tibial sections contaminated with bacteria and treated by irrigation showed that, in contrast to soft tissues, high-pressure lavage did drive bacteria into the intramedullary canal. In addition, the bone segments subjected to high-pressure lavage at 70 psi have shown visible and microscopic damage to the bone structure [15, 16].

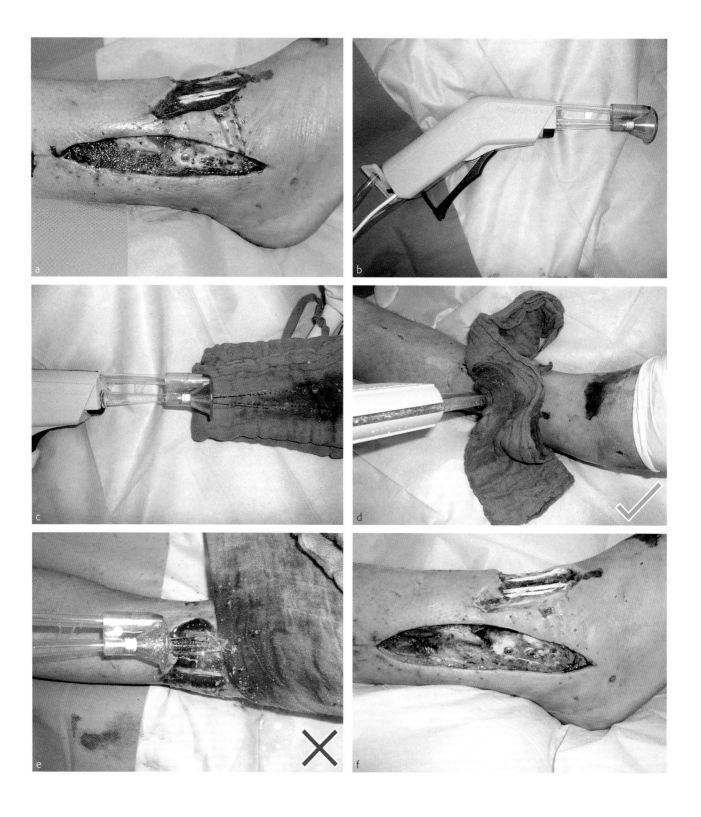

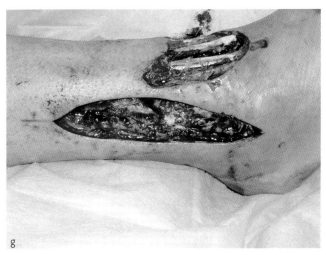
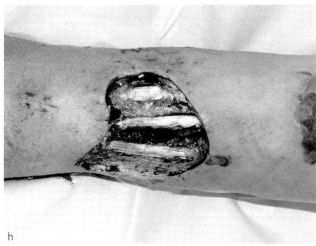

g

h

Fig 7.2-1a–h   Debridement of an open fracture of the distal right lower leg of a 45-year-old male patient after a high-energy motorcycle accident.
a   Skin loss at the anterior aspect of the distal lower leg and dorsal foot, respectively, as well as at the site of the surgical incision for the preceding open reduction and internal fixation (ORIF) of the fibula. Note the exposed extensor tendons and screws. Microbiological analyses confirmed the presence of bacterial contamination. Situation before debridement.
b   Irrigator that includes a tube connected to the irrigation solution and a tube connected to a suction device.
c   Once the handle of the irrigator is activated, a jet exits the rubber cone.
d   Correct handling of the irrigator while jet-lavaging the wound in order to prevent squirting.
e   Incorrect handling of the irrigator. Note the abundant squirting.
f   After both surgical debridement and irrigation. A tourniquet is being used at the level of the thigh.
g   Diffuse bleeding of healthy tissues after release of the tourniquet.
h   Close-up of the distal lower leg and dorsal foot, respectively.

At the same time, the efficacy of high-pressure lavage for cleansing bone tissue has been questioned. Bhandari and colleagues showed that bacterial removal from contaminated bone surfaces is improved with high-pressure lavage over low-pressure lavage, but only when there had been a delay to treatment—in their study, a period of more than 6 hours. In freshly contaminated specimens, low-pressure lavage performed as well as high-pressure lavage at removing bacteria [4]. A study using metaphyseal femoral cancellous bone contaminated with graphite particles revealed that low-pressure irrigation with a bulb syringe is equally effective in removing particles as high-pressure, pulsed irrigation [16]. In another experiment using cancellous bone slices, high-pressure lavage caused more tissue damage than low-pressure lavage or suction/brush treatment, but did not remove more particulate inorganic debris. Similarly, high-pressure lavage has been shown to penetrate deeper and cause more disruption of soft tissues when compared to low-pressure lavage [17].

Studies of high-pressure lavage seem to offer support for its use in cleansing soft-tissue wounds as well as simple, hard surfaces such as implant material and cortical bone as encountered in open fractures whenever treatment is delayed after contamination. In fresh fractures, particularly with exposed cancellous surfaces, it does not seem to offer the same advantages and may pose some risk. While there may be a pressure setting at which the advantages are retained and the risks are reduced, this has not yet been shown. If the lavage system offers a variety of settings, choosing a mid-level pressure of ~20 psi (1034 mmHg) seems to make sense.

7.2.5 Summary

Irrigation serves to mechanically dislodge and physically remove necrotic and foreign material, including pathogens, from wounds. There is little definitive scientific evidence to support one technique over another, but the data do suggest that irrigation is effective in reducing bacterial counts and consequently, the grade of wound contamination or infec-tion. It is also clear that proper irrigation should not be relegated to beginners. Too often, irrigation is left to a junior surgeon, who stands over the wound idly spraying water on a wound as though the mere presence of an irrigator would "sterilize" the wound. Rather, the surgeon should visualize any wound that has a sticky substance like honey on it, which can only be removed by deliberate irrigation of every nook and cranny within the wound.

7.3 Role of fracture stabilization

Author   Robert D Teasdall

7.3.1 Rationale and importance of fracture stabilization

Nowhere has the value of fracture stabilization in reducing morbidity and mortality of fracture patients been demon-strated more clearly than on the fields of World War I [18]. Hardly any evacuation of the wounded, patients lying around in the heavily contaminated soil, and the lack of any type of fracture immobilization in the field led to mortality rates of up to 90% from femur fractures caused by missiles. After the introduction and widespread use of the Thomas splint, the mortality rate dropped to less than 20%. While the de-bate goes on about the exact mortality figures and the con-tribution of more effective evacuation policies, it is clear that immobilization of fractures in the field played a major role.

Today, surgical stabilization of an underlying fracture is considered critical in the treatment of open wounds with soft-tissue damage. Available options for fracture fixation in open injuries include screws, plates, intramedullary nails, external fixators, or a combination of these techniques [19]. The goals of fracture fixation are to achieve an adequate reduction and fixation of the bone while preserving soft-tissue and bone viability, which allows for early motion and return to function of the injured limb and patient.

Stabilizing the fracture has been shown to prevent further damage to the soft tissues otherwise caused by mobile bone fragments, provided the soft tissues are handled gently. By correcting the bone deformity and alignment, the soft-tissue structures are subjected to tension, thereby reducing dead space and hematoma volume. The inflammatory response is dampened [20], exudation and edema reduced, and tissue revascularization encouraged. Furthermore, by providing sta-bility, access to the wound for further surgical soft-tissue pro-cedures is facilitated and the injured limb can more easily be mobilized. Stabilization of the fracture provides an optimal environment and conditions for tissue repair and recovery.

The balance of providing adequate fracture fixation and preservation of the soft tissue must be individually assessed in each case. It is important to stabilize the bone, and yet prevent further damage to the local blood supply and soft tissues [21]. Factors to be considered when planning for bone stabilization include:
- anatomical location and characteristics of the fracture
- state of the surrounding skin and soft tissues including the site and size of the open wound
- degree of contamination
- presence of other injuries
- overall condition of the patient.

When stabilizing the bone, it is important to follow the general principles of anatomical reduction of joint surfaces, achieving absolute stability of fixation, while in diaphyseal and metaphyseal fractures, the restoration of length and alignment appears sufficient, combined with a relatively stable type of fixation. In cases of high-energy injuries with fracture fragmentation and compromised soft tissues, min-imally invasive techniques may have advantages. However, respect for the soft tissues and careful preoperative planning are essential. Therefore, surgical approaches, as well as in-ternal or external fixation devices should be positioned and/ or introduced in such a way that they do not compromise later orthopaedic or plastic reconstructive procedures. The reconstructive surgeon should, therefore, be involved from the very beginning, when fracture fixation is being planned (chapter 6.2, 8.1).

It should be noted that definitive fixation should not neces-sarily be regarded as mandatory in the initial surgical intervention. Often, temporary stabilization of a limb is performed using an external fixator, if necessary bridging the injured zone or spanning across a joint in order to maintain length and alignment. The definitive fixation is performed at a later date, when swelling has settled and the full extent of the soft-tissue wound has been assessed and, hopefully, covered. Preliminary joint-spanning external fixators may be recommended for open supracondylar femur fractures with or without tibial plateau fractures, comminuted, open pilon fractures as well as comminuted, open tibial shaft fractures. Definitive fixation with plates and screws or intramedullary nailing will be performed at a later date, when the soft-tissue envelope permits internal fixation.

7.3.2   Methods of fracture stabilization

Fixation with plates and screws

Plates and screws providing absolute stability are commonly used for articular and simple metaphyseal fractures. Plates are also indicated in open diaphyseal fractures of the forearm as they provide the stability required to maintain the anatomical relationship between the radius and ulna. Similarly, plates may be indicated in open fractures of the humerus.

Intramedullary nailing

Intramedullary nails are state of the art for the fixation of diaphyseal fractures in the femur or tibia. Intramedullary nails are generally inserted "closed" or with minimally invasive reduction techniques, preserving the soft-tissue envelope, compared to "open" reduction and internal fixation with plates and screws. Reaming of the medullary canal has been shown to stimulate fracture healing, although insertion of solid nails without reaming has been recommended for open fractures in the hope of reducing the risk of infection. Current evidence shows no conclusive difference between nail insertion with or without reaming of the medullary canal in open fractures [22]. Thanks to new generations of nails and interlocking devices, the indications for intramed-

ullary fixation with or without reaming are being expanded to metaphyseal fractures and have become acceptable in most fractures of the Gustilo types I–IIIB (chapter 5.2).

External fixation

External fixation is the method of choice in severely soiled and contaminated fractures, including Gustilo type IIIC fractures, in which metal implants with their risk of bacterial adherence are best avoided. External fixators are particularly useful whenever wounds and their soft-tissue characteristics do not allow direct surgical access to the fracture. Properly placed external fixators have the great advantage of providing relatively stable fracture fixation without violating the injured zone. They must, however, be planned and applied in such a way as not to impede second-look debridement or any later reconstructive procedures of the soft tissues, especially if a free flap is to be used. The positioning of the microscope during surgery may be hampered by the fixator pins. The main disadvantage of external fixators is the significant risk of pin-track infections. It is important to insert the pins at a safe distance from the injured zone within areas of healthy tissue and—in the tibia—preferably where the bone lies subcutaneously. If a hybrid fixator is used, the placement of thin wire too close to the joint capsule must be avoided [23].

7.3.3   Summary

Stabilization of the fracture with plates, screws, intramedullary nails, or external fixators is a significant part of managing open wounds with extensive soft-tissue damage. By stabilizing the fracture, an optimal environment is provided for tissue repair and recovery, while the patient is more comfortable and the injured limb can be mobilized more easily, which improves the functional outcome. Fractures with complex soft-tissue injury need an early involvement of the plastic surgeon or the surgeon capable of restoring the soft tissues.

References and further reading

[1] **Noe A** (2006) Extremity injury in war: a brief history. *J Am Acad Orthop Surg;* 14(10):S1–6.

[2] **Helling T, Daon E** (1998) In Flanders Fields: The Great War, Antoine Depage, and the resurgence of débridement. *Ann Surg;* 228(2):173–181.

[3] **Scully RE, Artz CP, Sako Y** (1955) The criteria for determining the viability of muscle in war wounds. *Howard JM: Battle Casualties in Korea.* Washington, DC: Army Medical Service Graduate School, 181–187.

[4] **Bhandari M, Schemitsch EH, Adili A, et al** (1999) High and low pressure pulsatile lavage of contaminated tibial fractures: an in vitro study of bacterial adherence and bone damage. *J Orthop Trauma;* 13(8):526–533.

[5] **Owens BD, Wenke JC** (2007) Early wound irrigation improves the ability to remove bacteria. *J Bone Joint Surg Am;* 89(8):1723–1726.

[6] **Svoboda SJ, Bice TG, Gooden HA, et al** (2006) Comparison of bulb syringe and pulsed lavage irrigation with use of a bioluminescent musculoskeletal wound model. *J Bone Joint Surg Am;* 88(10):2167–2174.

[7] **Anglen JO** (2001) Wound irrigation in musculoskeletal injury. *J Am Acad Orthop Surg;* 9(4):219–226.

[8] **Samelson SL, Reyes HM** (1987) Management of perforated appendicitis in children–revisited. *Arch Surg;* 122(6):691–696.

[9] **Dashow EE, Read JA, Coleman FH** (1986) Randomized comparison of five irrigation solutions at cesarean section. *Obstet Gynecol;* 68(4):473–478.

[10] **Mathelier AC** (1992) A comparison of postoperative morbidity following prophylactic antibiotic administration by combined irrigation and intravenous route or by intravenous route alone during cesarean section. *J Perinat Med;* 20(3):177–182.

[11] **Anglen JO, Gainor BJ, Christensen G, et al** (2003) The use of detergent irrigation for musculoskeletal wounds. *Int Orthop;* 27(1):40–46.

[12] **Bhandari M, Adili A, Schemitsch EH** (2001) The efficacy of low-pressure lavage with different irrigating solutions to remove adherent bacteria from bone. *J Bone Joint Surg Am;* 83(3):412–419.

[13] **Anglen JO** (2005) Comparison of soap and antibiotic solutions for irrigation of lower-limb open fracture wounds. A prospective, randomized study. *J Bone Joint Surg Am;* 87(7):1415–1422.

[14] **Dirschl DR, Duff GP, Dahners LE, et al** (1998) High pressure pulsative lavage irrigation of intraarticular fractures: effects on fracture healing. *J Orthop Trauma;* 12(7):460–463.

[15] **Bhandari M, Adili A, Lachowski RJ** (1998) High pressure pulsatile lavage of contaminated human tibiae: an in vitro study. *J Orthop Trauma;* 12(7):479–484.

[16] **Lee EW, Dirschl DR, Duff G, et al** (2002) High-pressure pulsatile lavage irrigation of fresh intraarticular fractures: effectiveness at removing particulate matter from bone. *J Orthop Trauma;* 16(3):162–165.

[17] **Boyd Ji, Wongworawat MD** (2004) High pressure pulsatile lavage causes soft tissue damage. *Clin Orthop Relat Res;* 427:13–17.

[18] **Manring MM, Hawk A, Calhoun JH, et al** (2009) Treatment of war wounds: a historical review. *Clin Orthop Relat Res;* 467(8):2168–2191.

[19] **Rüedi TR, Buckley RE, Moran CG** (2007) *AO Principles of Fracture Management.* 2nd ed. Stuttgart New York: Thieme Verlag.

[20] **Pape HC, Schmidt RE, Rice J, et al** (2000) Biochemical changes after trauma and skeletal surgery of the lower extremity: quantification of the operative burden. *Crit Care Med;* 28(10):3441–3448.

[21] **Farouk O, Krettek C, Miclau T, et al** (1999) Minimally invasive plate osteosynthesis: does percutaneous plating disrupt femoral blood supply less than the traditional technique? *J Orthop Trauma;* 13(6):401–406.

[22] **Bhandari M, Guyatt G, Tornetta P 3rd, et al** (2008) Randomized trial of reamed and unreamed intramedullary nailing of tibial shaft fractures. The study to prospectively evaluate reamed intramedullary nails in patients with tibial fractures. *J Bone Joint Surg Am;* 90(12):2567-2578.

[23] **Hutson JJ Jr, Zych GA** (1998) Infections in periarticular fractures of the lower extremity treated with tensioned wire hybrid fixators. *J Orthop Trauma;* 12(3):214–218.

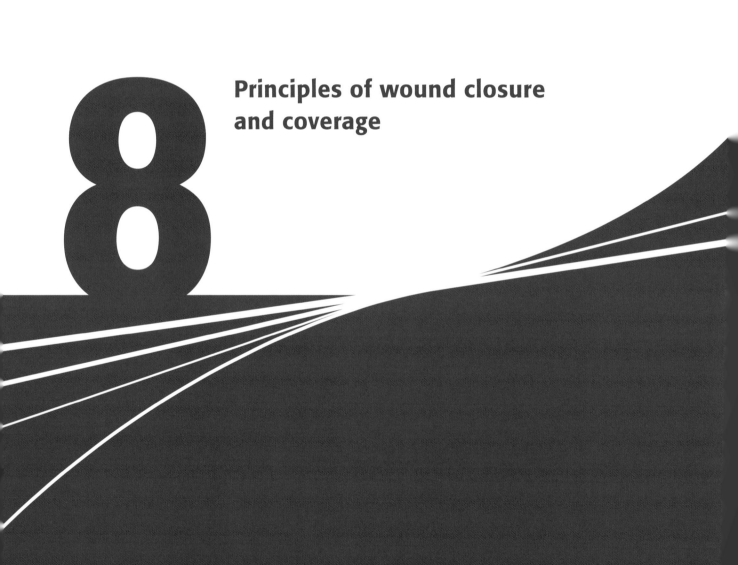

8

**Principles of wound closure
and coverage**

8.1 Principles of decision making

Authors Reto Wettstein, Daniel F Kalbermatten

8.1.1 Historical background of wound management

"Successful reconstructive surgery is measured in terms of safe defect coverage with simultaneous restoration of form and function and avoidance of donor site deformity" [1].

The history and evolution of wound management is closely related to the development of civilization and especially to warfare. The nature of war wounds has changed considerably from ancient times to present day in accordance with the technical progress of the weapons used. These changes constantly challenge all players involved in the treatment of casualties. They have led to improved techniques in both military and civilian surgical care and were the starting point of surgical specialties such as plastic and reconstructive surgery. In ancient Greek and Roman times, the options for managing wounds caused by arrows, spears or swords were sparse, and the mortality rate was high. This did not seem to change until the 16th century, when better patient selection (triage) (chapter 6), early surgical repair, the technique of vessel ligation, as well as the use of a tourniquet were introduced. This reduced the mortality rate of war wounds to extremities considerably. The treatment, of course, mainly consisted in amputation [2]. The fact that even by the end of the 19th century, infection and pus were considered an inevitable consequence of surgery indicates that undergoing an operation was still a hazard. While initially gunpowder was held responsible for any infection, the introduction of antiseptic and aseptic techniques, and the new theory that germs are responsible for infections were further milestones. Beside advances in imaging, improved surgical techniques, and higher respect for the soft parts, the introduction of antibiotics dramatically changed the outcome of surgery. Finally, the advances in reanimation and anesthesia spurred progress in wound management and decision making (chapter 6.2). While only a few decades ago the immediate and definitive stabilization of fractures as well as primary wound closure were the goal of treatment, today's trend is towards multistage procedures with repeated debridement and delayed wound closure, which appear to reduce wound-healing complications. This has opened the door for the salvage of complex extremity trauma that previously had to be subjected to amputation. Substantial improvements in fracture-fixation techniques in the second half of the 20th century were accompanied by the development of the soft-tissue reconstruction principles that are outlined in this book.

Currently, most wounds observed in orthopaedic and plastic surgery are either acute—by blunt (chapter 3.1) or penetrating (chapter 3.2) trauma—or chronic in nature such as in diabetic, neuropathic, or vasculopathic patients. Various environmental exposures, such as thermal and/or electrical insults, compression forces, radiation, or animal bites cause specific types of wounds that usually require special treatment and attention. A multitude of different dressing options exists, ranging from simple saline-soaked or paraffin-embedded gauzes to antimicrobial, fibrinolytic, or growth-factor-enhanced devices (chapter 9.1). Negative-pressure wound therapy is also a rather recent and promising treatment option that is enjoying wide-spread application (chapter 9.3). However, scientific evidence is still lacking for most of these treatment modalities and their respective indications. Nevertheless, many of these possibilities can positively enhance wound healing, but they cannot replace the need for sound knowledge of the basic principles of wound management.

8.1.2 Analysis of patient and wound

Most surgical and many traumatic wounds are considered "clean", allowing for primary wound closure with or without excision of the wound margins. This is described in chapter 10.1. Then again, a considerable part of the practice of plastic surgery deals with the reconstruction of defects. The armamentarium for the surgical techniques varies from simple procedures such as tissue advancement (chapter 10.1) or skin grafting (chapter 10.2) to sophisticated tissue transplantation (chapter 10.3 to 10.6). Regardless of the technical skills of the surgeon, it is paramount to include the patient and, possibly, even his or her relatives in the decision-making process. Therefore, the analysis of the patient and especially of the wound and/or defect as well as the evaluation of local and systemic parameters run in parallel and are inseparable processes.

The overall assessment of the patient needs to be based on a detailed medical history, including professional occupation, personal interests, and expectations. The compliance of the patient and his or her mental capacity to understand and follow complex reconstructive procedures must be evaluated. Furthermore, systemic factors that potentially influence wound healing (chapter 4.4) such as peripheral artery occlusive disease, diabetes mellitus, neuropathies, malnutrition, smoking, or steroid or drug intake have to be acknowledged and included within the decision-making process.

The medical history inquires into the etiology, the mechanism and energy of the injury as well as the age of the lesion, its location, size and any loss of function. Depending on the nature of the lesion, exposed and missing structures, the presence of foreign material, ischemic or necrotic tissue, fibrin and granulation tissue, quality and quantity of exudation, as well as signs of inflammation and infection have to be assessed. The viability of tissues can also change following radiotherapy, in the presence of a neoplasm, such as a Marjolin ulcer in a chronic unstable scar, or in the case of vasculitis.

After compiling the different findings necessary for decision making, the complex interdependence of all these factors is analyzed, pros and cons are balanced against each other and brought into relation with the therapeutic goals. The proposals can range from a conservative, nonoperative proposal to a complex multistage surgical reconstruction. Whereas in some situations the indication and the advantages for a patient are obvious, there is a gray zone where either a conservative or surgical, a simple or complex approach could eventually be successful and benefit the patient.

With regard to the safety of a procedure, ie, the success of wound closure, it is a commonly held misbelief that a simple procedure is a safe procedure. Wound-edge advancement and closure under tension is simple but will frequently result in delayed wound healing or wound breakdown. The success of a skin graft depends on multiple factors and cannot always be guaranteed. Thus, time to complete healing can be long, as reoperations and prolonged immobilization may be necessary. On the other hand, free tissue transfer is comparatively safe with a success rate of > 95% in most centers treating complex limb trauma on a regular basis, provided precise anatomical knowledge and technical skills in microsurgery are available (chapter 10.6). However, the loss of a split-thickness skin graft does not have such a catastrophic effect as the failure of a free flap.

In summary, decision making in plastic and reconstructive surgery is a very individual process that needs to consider a wide range of factors. The optimized preparation of both the patient and wound is necessary in order to obtain conditions for successful wound closure or coverage by a surgical intervention. Preoperative modification of the local and systemic factors that negatively influence wound healing can make a big difference.

A prerequisite for optimal patient management is that the decision-making process, the therapeutic approach, and follow-up are a multidisciplinary endeavor from beginning to end (chapter 6.2). The joint establishment of a treatment plan will substantially decrease the rate of morbidity, reduce the number of operations, shorten hospital stay and outpatient visits, improve patient satisfaction, and, last but not least, reduce costs.

8.1.3 Preoperative planning and timing

General considerations
Preoperative planning is the most important step in plastic and reconstructive surgery. It helps to reduce intraoperative hazards and, finally, improves the outcome. The time spent on preoperative planning will also reduce the length of surgery and increase the efficiency of the procedure. The entire team in the operating room appreciates a detailed preoperative plan as this facilitates positioning and draping of the patient as well as the preparation of the necessary instruments. While the classic tools of drawings, photographs, and x-rays may still be very useful today, the availability of computed tomography, magnetic resonance, and of even more modern tools like surface scanners, micro scanners, and computer animation as well as rapid prototyping permit a precise simulation of every surgical step (**Fig 8.1-1a–d**) [3].

The reconstructive ladder (chapter 8.2), introduced in orthopaedic trauma surgery in 1993 by Levin et al [4], helps to decide which level of surgical complexity to choose, from direct primary wound closure or skin graft to local, regional or distant flaps up to free-flap transfer with microvascular anastomosis. While the procedure itself should be kept as simple as possible, a low rung on the reconstructive ladder reflects the technical simplicity and not the likeliness of a good outcome of a procedure. More complex surgery often achieves better results without an increased rate of complications. A sound plan, therefore, has to address this issue as well as both functional and aesthetic aspects. It is recommended to adhere to a few basic principles in planning before embarking on any reconstructive procedure, in order to decrease morbidity as well as donor site deformity [5].

Principle I: Replace like with like
When filling a defect, it is preferable to replace the part lost with the same tissue, ie, bone for bone, fat for fat, muscle for muscle, and skin for skin in order to restore normal shape and contour in terms of function, thickness, texture as well as color and sensation of the skin. If this cannot be accom-

plished, the most similar tissue is chosen in order to reconstruct the defect with minimal donor site morbidity.

Principle II: Tissue bank

The human body is a precious "tissue bank", but with limited resources. Donor-site morbidity must always be included in the plan in order to insure that the damage caused by harvesting does not turn out to be more important than the original defect. In case of limb amputation, the removed part may provide valuable tissues for reconstruction.

Principle III: Functional and aesthetic aspects

While esthetic aspects are less important in extremity trauma than in facial reconstruction, the restoration of function in the weight-bearing zone has to be taken into consideration, and the exact placement of incisions should be thoroughly thought through in order to avoid scars within pressure zones.

Principle IV: Back-up plan

During the intervention, adjustment of the original plan may become necessary if an unexpected situation is encountered. Since any reconstructive procedure carries a risk of failure, it is important to always have an alternative plan.

Timing

Once the surgical plan is established, the timing of the procedure has to be determined. This obviously also depends on several factors. Since most reconstructive procedures can wait for 1 or 2 days, this time should be used for the planning and possibly correct any comorbidity factors such as nutritional supplementation, adjustment of diabetes, or even planning a vascular intervention. An interdisciplinary approach and good communication between the different teams is not only essential for setting priorities but also to decide on the best timing for treatment. Secondary bone grafting,

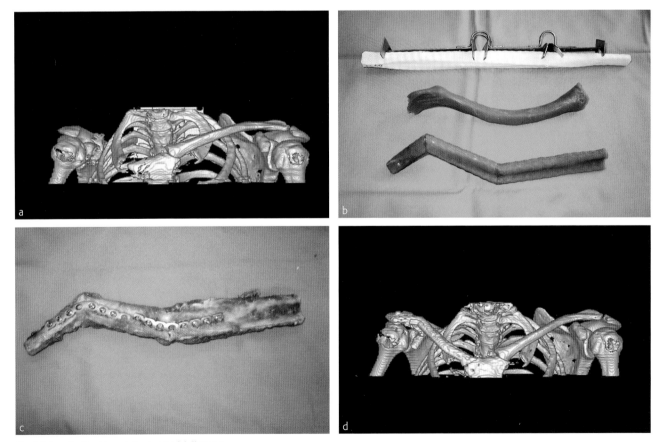

Fig 8.1-1a–d Rapid prototyping and follow-up.
a CT scan after resection of the right clavicle due to a tumor.
b Computer-aided, 3-D reconstruction of the middle third of the clavicle.
c Fibula autograft osteotomized to correspond to the shape of the clavicle before microsurgical transfer.
d CT scan 12 months after reconstruction.

for example, has to be done differently whether a fasciocutaneous or a muscle flap has been used for initial soft-tissue reconstruction, because the surgeon must know the location of the vascular pedicle when he or she returns to expose the fracture and place a graft. Ignoring this difference may lead to disastrous results.

8.1.4   Operative principles

Gentle soft-tissue handling and good knowledge of the regional anatomy are essential in order to avoid unnecessary trauma (chapter 1). Excessive tension on the skin margins or on a flap can result in wound breakdown, or partial or complete flap loss, and is a sign of poor operative technique and lack of planning. Meticulous and careful hemostasis is a prerequisite for the visualization of the flap pedicle(s) and neighboring structures. Unless contraindicated, flap and recipient site preparation may be performed under tourniquet control. The tourniquet should, however, be released before completion of the procedure both to enable evaluation of the flap and recipient vascular perfusion, and to check hemostasis. Hematoma formation under a flap may lead to flap failure secondary to tension or pedicle compression and can predispose to infection (chapter 11.3).

8.1.5   Outcome analysis

Patient satisfaction and the return to the previous lifestyle and occupation are the ultimate end points when assessing the success of a soft-tissue reconstruction. While economic aspects are turning into an ever more important issue, objective cost-benefit data are usually difficult to obtain, since wounds and defects can hardly be compared or standardized. The costs of reconstruction not only include the actual medical care and hospital stay, but also socio-economic aspects such as insurance contributions (eg, workmen's disability compensation) as well as costs incurred by long-term complications (eg, unstable scars, chronic osteomyelitis).

8.2   Aim of reconstruction

Authors   Daniel F Kalbermatten, Reto Wettstein

8.2.1   Introduction

The aim of any reconstructive procedure is to obtain a lasting wound closure or cover, while preserving or restoring function of the injured limb [1]. Once the basic decisions for the closure or coverage of a specific wound have been defined in an interdisciplinary process and the timing of treatment has been determined, the choice of the actual surgical procedure has to be established.

8.2.2   Linear concept versus new modular approach

The original idea of the reconstructive ladder [4, 6] was to provide a sequence of different surgical treatment options that can be applied according to their complexity (**Fig 8.2-1**). This principle was first applied to reconstruct complex orbitofacial defects. Two years later, the concept was taken over by orthopaedic surgeons to reconstruct bone [7] and soft-tissue defects [8]. The pitfall with this rather rigid reconstructive ladder, however, is that it implies that the simplest technique should be explored first and only to proceed to the next rung if the "simpler" one has failed [7]. Today, this has been modified, since the solution with the best chances of success should be applied, not the simplest one [8]. Wound closure or cover with questionable stability should be avoided—even though the procedure is technically easy to perform and appears as the least invasive for the patient—as it will most probably only postpone the need for major surgery to a less favorable point of time. As an example, a split-thickness skin graft for a considerable defect at the heel—a most important weight-bearing zone—may yet be an acceptable solution for a nonambulatory person. However, an athlete with a similar defect certainly will be much better served with a more demanding flap transfer that matches the local requirements, such as thickness, resistance, texture, and sensation. Poorly vascularized structures such as exposed bone and tendons were originally considered indications for reconstruction by a flap, since they do not provide the matrix for a skin graft in contrast to muscle, subcutaneous tissue and dermis. The availability of negative-pressure wound therapy combined with a skin graft has,

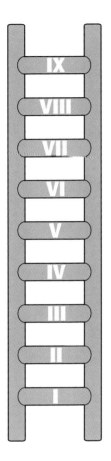

Fig 8.2-1 Classic reconstructive ladder. The simplest method which is likely to achieve stable closure or coverage should always be aimed at in order to avoid complications. The next rung is only climbed, if a simpler method fails. Primary, delayed primary, and secondary closure are not considered in this ladder.

I   Healing by secondary intention.
II   Primary closure.
III   Delayed primary closure.
IV   Split-thickness skin graft.
V   Full-thickness skin graft.
VI   Tissue expansion.
VII Random pattern flap.
VIII Pedicled flap.
IX   Free flap.

however, recently challenged this point of view. The decision, which of the two options to choose, not only needs to include an evaluation of the long-term result and stability, donor site morbidity and rehabilitation time, but also the patient's general condition as well as the available resources and the surgeon's skill. Unstable scar formation is a cumbersome condition and potential source of malignancy that can be prevented by early and interdisciplinary decision making.

Since one rung of the traditional ladder at best represents one option of the different reconstructive procedures, it is suggested that the single rungs of the ladder be replaced with reconstructive modules that may combine different techniques of wound cover (**Fig 8.2-2a–b**) in accordance with the proposal by Wong and Niranjan [9]. Partial primary closure, delayed closure, skin grafts, tissue expansion, local flaps, regional flaps, free flaps, and possibly tissue engineering can all be combined, arranged and used as modules, in order to provide an individually tailored solution for every case as considered necessary and adequate [8]. Decisions based on such a modular reconstructive ladder are better able to satisfy the needs of the patient in regard to the complexity of the injury and the procedure than such based on the classic reconstructive ladder (**Fig 8.2-1**).

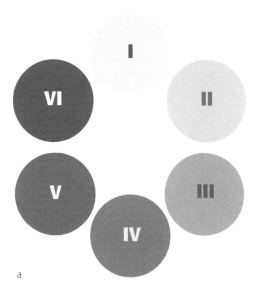
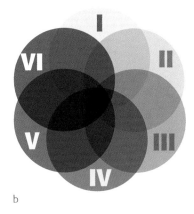

a

b

Fig 8.2-2a–b Reconstructive modules.
Reconstructive modules focus on an interaction of all methods to provide the best result.
I   Split-thickness skin graft.
II   Full-thickness skin graft.
III   Tissue expansion.
IV   Random pattern flap.
V   Pedicled flap.
VI   Free flap.
a   The different options of the reconstructive armamentarium are represented as circles.
b   Modular evolution: The different techniques of wound closure and cover interact to provide the best result.
        Different combinations are possible, eg, pedicled and free flap, split-thickness skin graft and free flap etc.

References and further reading

[1]   **Mathes SJ, Nahai F** (1997)
      *Reconstructive Surgery: Principles,
      Anatomy, and Technique.* 1st ed. St.
      Louis London: Quality Medical
      Publishing, Churchill-Livingstone,
      Vol. 3, 1193–1206.

[2]   **Manring MM, Hawk A, Calhoun JH,
      et al** (2009) Treatment of war wounds:
      a historical review. *Clin Orthop Relat
      Res;* 467(8):2168–2191.

[3]   **Kalbermatten DF, Haug M,
      Schaefer DJ, et al** (2004) Computer
      aided designed neo-clavicle out of
      osteotomized free fibula: case report.
      Br J Plast Surg; 57(7):668–672.

[4]   **Levin PS, Ellis DS, Stewart WB, et al**
      (1991) Orbital exenteration. The
      reconstructive ladder. *Ophthal Plast
      Reconstr Surg;* 7(2):84–92.

[5]   **Millard DR** (1986) *Principlization of
      Plastic Surgery.* 1st ed. Boston: Little,
      Brown and Company.

[6]   **Lineaweaver WC** (2005) Microsurgery
      and the reconstructive ladder.
      Microsurgery; 25(3):185–186.

[7]   **Levin LS** (1993) The reconstructive
      ladder. An orthoplastic approach.
      Orthop Clin North Am; 24(3):393–409.

[8]   **Levin LS, Condit DP** (1996) Combined
      injuries—soft tissue management.
      Clin Orthop Relat Res; (327):172–181.

[9]   **Wong CJ, Niranjan N** (2008)
      Reconstructive stages as an
      alternative to the reconstructive
      ladder. *Plast Reconstr Surg;*
      121(5):362–363.

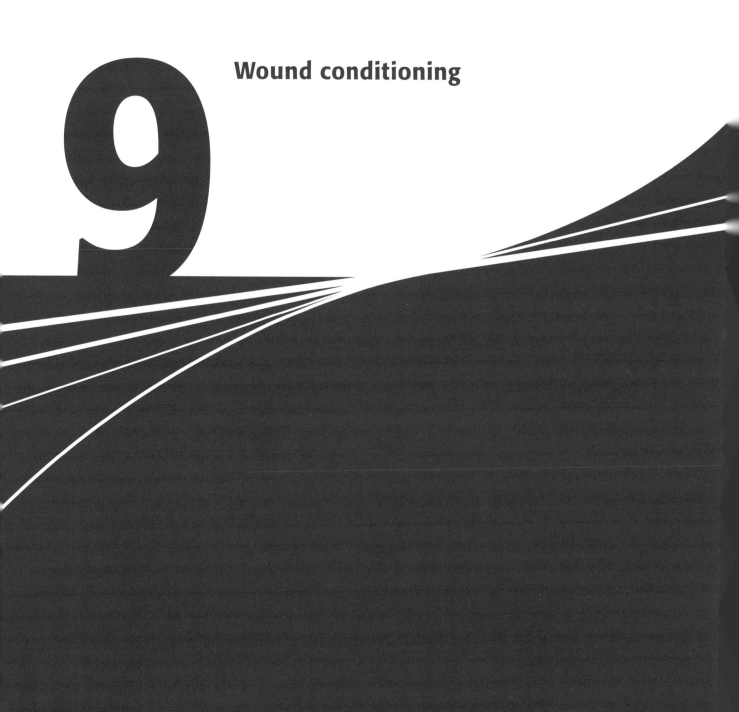

9

Wound conditioning

9.1 Dressings

Author   David A Volgas

9.1.1   Goals of wound dressing

The skin serves as a barrier (mechanical, chemical, and thermal) that is vital to preventing infection and to maintaining homeostasis (chapter 2.1 to 2.3). Whenever the skin is violated, whether by trauma or by surgery, the protective function, which skin provides, is compromised. Dressings are used to cover wounds until the skin is functionally restored. In many cases, dressings are also used to condition the wound, ie, to prepare it for a definitive procedure designed to restore the integrity of the integument.

Dressings are used for various purposes, depending on the wound environment:
- moisten or dry a wound
- prevent further contamination of a wound
- deliver antibiotics to a wound
- avoid further trauma to a wound
- debride and condition a wound
- promote healing.

Most recent literature affirms that for traumatic wounds, a moist wound environment that removes heavy exudates is optimal for wound healing, especially, if migration of fibroblasts to and ingrowth of vessels into the wound is enabled (chapter 4.1). While the formation of an eschar may prevent infection, it will undoubtedly impede reepithelialization. Dressings should ideally limit the moist environment to the wound, and keep the adjacent skin rather dry in order to avoid maceration.

The application of dressings is often relegated to the less experienced members of the treatment team or to outside personnel (with a high turn-over rate) that prevents a regular and good follow-up. Especially complicated or chronic wounds may benefit from specialized personnel known as wound specialists. Otherwise, this may easily result in wounds, which are not adequately monitored. Yet, it is the continuous assessment of wound healing, which is critical to successful outcomes.

There are many types of dressings from the simple to the exotic (**Table 9.1-1**). The range of dressing materials is ever-expanding. While there are many different opinions on which dressings are most appropriate for which wounds, neither in literature nor in practice is there consensus or evidence as to the ideal dressing for a given wound environment. The choice of dressing depends on the surgeon's assessment of the wound environment and preferences. The following discussion represents what the authors feel is the preponderance of evidence in literature and common practice. Principles will be discussed, rather than attempting to discuss every type of dressing.

9.1.2   Traditional dressings

Traditional dressings include various types of gauze dressings, wet or dry nonadherent dressings, and bulky dressings. They are considered to be low-tech, but they are not necessarily less expensive over the course of treatment than more modern, higher-tech solutions. Such dressings often require more experience than is commonly assumed if they are to be applied correctly. However, they are more generally available than advanced dressings. Gauze dressings come in a variety of sizes and patterns. They are usually made of cotton and have a loose weave, whose size may vary. In the acute setting, gauze dressings are used to absorb drainage from surgical wounds. They are quite effective at wicking away moisture from surgical or traumatic wounds, keeping it away from intact skin. In the setting of an open wound with heavy exudate, gauze dressings are used as a wet-to-dry dressing. In recent years, these dressings have fallen out of favor because of significant pain accompanying the changing of dressing as well as the fact that they are indiscriminate in terms of what adheres to the gauze and is thus debrided. Both exudate and granulation tissue may be eliminated and debrided, respectively. Wet and dry, nonadherent dressings include dressings such as saline-moistened and/or petroleum-based gauzes as well as fenestrated plastic-covered gauze dressings. These may be used in wounds that are clean and have a good granulation bed, in wounds with slight drainage after surgery, or over skin grafts and split-thickness skin graft donor sites. They help lessen the pain of changing dressing, but do not completely prevent adherence of the dressing to dried exudate or blood. This dried material will generally fall off when this type of dressing is changed, resulting in debridement, sometimes causing bleeding and pain. Bulky dressings, often consisting of loose cotton fiber material, may be used to pad casts, to immobilize a joint, or to provide relief from pressure on flap pedicles, or pressure sores on extremities. They are often placed under a splint, which may also be used.

Class	Type	Available dressings*	Indications
Traditional	Gauze	Kerlix™, ABD	Surgical dressing
Modern	Alginate	Algicell™, Curasorb™	Moderately exudative wounds, chronic wounds
	Hydrocolloid	DuoDerm™, TegaSorb™, Comfeel™	Chronic wounds with low to moderate exudate
	Hydrofiber	Aquacel™, Aquacel Ag™	Partial-thickness burns, chronic wounds
	Paraffin gauze	Jelonet®	Surgical dressings, interfaces, burns
	Petroleum gauze	Adaptic®, Xeroform®	Surgical dressings, interfaces, burns
	Polymer	Op-Site™, TegaDerm™	Dressing at venous-catheter sites
	Silicone	Mepitel™, Mepilex™	Acute surgical wounds, dressing at venous-catheter sites
Antimicrobial (bacteriocidal, bacteriostatic)	Acetic acid	Various suppliers	Contamination with *Pseudomonas aeruginosa*
	Mafenide	Sulfamylon™	burns, combat wounds
	Povidone - iodine	Betadine™	Surgical preparation, some open traumatic wounds, colonized traumatic wounds
	Sodium hypochlorite	Dakin's solution	Suspected *Pseudomonas aeruginosa* colonization
	Silver	Silvadene™, Acticoat™, Actisorb™, Aquacel Ag™	Burns, colonized traumatic wounds
Hemostatic	Chitosan	HemCon™, Celox™,	Acute hemorrhage
	Fibrin-thrombin based	TachoComb-S™, Red Cross hemostatic dressing	Acute hemorrhage
	Poly-n-acetylglucosamine	RDH™ dressing	Acute hemorrhage
	Zeolite	QuikClot™	Acute hemorrhage
Biologic	Allograft, xenograft	Various suppliers	Burns
	Collagen matrix	Integra™, Matriderm™	Burns, wounds with exposed tendon or nerve, chronic wounds

Table 9.1-1 Different classes and types of dressings.
* The names of dressings might vary from one country to another, particularly between Europe and the US.

9.1.3 Modern dressings

Modern dressings include some form of hydrogel (jelly-like material with properties ranging from soft and weak to hard and tough), alginate (naturally occurring biopolymer derived from seaweed), or thin covers such as polymer or silicon dressings. They are mostly used for burn patients, chronic wounds such as diabetic ulcers, or the donor site of split-thickness grafts. There does not seem to be a large role for them in the acute trauma setting.

Thin-film, semipermeable dressings are made of polymers, which allow passage of water vapor from the wound and oxygen into the wound, but prevent liquids and bacteria from getting into the wound. These dressings may be used for small surgical wounds and at venous-catheter sites. They are also rather popular to cover donor sites of split-thickness skin grafts, sometimes in combination with alginates to reduce pain.

Silicon dressings have been used to help reduce scar and keloid formation. These dressings are not absorbent and should not be used on moderately or heavily exudating wounds. If used in an acute setting, these dressings are typically applied for surgical wounds with excellent hemostasis. Another major type of modern dressing is negative-pressure wound therapy (NPWT). This system is thoroughly discussed in chapter 9.3.

9.1.4 Antimicrobial dressings

Antimicrobial agents may either act as a bactericide or bacteriostatic agent and can be incorporated directly into gauze or hydrogel dressing, or—as a cream—may be applied beneath another type of dressing. These agents are also used to treat open and septic wounds. However, one should take into consideration that these agents may be harmful to tissues and may reduce the activity of the body's natural defenses. Silver has been used as a broad-spectrum topical agent with antimicrobial properties for decades. The elution properties of several preparations have been studied and proved to be effective for several days to weeks. Silver has good biologic activity against many common pathogens including *Escherichia coli, Staphylococcus aureus,* streptococci, *Pseudomonas aeruginosa, Candida albicans* and *Enterococcus faecalis* as well as antibiotic-resistant bacteria, such as methicillin-resistant *Staphylococcus aureus* (MRSA) and vancomycin-resistant enterococcus (VRE) [1]. Interestingly, *Acinetobacter baumanii* seems to be naturally resistant to topical silver dressings [2]. Susceptible bacteria do not seem to develop resistance to silver due to its activity at multiple bacterial target sites, making it suitable for long-term use [3]. However, it is less effective against bacteria in the biofilm state. There is evidence that the adjunctive use of silver with systemic antibiotics is additive and, in some cases, even synergistic. However, there is evidence that silver is toxic to fibroblasts and keratinocytes both in in vitro and in animal studies [4]. Furthermore, it could inhibit cellular proliferation and leukocyte activity. In mammalian cells, however, silver has only been associated with minimal toxicity at low concentrations [5]. There are few studies that examine the systemic absorption of silver from silver-impregnated dressings. Silver nanoparticles also affect the DNA of fibroblasts and stem cells in mouse cell lines [6].

There are many types of dressings and topical creams containing silver. The method of delivery and the quantity of free silver released into tissues is different in each. Silver sulfadiazine has been used extensively in burn patients, but does not offer sufficient activity against gram-negative organisms. Accordingly, cerium nitrate has been added to silver sulfadiazine to augment its effectiveness in burn patients. One drawback of prolonged local use of silver-containing agents may be the permanent deposition of silver molecules within the dermal layers of the skin, resulting in tattoo-like discoloration. More recently, silver has been applied in nanocrystalline form to an effective absorbent dressing, which can be used to treat wounds being prepared for staged coverage (eg, silver-containing alginate). These dressings must be removed before an MRI is performed and should not be used in combination with petroleum dressings. They may be left in place for 3–7 days, depending on the product (**Fig 9.1-1a–d**).

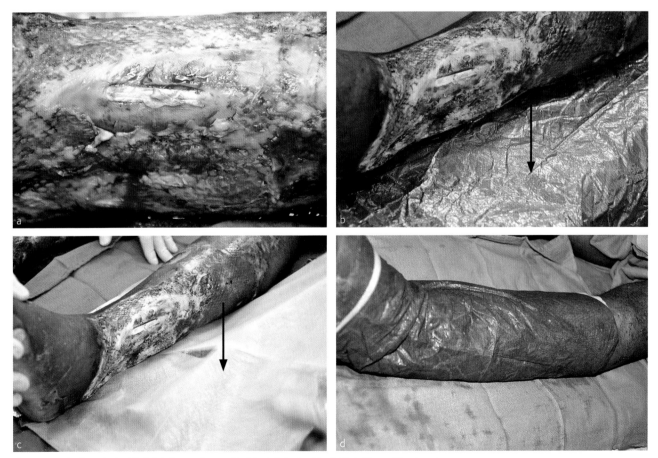

Fig 9.1-1a–d A patient with third-degree burns. Residual defects after initial skin grafting by a burn surgeon.
a   Defect over exposed tendons.
b   Silver-impregnated dressing (arrow) will be used to decontaminate the wound in preparation for a bilayer collagen graft.
c   Note the layer of petroleum dressing (arrow) between the silver dressing and skin.
d   Lower extremity covered by moistened silver-impregnated dressing.

Povidone-iodine-impregnated dressings were commonly used in the past for military wounds and burns. The substance exhibits excellent activity against most bacterial, fungal, and viral pathogens. There are varying reports concerning the tissue toxicity and effect on wound healing of povidone-iodine preparations [7], although more recent methods of application may have ameliorated this concern. Povidone-iodine has been shown to be toxic to synovium and cartilage and should, therefore, be handled with care or even avoided in the setting of complex bone or articular injuries [8]. In the acute setting, most surgeons now consider it to be useful for cleansing a surgical site, but not for packing traumatic wounds, because of the presumed tissue toxicity and the availability of alternative, less-toxic solutions.

Dakin's solution (sodium hypochlorite), a chlorine-releasing solution originally consisted of concentrations of 0.4–0.5% sodium hypochlorite and boric acid (4%). However, in recent years, it has been diluted to half-strength (0.25%), quarter-strength (0.125%), and down to 0.0125% solutions in order to reduce the tissue toxicity of the original solution. It exhibits relatively broad antibacterial activity, including MRSA, VRE, and Pseudomonas species. It has been shown in vitro that diluted solutions (0.0125%) continue to show antibiotic properties, without any detrimental effect on keratinocytes. Dakin's solution is inherently unstable and so must be made up as needed.

Mafenide acetate and mafenide hydrochloride are antibacterial agents, though the hydrochloride solution is more potent. They both exhibit wide antimicrobial activity and are uniquely effective against *Acinetobacter baumanii*. Their usefulness in burn patients has been well established [9]. As mafenide acetate has been shown to inhibit DNA and protein synthesis in wounds and to delay reepithelialization, prolonged use in open wounds is not indicated. However, as an initial treatment of open wounds, it appears to be useful.

Finally, hydrogen peroxide has successfully been used as an antiseptic and antibacterial agent for a long time due to its oxidizing effect. While its use has decreased in recent years with the popularity of readily available over-the-counter products, it is still used by many hospitals and doctors.

9.1.5 Hemostatic dressings

The major cause of early mortality in trauma victims, military or civilian, is uncontrolled hemorrhage. Dressings have been developed, largely for military use, which can be applied directly to hemorrhagic wounds in order to immediately stop bleeding. These dressings are typically made of chitosan, zeolite or derivatives of marine algae.

A number of dressings are currently based on chitosan, a derivative of chitin. Chitin forms the exoskeleton of crustaceans. Chitosan is produced by the deacetylation of chitin. It is provided in granules or on a sponge. It acts by binding to receptors on red blood cells, forming a gel. It works regardless of hypothermia, the presence of anticoagulants, or depletion of coagulation factors. Unlike zeolite dressings, it does not produce an exothermic reaction. Zeolite is an aluminosilicate substance similar to that found in volcanoes. It acts by rapidly absorbing water from blood, thus concentrating coagulation factors and potentiating the coagulation cascade. It may be applied as a powder or on a sponge. It must be applied directly to the source of bleeding and, therefore, may be difficult to apply directly to deep arteries. The major drawback is that it creates an exothermic reaction, which can cause burns. It has recently been combined with silver to form an antimicrobial dressing and has been successfully applied for the treatment of combat wounds.

Poly-n-acetylglucosamine is derived from marine algae. It appears to work by sealing the wound and facilitating the coagulation cascade. The procoagulative effect abates within a few hours, but by then, the patient can hopefully receive definitive care. This dressing is currently in use by the US military. Dressings that are saturated with fibrin, thrombin, or calcium have also been used, but appear to be less effective, with considerably more bleeding seen in clinical practice than with those mentioned before.

9.1.6 Biological dressings

Biological dressings are being used more and more in acute trauma. While generally considered temporary dressings, they work in concert with the natural healing process until the wound is prepared to accept definitive coverage, such as a split-thickness skin graft. They may be composed of allograft skin, xenograft skin, or collagen matrices (chapter 10.2). The goal of these dressings is to conserve water, protein and electrolytes, and reduce infection. By providing a substrate that allows ingrowth of fibroblasts and promotes angiogenesis, these dressings prepare the wound to accept skin grafts.

For many years, xenografts, particularly porcine grafts, have been used for burn patients to temporarily cover wounds and allow time for skin to be reharvested or for the patient to stabilize before split-thickness skin grafting. To prevent rejection by the host, these grafts are processed to remove most antigens. Nevertheless, in time, they will be rejected, necessitating replacement by native skin. Similarly, allograft skin can be used.

Bilayer collagen matrix dressings (**Fig 9.1-2a–d**) are composed of bovine type I collagen, which has been processed to provide cross-linked collagen fibers. These degrade slowly and are replaced by neodermis [10]. This layer of collagen is covered by a thin silicone layer, which helps to prevent the colonization of the collagen matrix by bacteria and the loss of water. It is transparent, so the wound can still be visualized. These dressings may be combined with negative-pressure wound therapy to foster angiogenesis and decrease the period before split-thickness skin grafting from 2–3 weeks to 7–10 days. Once the collagen matrix is ready to accept a skin graft, it will change to a salmon color. Nowadays, single-layer matrices are available that allow a one-stage surgical procedure, ie, simultaneous application of both matrix and skin grafts. With each of these dressings, it is important that the wound bed be rendered as sterile as possible. Bacterial colonization will significantly decrease the survival rate of such grafts.

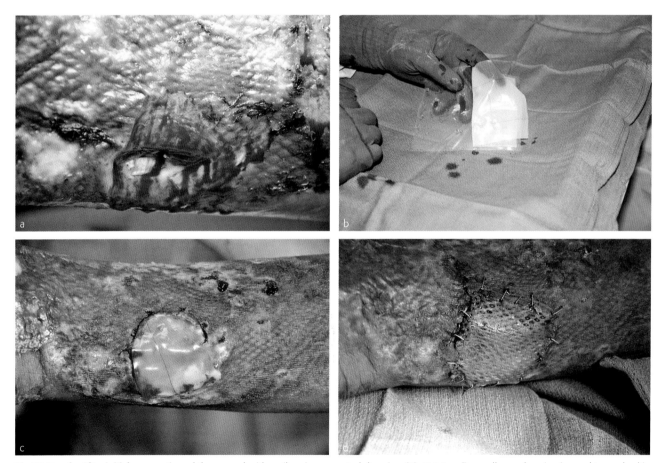

Fig 9.1-2a–d   After initial preparation of the wound with a silver-impregnated dressing (**Fig 9.1-1a–d**), a collagen dressing is used to apply skin grafting over tendons.
a   Residual defect over the fibular tendon.
b   Bilayer collagen with silicone top layer before application.
c   Dressing in place.
d   Split-thickness skin grafting after 10 days.

9.2 Local antibiotic therapy

Author   James P Stannard

9.2.1 Nonresorbable antibiotic bead therapy

Local antibiotic therapy is frequently used to prepare contaminated dead space for eventual bone grafting or substitution with vascularized bone or muscle and coverage. Antibiotic beads are frequently made by mixing polymethyl methacrylate (PMMA) with an appropriate antibiotic. The beads are packed into the open or dead space and then the wound is either closed or covered with a semipermeable membrane, which is the so-called bead-pouch technique

(**Fig 9.2-1a–d**). The majority of the drug is eluted over the first 24 hours. However, some studies suggest elution may occur in small doses for as long as 90 days [11, 12]. Antibiotic elution is related to the surface area of the antibiotic spacer used. Therefore, small beads arrayed in chains will elute more than larger beads, which will elute more than a block spacer. There are many considerations that may guide the choice of the shape and the size of the antibiotic beads, but if elution of antibiotics is the primary aim and all other factors are the same, the use of small beads is advised.

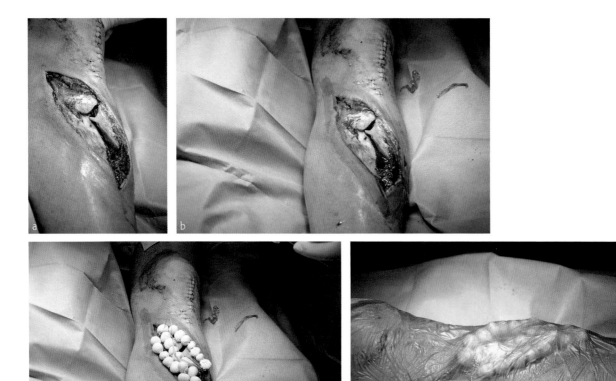

Fig 9.2-1a–d   Antibiotic bead-pouch technique consisting of Palacos® bone cement with 2.0 g vancomycin and 2.4 g tobramycin.
a   Clinical photograph of a Gustilo type IIIB fracture after debridement.
b   The edge of the wound is protected by first applying collodion or benzoin, and a thin rim of occlusive dressing in order to prevent maceration of the wound edges.
c   Small 5–8 mm beads strung on a suture are placed over the wound.
d   Coverage by an occlusive dressing.

There are a number of ways in which local antibiotics can be used. Antibiotic-coated implants such as intramedullary nails are currently available in some locations in Europe, but are not available in the United States at this time. Antibiotic beads are often applied using the bead-pouch technique to provide large concentrations of antibiotic in an area of bone deficit that has been severely contaminated. Finally, some surgeons now prefer to use a block of cement covered with antibiotics in order to provide a high concentration of antibiotic and also to allow the formation of a biologically active membrane around the cement block. Furthermore, the block of cement acts as a spacer and eases subsequent reconstruction of the bone and/or soft tissues, eg, nonvascularized or vascularized bone and/or fasciocutaneous flap, muscle or musculocutaneous flap.

A wide variety of antibiotics have been used in beads, ranging from aminoglycosides to vancomycin to a third-generation fluoroquinolone [11–13]. The requirements of an antibiotic to be used in beads include:
- water solubility
- broad spectrum
- good tolerance
- heat stability
- bactericidal in low concentrations
- availability in powdered form [11].

The most commonly used antibiotics are tobramycin and vancomycin. We frequently combine 2.4 g of powdered tobramycin or 2.0 g of vancomycin with a 40 g pouch of Palacos® Bone Cement (Biomet Orthopedics, Inc., Warsaw, IN, USA). It is important to select a type of cement that keeps a dough-like consistency for a number of minutes in order to allow the formation of the beads. If the wound contains multiple organisms or a broad spectrum of coverage is required, both 2.4 g of tobramycin and 1.0 g of vancomycin can be combined with a single packet of polymethyl methacrylate cement. Beads can be created either using commercially available molds or by hand rolling the beads. Regardless of which technique is used to create the beads, they should be strung on a strong nonresorbable suture. Commercial formulations of antibiotic beads are available outside the United States, but are not currently available within the United States. Precise mixing directions and uniformity of size cannot be achieved with hand rolled beads, leading to differences in drug elution from the varying surface areas of the beads [14]. It should be noted that rarely systemic levels of antibiotics have been detected in patients. Therefore, this technique should be used with caution in patients with antibiotic allergies or severe renal disease.

There is a large body of evidence from animal studies documenting successful use of antibiotic beads for both the treatment of contaminated wounds and chronic osteomyelitis [12, 14]. However, the clinical data is limited due to studies that are primarily retrospective and/or have a small sample size. There are no well-designed prospective randomized clinical trials to document the efficacy of polymethyl methacrylate beads. Despite this shortcoming, the combination of solid animal data and suggestive clinical data has led to the widespread use of antibiotic beads and the bead-pouch technique [11, 12, 14–16].

9.2.2 Resorbable antibiotic bead therapy

Resorbable antibiotic bead pellets and other resorbable antibiotic delivery systems have been the subject of a multitude of studies in recent years. Numerous substances have been used in biodegradable systems including:
- lyophilized human fibrin
- polyglycolic acid
- polylactic acid (PLA)
- polycaprolactone
- calcium sulfate pellet.

The latter is the most commonly used biodegradable material by far.

Animal studies have used rabbit, canine, and goat models to demonstrate the effectiveness of calcium sulfate as a biodegradable carrier for antibiotics [14, 17, 18]. There have also been a limited number of studies documenting the use of calcium sulfate pellets in humans [11, 19]. The early experience has been encouraging, but data is extremely limited. One problem that can occur with the use of calcium sulfate pellets is the development of a sterile draining sinus [14]. Additional work is needed on both calcium sulfate pellets and antibiotic polylactic acid microspheres, but the future of local antibiotic delivery may be marked by biodegradable carriers.

9.3 Negative-pressure wound therapy

Author   James P Stannard, William J Harrison

9.3.1 Basic physiological concepts

Negative-pressure wound therapy (NPWT) is a relatively new therapy for enhancing soft-tissue healing following trauma. It was initially developed by a plastic surgeon and basic scientist and was intended to treat chronic, nonhealing wounds in patients, who were not good candidates for surgery [20]. The therapy initially received clearance from the Food and Drug Administration (FDA) for use in the United States in 1995. The vast majority of the research and clinical application of negative-pressure wound therapy has currently involved the Vacuum Assisted Closure (VAC®) system (Kinetic Concepts Inc. (KCI), San Antonio, TX, USA). This system works by using an open cell-foam dressing over soft tissues, with a fenestrated evacuation tube connected to an adjustable vacuum source that creates a controlled subatmospheric pressure environment under the foam dressing (**Video 9.3-1a–d**). Although first described by a European team of trauma surgeons [21], clinical use of this device was initiated on a large scale in patients undergoing plastic surgery in the US. In the last few years, the application of negative-pressure wound therapy has progressively spread to include the treatment of acute wounds of skeletal trauma patients that could not be closed or wounds that had undergone breakdown in the postoperative period (**Fig 9.3-1a–d**). Negative-pressure wound therapy is also useful in exudative wounds to draw off fluids and stimulate the formation of granulation tissue [22]. As such, this method helps to avoid infection and to cover open wounds, even over exposed bone. In the majority of the hospitals throughout the world, patients who have sustained orthopaedic trauma—including soft-tissue wounds—are now the most common recipients of negative-pressure wound therapy.

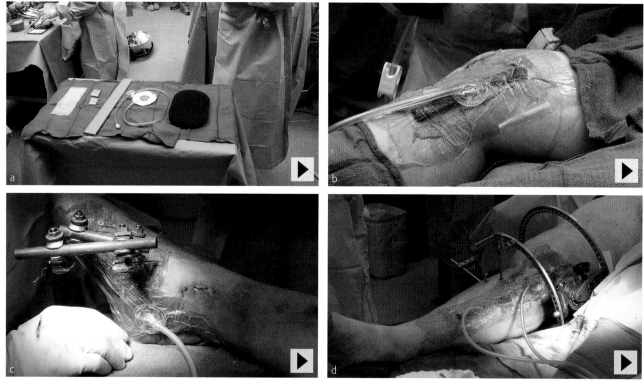

Video 9.3-1a–d   Negative-pressure wound therapy.
a   Components of the Vacuum Assisted Closure (VAC®) system distributed by Kinetic Concepts Inc. (KCI), San Antonio, TX, USA.
b   Application on a closed high-risk surgical incision.
c   Application on an open wound and around an external fixator.
d   Application on a split-thickness skin graft and an adjacent closed surgical incision.

Basic science studies suggest that negative-pressure wound therapy works by at least three primary mechanisms:
1. increased blood flow and/or angiogenesis
2. mechanical stretching of cells, leading to the secretion of cytokines and growth factors associated with wound healing
3. reduction of edema formation.

Animal studies performed at the laboratories of Argenta and Morykwas et al using porcine models suggested that negative-pressure wound therapy led to increased blood flow and the production of abundant vascular granulation tissue in wounds. Blood flow increased 4-fold while granulation tissue increased by 63% with continuous topical negative pressure and by 103% with intermittent pressure. The porcine models were used to establish the ideal cycle of 5 minutes of subatmospheric pressure followed by two minutes off for the intermittent mode [20]. Timmers et al published a study looking at blood flow over intact forearm skin in healthy individuals [23]. Their results demonstrated up to a 5-fold increase in blood flow under the sponge, even with intact skin. The increase in blood flow depended on the amount of subatmospheric pressure applied, and increased all the way up to a pressure of 300 mmHg. Several published studies using laser Doppler technology suggest that negative-pressure wound therapy alters blood flow to the wound edges when applied to healing wounds. One of the studies used an inguinal wound porcine model. This study suggested relative hypoperfusion immediately adjacent to the wound edges, with hyperemia and marked increased blood flow when the negative-pressure wound therapy was terminated [24]. This study suggests that intermittently applied subatmospheric pressure may be superior to constant pressure

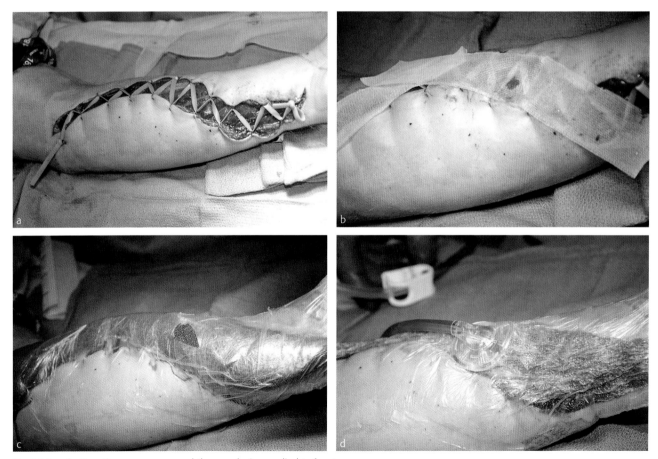

Fig 9.3-1a–d Negative-pressure wound-therapy device applied to forearm.
a Forearm fasciotomy partially closed with an elastic vessel loop.
b A petroleum-based semi-permeable dressing is applied to the wound.
c The sponge for negative-pressure wound therapy is cut to size and secured at the edges with staples.
d The negative-pressure wound-therapy device is activated, collapsing the sponge.

application for blood flow. Other studies suggested increased blood flow in both situations [25].

The second proposed mechanism of action of negative-pressure wound therapy is the mechanical stimulation of cells, leading to the production of factors that support wound healing. It is postulated that such stresses to the surrounding soft tissues deform the extracellular matrix and cell cytoskeleton, enhancing tissue growth and expansion. The principle of mechanical stimulation leading to tissue genesis, be it regeneration or repair, is already well established with the Ilizarov method of distraction osteogenesis in orthopaedics as well as with the use of tissue expanders. Integrins link the extracellular matrix to the cell cytoskeleton, and are the modulator of force transmission to the internal cytoskeleton. This is believed to cause the release of intracellular second messengers and up-regulation of the immediate early response of oncogenes associated with cell growth, proliferation, and differentiation [26].

The final proposed mechanism of action of negative-pressure wound therapy is edema reduction. This mechanism is particularly important in specific conditions associated with fluid production including burns, compartment syndromes, and soft-tissue shear injuries such as the Morel-Lavallée lesion as they are seen in run-over accidents (chapter 3.3). Excess fluid is thought to hamper wound healing both by decreasing blood flow and tissue oxygenation as well as by accumulating deleterious substances as chronic exudates. Increases in interstitial pressure may lead to occlusion of the microvasculature and lymphatics, leading to tissue hypoxia and eventually necrosis. Additionally, interstitial fluid of chronic wounds contains elevated levels of enzymes such as collagenases and elastases, which catabolize extracellular matrix proteins, producing degradation products which may retard cell adhesion, migration, proliferation and differentiation [26]. This mechanism of action may be the least important of the three proposed mechanisms for the majority of skeletal trauma patients.

9.3.2 Indications and contraindications

Indications for the use of negative-pressure wound therapy for orthopaedic trauma patients are still being developed, due to the lack of level I clinical research data available. As more quality studies are published, the ideal indications for negative-pressure wound therapy will become clearer. Initially, negative-pressure wound therapy was primarily used for chronic wounds, wound complications and breakdown, the management of open fractures with considerable soft-

tissue defect, as well as the treatment of fasciotomy wounds following compartment syndrome. To date, several authors have reported retrospective series using negative-pressure wound therapy with open fractures. All authors either conclude that negative-pressure wound therapy appears to decrease the risk of infection or that it helps surgeons to obtain soft-tissue coverage following fracture treatment [27–29]. The author has completed a prospective randomized study of severe open fractures comparing negative-pressure wound therapy with saline wet-to-moist dressings and observed that there was a significant decrease in infection rate in the patients treated with negative-pressure wound therapy [30]. Recently, published reports have demonstrated good results with the use of negative-pressure wound therapy following high-energy combat wounds in Iraq [29]. Negative-pressure wound therapy has also been successfully used with complex skeletal trauma to decrease the need for free tissue transfers, allowing coverage using local techniques that are more easily obtainable, especially if specialized surgeons are not available. Parrett et al reported on open tibial fractures (Gustilo type IIIB fracture) in the Boston area, noting a decrease in the need for free flaps from 42% from 1992–1995, to 26% between 1996–1999, and finally to only 11% between 2000–2003 [31]. There was no change in the incidence of postoperative infection over the study period. The study, however, does not report the median and long-term follow-up with regard to wound breakdown, unstable scars, or fistulas that may indicate osteomyelitis or deep soft-tissue infection. Neither does it report the comparability of the cases assigned to those time periods.

Another innovative application involves subatmospheric pressure dressings placed at the site of a surgical incision over closure in high-risk wounds. Timmers et al demonstrated that negative-pressure wound therapy leads to increased blood flow under the sponge in closed skin [23]. Based on that finding, the author and his coworkers have recently presented data (unpublished) showing a significant decrease in infections and wound dehiscence in surgical incisions treated by negative-pressure wound therapy compared with those with a standard postoperative dressing following calcaneus, pilon, or tibial plateau fractures. The data suggests that negative-pressure wound therapy may play a considerable role in the prevention of wound complications in high risk situations. However, additional study will be needed to confirm these findings.

Finally, studies have been presented or published documenting the use of negative-pressure wound therapy for split-thickness skin grafts (STSG) (chapter 10.2), as recently published in two prospective studies. Llanos et al published a prospective, randomized, double-blind study comparing foam dressing with or without negative pressure [32]. They demonstrated significant benefits in regard to total graft survival rates and hospitalization time in patients undergoing negative-pressure wound therapy. Kim et al demonstrated significant improvements in engraftment time, total graft take, and complete healing time in a prospective, nonrandomized study of patients treated with negative-pressure wound therapy compared to patients treated with a classic tie-over dressing [33].

There are two contraindications to the use of negative-pressure wound therapy. The first, primary and most important contraindication is that it should not be used in wounds with uncontrolled bleeding, over exposed major vessels, or in patients who take anticoagulant drugs or are known to suffer from coagulopathy. If excessive bleeding develops while negative-pressure wound therapy is being used, it should be discontinued immediately. Bleeding problems are very rare, but there has been at least one case of a fatality associated with bleeding to death in a patient treated with negative-pressure wound therapy, as recently reported in the UK due to the inadequate use of negative-pressure wound-therapy devices. The second, yet relative contraindication is infection. It is acceptable to use negative-pressure wound therapy combined with debridement and irrigation of devitalized and/or grossly contaminated tissue, but it should not be used as the primary treatment of infection. In such cases, the foam should rather be applied over gauze that has been impregnated with a bacteriostatic or bactericidal agent.

9.3.3 Wound management

There are two methods of managing wounds with negative-pressure wound therapy. The first is the method for patients with open wounds that will be treated either with delayed primary closure, a skin graft, or a flap. In these cases, the black foam with large pores and the VAC® system (**Video 9.3-1a**) should be cut to fit within the wound. After placing the sponge in the wound, an airtight seal should be created using the drapes included with the system. A hole is cut into the drape and the suction is attached. In most cases, we recommend using intermittent negative pressure at 125–150 mmHg or just below the level of pain. The foam should ideally be changed every 48–72 hours in order to prevent infection and excessive ingrowth of the granulation tissue into the sponge. If changing the dressing causes too much pain, instilling the foam that has been disconnected from suction with a sterile solution containing a local anesthetic

~20 minutes in advance may relieve the pain. An exception to the recommendation of intermittent pressure is when negative-pressure wound therapy is used over split-thickness skin grafts. In this case, the skin graft should be covered with a dressing acting as an interface (eg, paraffin gauze (Jelonet®)) between the skin graft and foam in order to prevent graft disruption whenever the foam is changed or discarded. In this case, we recommend the use of continuous negative pressure between 75–125 mmHg. The white foam with smaller pores is indicated in superficial, chronic wounds.

The second method of wound management involves the use of negative-pressure wound therapy over surgically closed wounds (**Video 9.3-1b**). Following suture or staple closure, a nonadhering petroleum gauze (eg, Adaptic® or Xeroform®) should be positioned with the suture line in the middle of the dressing. The black foam dressing is placed over the petroleum gauze, with an airtight dressing covering both. This negative-pressure dressing can be safely maintained for up to 4–5 days since the soft-tissue envelope it covers is closed. The use of negative-pressure wound therapy around an external fixator (**Video 9.3-1c**) or in cases of two wounds in close proximity (**Video 9.3-1d**) presents special problems.

The efficacy of negative-pressure wound therapy has motivated many professionals to use these kits, even in developing countries. Unfortunately, commercially marketed negative-pressure wound therapy closure kits, which are nowadays supplied by various manufacturers, are very expensive. Therefore, Harrison et al have successfully used a homemade version of a low-budget, negative-pressure wound-therapy device with excellent effect in low to medium resource scenarios (chapter 9.4). The dressing system is based on a layer of vaseline gauze applied on the wound, followed by a piece of foam cut to size. A length of suction tubing is placed within the foam, which is then connected to a standard mobile suction unit. The dressing is sealed with an adhesive sealant-film dressing. The foam that is used is pressure-relieving foam, which comes clean rather than sterile and is often available in donations. Foam may be autoclaved, but it shrinks somewhat and the pore size decreases, which in turn slows the rate of development of granulation tissue. Standard mobile suction machines are not designed for continuous use and, therefore, are run in cycles of 30 minutes on, then 30 minutes off, during which time the suction tubing is clamped. In this system the only significant consumable cost is that of the adhesive film. If the dressing is airtight and the wound judged clean, the dressings may be left in situ for up to a week. If the foam is applied without vaseline gauze, or with a larger pore size, dressings should be changed more frequently as otherwise granulation tissue will grow into the foam (**Fig 9.3-2a–d**).

Experience demonstrates that homemade negative-pressure wound therapy is ideal both as a containment procedure pending more aggressive surgical treatment (eg, stabilization of open fractures) where necessary, and as a therapeutic component in combating an infected. Comparable to the VAC®, this homemade device dramatically reduces the need for assistance by a plastic surgeon and increases the speed and rate of successful wound healing (**Fig 9.3-3**).

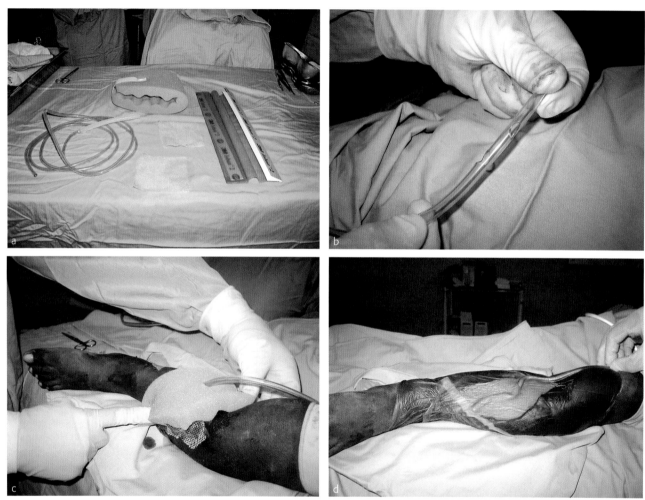

Fig 9.3-2a–d   Homemade negative-pressure wound-therapy device.
a   The basic setup for a homemade negative-pressure wound-therapy device.
b   Side ports are cut into the plastic tubing using a knife.
c   The sponge is placed over the wound.
d   Suction is applied to the sponge covered by an air-tight dressing.

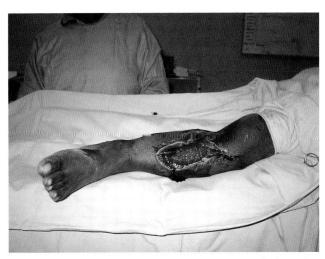

Fig 9.3-3 Effective treatment of a soft-tissue defect at the lower leg with a homemade, negative-pressure wound-therapy device. Note the abundant granulation tissue in the wound bed.

9.4 Alternative options

Author   William J Harrison, Yves Harder

9.4.1   **Oncotic pressure dressings**

Sugar or honey dressings are frequently used in countries with limited resources. Oncotic pressure dressings do not require any special preparation for wound conditioning, except that the wound should macroscopically be cleared of all necrotic tissues and surface slough prior to application.

Honey was popularized by Molan, who described its inhibitory effect to ~60 species of bacteria, including aerobe and anaerobe, gram-positive and gram-negative bacteria [34]. It plays an active role in wound healing in three different ways:

1. The high osmolarity is sufficient to inhibit microbial growth or even kill bacteria [35]. Paradoxically, the antibacterial properties increase once honey is diluted by wound exudate, which appears to contain an enzyme that produces hydrogen peroxide [36]. Hydrogen peroxide acts as a local antiseptic with presumably cytotoxic properties. As the concentration of the antibacterial solution produced after application of honey is known to be approximately a thousand times less than in a commonly used 3% antiseptic solution of hydrogen peroxide, it does not have the same harmful effect on fibroblasts of human skin [37]. Moreover, some kinds of honey have even been treated with catalase in order to eliminate the hydrogen-peroxide activity, as in Manuka honey. However, additional nonperoxide, antibacterial phytochemical components have been identified [38].

2. Honey has also been associated with an activation of the immune response to infection, including the proliferation of lymphocytes and monocytes, and the release of cytokines (ie, tumor necrosis factor (TNF-) β, interleukin (IL)-1 and IL-6) [39].

3. Furthermore, the high glucose content of honey and low pH environment, with a pH of 3–4, may assist in the bacteria-destroying macrophage activity [40].

Commercially available honey may simply be applied in a runny form, poured onto sterile gauze, which is then placed onto wounds (**Fig 9.4-1a–f**). Lately, there has also been a resurgence of interest in honey dressings in developed countries, where the increasing prevalence of antibiotic-resistant microbial species is a growing problem. Its utilization, however, is difficult to implement, especially if the honey is not introduced or confected by the pharmacy of the hospital (**Table 9.4-1**).

Adverse effects to honey are rare and rather irrelevant and comprise local allergic reactions—attributed to specific pollen in the honey—as well as localized stinging sensation due to its acidity [41].

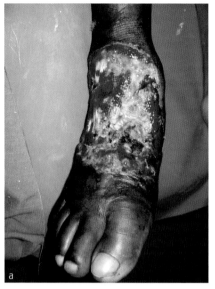
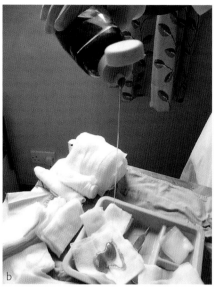
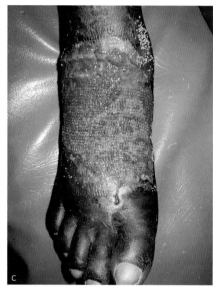
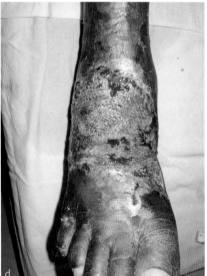
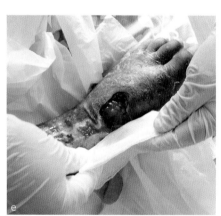
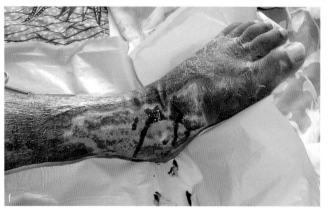

Fig 9.4-1a–f Wound conditioning with honey, with or without skin graft.

a Crush injury of the anterior aspect of the right foot with considerable soft-tissue defect, necrotic tissue, and exposed extensor tendons. State before conditioning.

b Pouring of honey onto dry, sterile gauzes.

c After 4 weeks of wound conditioning with honey. The wound is now covered by abundant granulation tissue and is ready to receive a skin graft.

d After application of a meshed split-thickness skin graft.

e Application of dry gauzes soaked with honey.

f Incomplete secondary healing with slough, hypergranulation, and inhomogeneous pigmentation.

Sugar has the advantage of being even cheaper than honey (**Fig 9.4-2a–b**). It exerts an osmotic effect and may stimulate macrophages. It can be purchased as table sugar and simply poured onto wounds. Alternatively, a paste can be made by mixing sugar with petroleum jelly and glycerin (**Table 9.4-1**). Mphande et al regularly use honey in clinical practice for the treatment of open and/or septic wounds [42]. In their study comparing honey and sugar dressings, they found that honey had an advantage over sugar in reducing bacterial wound contamination, and accelerating healing times. From a practical point of view, substantial amounts of honey need to be applied to a wound in order to achieve adequate potency. Although it may be very viscous or even solid at room temperature, honey becomes rather fluid at body temperature and even more fluid if diluted with small volumes of wound exudate. It is therefore very important that sufficient honey is applied to a wound and that it is kept in place if a good therapeutic effect is to be obtained.

9.4.2 Maggot-debridement therapy

Ideally, wound debridement is undertaken surgically. Occasionally, if safe anesthesia is unavailable, the environment is inadequate, and/or the surgical expertise is lacking, surgical debridement may be by-passed by "bio-surgical" debridement, using maggots as an attractive and effective alternative (**Table 9.4-1**) [43]. Maggot therapy, also known as maggot-debridement therapy, involves the intentional

Type of treatment	Advantages	Disadvantages	Comments
Honey	Cheap, available, biological, nontoxic	Requires adjunctive surgical debridement	Very helpful in developing countries
Sugar	Very cheap, available, nontoxic	Requires adjunctive surgical debridement, moderate efficacy	Alternative if honey is unavailable
Iodine (chapter 9.2)	Available, strong antiseptic	Toxic to tissues, unproven efficacy	Not recommended
Maggots	Excellent debridement of dead tissue	No debridement of dead bone, needing production capacity, variable patient acceptance	Only method that includes debridement
Negative-pressure wound therapy (chapter 9.3)	Highly effective even to cover exposed bone	Requires suction pump, power, adhesive films	Very helpful, especially if plastic surgery is unavailable

Table 9.4-1   Advantages and disadvantages of alternative wound-conditioning methods in comparison to antiseptics and closure by negative-pressure wound therapy.

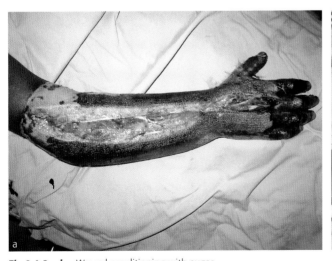 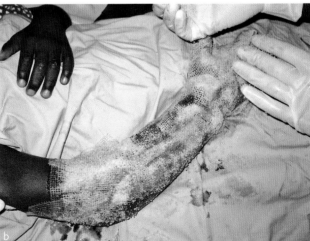

Fig 9.4-2a–b   Wound conditioning with sugar.
a   After fasciotomy of the right forearm and hand (compartment syndrome).
b   Sugar dressing with paraffin gauze.

introduction of viable, disinfected larvae of the common green bottle fly, ie, *Lucilia sericata,* that evolve into maggots within necrotic, contaminated or nonhealing wounds. Larvae may be cultivated quite simply, but it is important to disinfect them correctly. Larvae produced by contaminated flies may debride the wound effectively, but may also introduce tetanus. The efficacy of tetanus immunization is often questionable in developing countries, and a tetanus antibody cover or tetanus-toxoid immunization boost must be considered in case of accidental contamination by maggots. Maggots develop three principal modes of actions. The combination and interactions of these actions make maggots an extremely potent tool in specific wound-care problems:

1. **Selective wound debridement by dissolving necrotic tissue:** Maggots operate precisely at the boundary between healthy and necrotic tissue by secreting a broad spectrum of proteolytic enzymes that liquefy necrotic tissue (ie, extracorporeal digestion) and by ingesting the resulting semi-liquid within a few days [44]. As maggots do not debride bone, they are not useful or suited for the elimination of dead or infected fracture fragments, or osteomyelitic sequestra.

2. **Wound disinfection:** The antibacterial effect of maggots is based on the secretion of specific antibacterial factors (ie, allantoin, urea, phenylacetic acid, phenylacetaldehyde, calcium carbonate, and proteolytic enzymes). Bacteria that have not been killed by these secretions will subsequently be ingested and digested by the maggots. Maggots are able to inhibit and destroy a wide range of bacteria, including group A and B streptococci, gram-positive aerobic and anaerobic strains as well as methicillin-resistant *Staphylococcus aureus* (MRSA) [45].

3. **Stimulation of wound healing:** Last but not least, maggot therapy has shown to enhance wound healing by releasing growth factors and cytokines as well as by stimulating the growth of human fibroblasts. Furthermore, micromassaging of the wound by maggot movement is believed to stimulate the formation of granulation tissue and wound exudates by the host [46].

A moist and exudating wound with sufficient oxygen supply is a prerequisite for maggot therapy, whereas dry or open wounds in body cavities do not provide a good environment for maggots to feed. In some cases, it may be possible to make a dry wound suitable for maggot therapy by moistening it with saline soaks, applied for 48 hours. Maggots have a short shelf life, which prevents long-term storage before use. Patients, their relatives, and physicians may find maggots distasteful. Bandages must be applied in order to prevent any maggots from escaping, while allowing sufficient air to reach the maggots. Finally, bandages help to minimize the uncomfortable tickling sensation that the maggots often cause.

9.4.3 Other approaches

Some wounds of trauma patients can become chronic and even problematic, especially in the growing group of aging people with multiple comorbidities. This is a challenge not welcomed at all by health-care providers. Many of these patients will first undergo nonsurgical treatment in order to prepare the wound, so that a smaller surgical intervention may be performed with a greater chance for success. To date, the following methods have been tried and are more or less successful:

- hyperbaric oxygen
- electrical stimulation
- negative-pressure wound therapy (chapter 9.3)
- exogenous application of growth factors
- cultured keratinocyte grafts [22].

References and further reading

[1] **Lansdown AB** (2002) Silver. I: Its antibacterial properties and mechanism of action. *J Wound Care;* 11(4):125–130.

[2] **Davis SC, Pisanni F, Montero RB** (2008) Effects of commonly used topical antimicrobial agents on Acinetobacter baumannii: an in vitro study. *Mil Med;* 173(1):74–78.

[3] **Percival SL, Bowler PG, Russell D** (2005) Bacterial resistance to silver in wound care. *J Hosp Infect;* 60(1):1–7.

[4] **Hsin YH, Chen CF, Huang S, et al** (2008) The apoptotic effect of nanosilver is mediated by a ROS- and JNK-dependent mechanism involving the mitochondrial pathway in NIH3T3 cells. *Toxicol Lett;* 179(3):130–139.

[5] **Demling RH, DeSanti L** (2001) Effects of silver on wound management. *Wounds;* 13(Suppl 1):5–14.

[6] **Ahamed M, Karns M, Goodson M, et al** (2008) DNA damage response to different surface chemistry of silver nanoparticles in mammalian cells. *Toxicol Appl Pharmacol;* 233(3):404–410.

[7] **Wilson JR, Mills JG, Prather ID, et al** (2005) A toxicity index of skin and wound cleansers used on in vitro fibroblasts and keratinocytes. *Adv Skin Wound Care;* 18(7):373–378.

[8] **Kataoka M, Tsumura H, Kaku N, et al** (2006) Toxic effects of povidone-iodine on synovial cell and articular cartilage. *Clin Rheumatol;* 25(5):632–638.

[9] **Brown TP, Cancio LC, McManus AT, et al** (2004) Survival benefit conferred by topical antimicrobial preparations in burn patients: a historical perspective. *J Trauma;* 56(4):863–866.

[10] **Jeng JC, Fidler PE, Sokolich JC, et al** (2007) Seven years' experience with Integra as a reconstructive tool. *J Burn Care Res;* 28(1):120–126.

[11] **Anglen JO, Watson JT** (2007) Musculoskeletal infection associated with skeletal trauma. *Stannard JP, Schmidt AH, Kregor PJ (eds), Surgical treatment of orthopaedic trauma.* 1st ed. New York: Thieme Publishers, 20–43.

[12] **DeCoster TA, Bozorgnia S** (2008) Antibiotic beads. *J Am Acad Orthop Surg;* 16(11):674–678.

[13] **Efstathopoulos N, Giamarellos-Bourboulis E, et al** (2008) Treatment of experimental osteomyelitis by methicillin resistant Staphylococcus aureus with bone cement system releasing grepafloxacin. *Injury;* 39(12):1384–1390.

[14] **Kent ME, Rapp RP, Smith KM** (2006) Antibiotic beads and osteomyelitis: Here today, what's coming tomorrow? *Orthopedics;* 29(7):599–603.

[15] **Diefenbeck M, Mückley T, Hofmann GO** (2006) Prophylaxis and treatment of implant-related infections by local application of antibiotics. *Injury;* 37(Suppl 2):95–104.

[16] **Murray CK, Hsu JR, Solomkin JS, et al** (2008) Prevention and management of infections associated with combat-related extremity injuries. *J Trauma;* 64(Suppl 3):239–251.

[17] **Beardmore AA, Brooks DE, Wenke JC, et al** (2005) Effectiveness of local antibiotic delivery with an osteoinductive and osteoconductive bone-graft substitute. *J Bone Joint Surg Am;* 87(1):107–112.

[18] **Thomas DB, Brooks DE, Bice TG, et al** (2005) Tobramycin-impregnated calcium sulfate prevents infection in contaminated wounds. *Clin Orthop Relat Res;* 441:366–371.

[19] **Chang W, Colangeli M, Colangeli S, et al** (2007) Adult osteomyelitis: debridement versus debridement plus Osteoset T pellets. *Acta Orthop Belg;* 73(2):238–243.

[20] **Morykwas MJ, Argenta LC, Shelton-Brown EI, et al** (1997) Vacuum-assisted closure: a new method for wound control and treatment: animal studies and basic foundation. *Ann Plast Surg;* 38(6):553–562.

[21] **Fleischmann W, Strecker W, Bombelli M, et al** (1993) [Vacuum sealing as treatment of soft tissue damage in open fractures]. *Unfallchirurg;* 96(9):488–492. German.

[22] **Morykwac MJ, Argenta LC** (1997) Non-surgical modalities to enhance healing and care of soft tissue wounds. *J South Orthop Assoc;* 6(4):279–288.

[23] **Timmers MS, Le Cessie S, Banwell P, et al** (2005) The effects of varying degrees of pressure delivered by negative-pressure wound therapy on skin perfusion. *Ann Plast Surg;* 55(6):665–671.

[24] **Wackenfors A, Sjögren J, Gustafsson R, et al** (2004) Effects of vacuum-assisted closure therapy on inguinal wound edge microvascular blood flow. *Wound Repair Regen;* 12(6):600–606.

[25] **Lindstedt S, Malmsjö M, Ingemansson R** (2007) Blood flow changes in normal and ischemic myocardium during topically applied negative pressure. *Ann Thorac Surg;* 84(2):568–573.

[26] **Banwell PE, Téot L** (2003) Topical negative pressure (TNP): the evolution of a novel wound therapy. *Journal of Wound Care;* 12(1):22-28.

[27] **Herscovici D Jr, Sanders RW, Scaduto JM, et al** (2003) Vacuum-assisted wound closure (VAC therapy) for the management of patients with high-energy soft tissue injuries. *J Orthop Trauma;* 17(10):683–688.

[28] **Dedmond BT, Kortesis B, Punger K, et al** (2007) The use of negative-pressure wound therapy (NPWT) in the temporary treatment of soft-tissue injuries associated with high-energy open tibial shaft fractures. *J Orthop Trauma;* 21(1):11–17.

[29] **Leininger BE, Rasmussen TE, Smith DL, et al** (2006) Experience with wound VAC and delayed primary closure of contaminated soft tissue injuries in Iraq. *J Trauma;* 61(5):1207–1211.

[30] **Stannard JP, Volgas DA, Stewart R, et al** (2009) Negative pressure wound therapy after severe open fractures: a prospective randomized study. *J Orthop Trauma;* 23(8):552–557.

[31] **Parrett BM, Matros E, Pribaz JJ, et al** (2006) Lower extremity trauma: trends in the management of soft-tissue reconstruction of open tibia-fibula fractures. *Plast Reconstr Surg;* 117(4):1315–1322; discussion 1323–1324.

[32] **Llanos S, Danilla S, Barraza C, et al** (2006) Effectiveness of negative pressure closure in the integration of split thickness skin grafts: a randomized, double-masked, controlled trial. *Ann Surg;* 244(5):700–705.

[33] **Kim EK, Hong JP** (2007) Efficacy of negative pressure therapy to enhance take of 1-stage allodermis and a split-thickness graft. *Ann Plast Surg;* 50(5):536–540.

[34] **Molan PC** (1999) The role of honey in the management of wounds. *J Wound Care;* 8(8):415–418.

[35] **Chirife J, Herszage L, Joseph A, et al** (1983) In vitro study of bacterial growth inhibition in concentrated sugar solutions: microbiological basis for the use of sugar in treating infected wounds. *Antimicrob Agents Chemother;* 23(5):766–773.

[36] **White JW, Subers MH, Schepartz AI** (1963) The identification of inhibine, the antibacterial factor in honey, as hydrogen peroxide and its origin in a honey glucose-oxidase system. *Biochim Biophys Acta;* 73:57–70.

[37] **Hyslop PA, Hinshaw DB, Scraufstatter IU, et al** (1995) Hydrogen peroxide as a potent bacteriostatic antibiotic: implications for host defense. *Free Radic Biol Med;* 19(1):31–37.

[38] **Allen KL, Molan PC, Reid GM** (1991) A survey of the antibacterial activity of some New Zealand honeys. *J Pharm Pharmacol;* 43(12):817–822.

[39] **Tonks A, Cooper RA, Price AJ, et al** (2001) Stimulation of TNF-alpha release in monocytes by honey. *Cytokine;* 14(4):240–242.

[40] **Ryan GB, Majno G** (1977) Inflammation. A scope. Klamazoo, MI: The Upjohn Co.

[41] **Kiistala R, Hannuksela M, Makinen-Kiljunen S, et al** (1995) Honey allergy is rare in patients sensitive to pollens. *Allergy;* 50(10):844–847.

[42] **Mphande AN, Killowe C, Phalira S, et al** (2007) Effects of honey and sugar dressings on wound healing. *J Wound Care;* 16(7):317–319.

[43] **Thomas S, Jones M** (1998) The use of larval therapy in wound management. *J Wound Care;* 7(10):521–524.

[44] **Reames MK, Christensen C, Luce EA** (1988): The use of maggots in wound debridement. *Ann Plast Surg;* 21(4):388–391.

[45] **Pavillard ER, Wright EA** (1957) An antibiotic from maggots. *Nature;* 180(4592):916–917.

[46] **Sherman RA, Pechter EA** (1988) Maggot therapy: a review of the therapeutic applications of fly larvae in human medicine, especially for treating osteomyelitis. *Med Vet Entomol;* 2(3):225–230.

10

Wound closure and coverage techniques

10.1 Primary and secondary wound closure

Authors   Robert D Teasdall, James Long

10.1.1   Introduction

Wound closure is one of the more challenging aspects in trauma care. In general, the goal of treatment is to obtain a clean, closed wound involving as little time and the least possible physical and emotional commitment for the patient. It is important to remember that no method of wound closure or treatment is able to guarantee success and other options may have to be implemented should initial attempts fail. The advantage of primary or early wound closure is not only a psychological benefit, but also shortens the wound-healing process and thus also helps to spare health-care costs.

Wound healing occurs in three phases: inflammatory, proliferative, and remodeling and maturation (chapter 4). The inflammatory and proliferative phases of wound healing are considerably shortened if primary or early closure of clean wounds is obtained. This saves significant metabolic energy, causes less pain, and improves overall medical rehabilitation.

10.1.2   Primary closure

Indications

Once the wound has been debrided and irrigated, the physician must determine whether it is amenable to closure based on the time since injury, location, availability of tissue for a tension-free suture as well as the level of contamination. The decision in favor of closing the skin or of open wound management depends on the likely success of primary closure, which in turn heavily depends on the surgeon's experience. Failure of primary closure can lead to even more

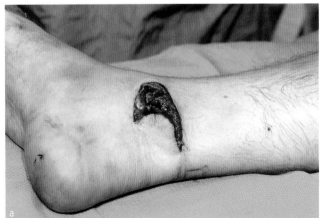

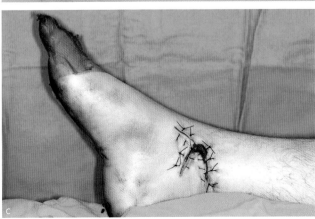

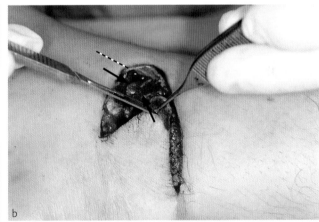

Fig 10.1-1a–c   Clinical photographs of an open wound on the ankle.
a   The cutaneous injury is not associated with a fracture.
b   The wound underwent debridement of the skin edges. An incision (dotted line) will be placed to allow closure of the wound (arrows).
c   Primary closure using Donati sutures. Note that the knots lie outside the flap.

damage and a worse outcome than open-wound care with delayed or secondary wound closure.

While in general, surgical incisions should always be closed primarily, this does not apply to all wounds not associated with a fracture, although many of them may also be closed primarily (**Fig 10.1-1a–c**). In the past, surgeons have been taught to leave wounds associated with internally fixed fractures open at the time of the first debridement and irrigation. Many surgeons today believe that wounds of open fractures—up to Gustilo type IIIA fracture—may be closed primarily, which is, however, still controversial [1, 2]. Absolute indications and contraindications to primary wound closure are shown in **Table 10.1-1**. Relative contraindications to primary closure include human and animal bites—with the exception of facial bites—and the presence of foreign material.

Absolute contraindications	Relative contraindications
Heavily contaminated wounds (stagnant water, farmyard, etc)	Wounds older than ~12 hours
Large soft-tissue defects (high-energy weapons, shotgun)	Animal or human bites (except facial bites)
Closure requiring excessive tension	Underlying fractures (controversial)
Puncture wounds	Acute fasciotomy wounds

Table 10.1-1 Absolute and relative contraindications for primary wound closure.

A common scenario is to extend the traumatic wound in order to provide better exposure for the debridement of recesses and the removal of debris, but also for the insertion of implants. In such cases the clean surgical extension may be closed primarily, while the traumatic portion of the wound is often left open for secondary closure.

Systemic factors and associated conditions must also be taken into consideration when deciding whether to close a wound primarily or not (chapter 4.4). These include:
- history and mechanism of injury
- associated injuries
- patient age
- vascular status and/or diabetes mellitus
- immune function
- coagulation status.

Questionable viability of adjacent tissues including compartment syndrome should preclude primary closure. This is an important consideration in:
- crush or missile injuries
- thermal burns
- electrical injury.

In each of these situations there frequently is an extensive zone of injury beyond the central area of nonviable tissue, and a zone of questionable tissue viability in between (chapter 3, 10.3.3). As a result, in many injuries with underlying muscle damage, serial debridements may be necessary before the extent of the lesion is fully demarked and wound closure can be considered. The degree of contamination, either based on history, mechanism of trauma or examination, is another important variable to assess.

Too much tension on the wound edges is the greatest enemy of primary wound closure. If in doubt, it is often better to leave the wound open and only close it secondarily. A good measure to judge the tension of skin edges is impaired vascular perfusion or lack of capillary refill when tying the sutures, as may best be seen when the skin appears blanched between stitches. Approximation of the subcutaneous fascia (superficial fascia of the fat) may be helpful in order to reduce the tension of a primary skin suture, but depending on the trauma mechanism (eg, avulsion injury) or the region of the body (eg, lower leg) this is not always possible.

Timing

An important factor to include in the decision for primary closure is the time interval since the injury. In general, the likelihood of infection rises with the length of time the wound is left without debridement. Most surgeons believe that wound debridement and irrigation should occur within 6–8 hours, although some would consider 12 hours to be acceptable. The more heavily contaminated the wound, the more important a shorter time to debridement (chapter 7.1) becomes.

Some surgeons believe that no open fracture wound should be closed primarily, but among those who do close open fractures primarily, debridement within the above guidelines is a prerequisite.

Characteristics of suture materials

There are numerous suture materials available for wound closure. These sutures possess many characteristics, among which size, configuration and resorbability are the most important. Size denotes the diameter of the suture material. The accepted surgical practice is to use the smallest diameter suture that will adequately hold the mending wounded tissue. This practice minimizes trauma while the suture is passed through the tissue to effect closure. It also ensures that the minimum mass of foreign material is left in the body. Suture size is stated numerically; as the number preceding the zero in the suture size increases, the diameter of the strand decreases, eg, 4-0 is much smaller than 1-0 or even 1.

Sutures may generally be classified according to the number of strands of which they consist. Monofilament sutures are made of a single strand of material. Because of their simplified structure, they encounter less resistance as they pass through tissues than multifilament suture material consisting of several twisted or braided strands. Although multifilament strands possess greater tensile strength, pliability, and flexibility, the multitude of filaments of braided sutures may more easily harbor organisms that may cause infection. Sutures may also be classified according to their degradation properties. Sutures that undergo degradation and resorption in tissues are considered resorbable sutures. Sutures that generally maintain their tensile strength and are resistant to resorption are nonresorbable sutures.

As a general rule, resorbable sutures are used for closure of fascial layers, subcutaneous tissue (ie, the approximation of the superficial fascia of the fat), and joint capsules. Nonresorbable sutures are typically used for skin and tendon repair. Synthetic suture materials are resorbed by hydrolysis. Natural suture materials, such as catgut, are resorbed by proteolysis. Monofilament sutures cause less tissue damage. They also resist infection better than braided suture. However, monofilament sutures do not hold a knot as well as braided suture.

Table 10.1-2 shows representative suture types and their characteristics. Needles should be chosen based on the tissue, which is being sutured. Tapered needles are used for easily penetrated tissues, whereas cutting or reverse-cutting needles are used for skin or heavy fascia.

Material	Source	Type	Coating (if applicable)	Retention profile or tensile strength	Absorption time	Absorption process
Catgut (sheep submucosa)	Natural	Monofilament	n/a	100% at 7–10 days	~70 days	Proteolytic, enzymatic digestion
Polyglactin (eg, Vicryl®, Vicryl rapide®, Vicryl plus®)	Synthetic	Braided	Polyglactin 370 Calcium Sterate	50% at 5 days 0% at 10–14 days	42 days	Hydrolysis
			Polyglactin 370 Calcium Sterate	75% at 14 days 50% at 21 days 25% at 28 days	56–70 days	Hydrolysis
			Polyglactin 370 IRGACARE MP** (triclosan)	75% at 14 days 50% at 21 days 25% at 28 days	56–70 days	Hydrolysis
Poliglecaprone (eg, Monocryl®)		Monofilament	n/a	60–70% at 7 days 30–40% at 14 days	91–119 days	Hydrolysis
Polydioxanone (PDS)			n/a	70% at 14 days 50% at 28 days 25% at 42 days	180–210 days	Slow hydrolysis
Nylon			n/a	20% loss per year	Nonresorbable	n/a
Polypropylene (Prolen®)			n/a	Indefinite	Nonresorbable	n/a

Table 10.1-2 Suture materials and their characteristics. Table modified according to Ethican Products Worldwide a Johnson & Johnson Company, GA, USA.
**Trademark of Ciba Specialty Chemicals Corp.

Suture techniques

Wounds are closed in layers, from deep to superficial. Sutures (**Video 10.1-1a–h**) are used to close dead space in a wound and to close the skin. Joint capsules and fascia are usually closed using a simple interrupted suture (**Fig 10.1-2**), figure-of-eight suture (**Fig 10.1-3**) or a running suture (**Fig 10.1-4**). Both fascia and joint capsules should be closed to form a water-tight layer in order to prevent bacteria from gaining access to underlying joints. Tendons may be sutured using a number of different techniques, such as a modified Krakow, Bunnell or any of a myriad of specialty-specific sutures. These sutures have been adequately described in numerous textbooks or specialized manuals and do not need repeating here. Furthermore, there is no set rule that postulates: this layer needs this specific suture technique and this specific suture material. Often, suture techniques and suture material go with the personal preference and experience of the surgeon.

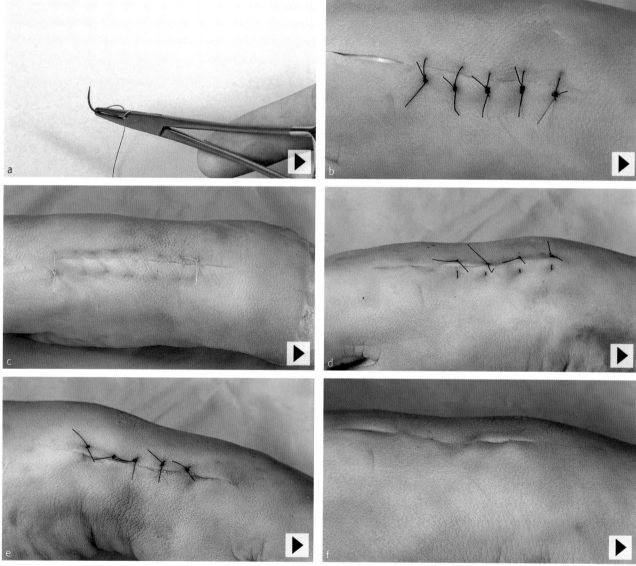

Video 10.1-1a–h   Suture techniques shown on a porcine foot.
a   General handling of instruments.
b   Simple, interrupted suture technique.
c   Simple, running suture technique.
d   Vertical mattress (Donati) suture technique, interrupted and running.
e   Allgöwer-Donati suture technique, interrupted and running.
f   Simple, buried, interrupted suture technique.

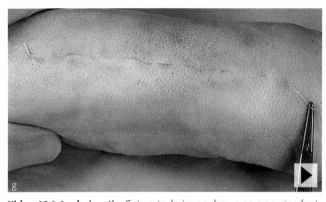 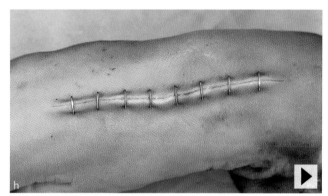

Video 10.1-1a–h (cont) Suture techniques shown on a porcine foot.
g Intradermal, running suture technique.
h Skin closure with staples.

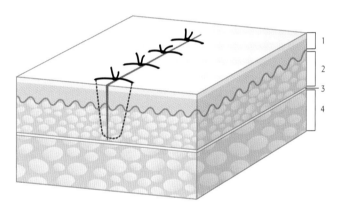

Fig 10.1-2 Simple, interrupted suture technique. The standard wound closure.
1 Epidermis and dermis.
2 Superficial fat compartment.
3 Superficial fascia of the fat (hypodermis/subcutaneous tissue).
4 Deep fat compartment.

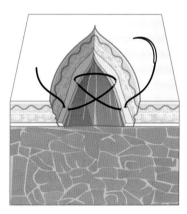

Fig 10.1-3 Figure-of-eight suture technique. This is often used in closure of heavy tissue such as fascia or joint capsules.

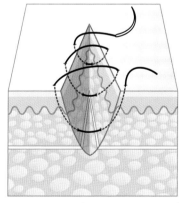

Fig 10.1-4 Simple, running suture technique.

The goal of all these different techniques of suturing the skin is to provide a mechanical closure of the wound without putting too much tension on the wound edges, allowing for uneventful reepithelialization within 24 hours. Excessive tension at the skin edges can compromise local blood supply as well as the healing process, but placing too many sutures may also result in local hypoxia and hence compromise vascularity, making wound closure a balancing act. While appropriate tension on the skin is difficult to judge clinically, signs that there is too much tension on the skin include blanching of the skin between sutures due to a lack of capillary refill, indentation of the suture into the skin, and loosening of the suture. Keep in mind that edema is common after injury or surgery, so the degree of tension on the skin will often increase during the first few days after closure. This should be anticipated when closing a wound. Soft-

tissue edema and contamination of the wound are two major reasons not to use running sutures for skin closure, but rather interrupted sutures. The latter allows to selectively remove some sutures in case of undue tension, hematoma or seroma formation and/or local inflammation and infection, respectively.

Techniques which reduce strain on the dermis without further damaging the blood supply to the skin involve separate closure of deep layers, such as muscle fascia and subcutaneous fascia (ie, superficial fascia of the fat), the use of horizontal (**Fig 10.1-5**) or vertical mattress (Donati) suture (**Fig 10.1-6**), and the careful placement of an appropriate number of stitches. A simple buried suture (**Fig 10.1-7a–b**) may be used for the fascia within the subcutaneous tissue or the dermis.

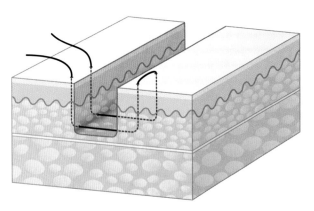

Fig 10.1-5 The horizontal mattress suture technique may be used cautiously in thick skin, which is not in danger of being closed under too much tension, such as that of the thigh or back. Care must be taken to avoid over-tightening these sutures.

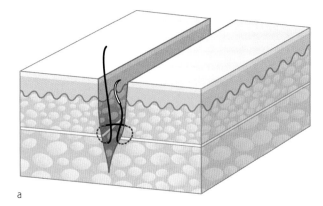

a

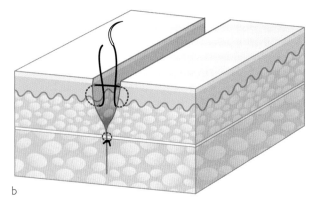

b

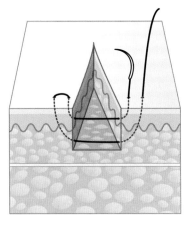

Fig 10.1-6 The vertical mattress (Donati) suture technique is often used to reapproximate thick subcutaneous tissue, with the knots buried. The technique may also be used to reapproximate the skin, as shown here.

Fig 10.1-7a–b Simple, buried suture technique, which can be used in different layers.

a   Reapproximation of the subcutaneous fascia of the fat. This suture may be performed by placing the knot upside down. Note that the fat itself is not sutured.

b   Reapproximation of the dermis. This suture is usually applied by placing the knot upside down.

Cutaneous edges may be closed in many ways. The strongest is closure of the deep dermis with a figure-of-eight suture using a resorbable suture (ie, polyglycolic acid) followed by closure of the dermis with intradermal suture (**Fig 10.1-8**). The least amount of observable scar is created with a running, nonresorbable, intradermal suture with the least inflammatory response (ie, polypropylene) (**Fig. 10.1-8**). However, this suture does require removal. It is usually recommended to remove the sutures from extremities within 10–14 days. In doubtful cases or specific regions such as the thigh or the calcaneus, removal after 3 weeks is reasonable. A resorbable intradermal suture (ie, poliglecaprone 25) can be used, but involves a prolonged inflammatory phase during suture degradation.

Instead of using Donati-type mattress suture, Allgöwer described a modification called the Allgöwer-Donati suture (**Fig 10.1-9**), where the opposite skin edge is caught and ex-

ited within the dermis. This technique with 3-0 or 4-0 nonresorbable suture material allows to approximate the skin edges at equal level without eversion or bulging, which cosmetically leaves almost invisible scars. The skin edge with the more problematic vascular supply, eg, the side of a flap and not the side of the local skin, is chosen for the intradermal part of the backstitch in order to have the knot lying on the well-perfused side of the wound.

In wounds forming angles—particularly if there is a T-shape—a corner suture (**Fig 10.1-10**) may be used. A special suture called an over-and–under or far-near-near-far suture (**Fig 10.1-11**) may be used as a retention suture whenever temporary swelling precludes primary closure. Such sutures must be used with care, since they may exert a tremendous amount of tension on the skin. If swelling does not abate quickly, they may even lead to tissue necrosis. At corners or apices of flaps, it is important to avoid placing sutures,

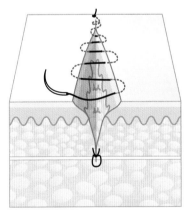

Fig 10.1-8 The intradermal running suture technique is applied whenever cosmesis is important. Tension on the suture from below is avoided by separately closing the subcutaneous tissue first at fascia level (as shown here), or at a dermal level.

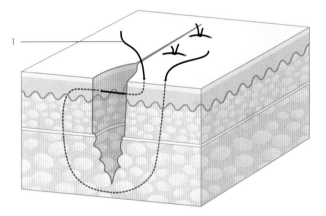

Fig 10.1-9 Allgöwer-Donati suture technique. Note that the far limb of the suture (1) remains within the dermal layer.

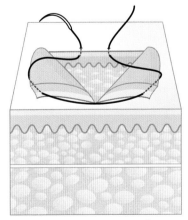

Fig 10.1-10 Corner suture technique.

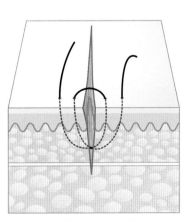

Fig 10.1-11 Far-near-near-far suture technique.

particularly the ones that are on a dermal level, so as not to compromise perfusion. Rather place single sutures at an adequate distance from the corner or apex of the flap. Fine approximation of the corner or apex can be performed with single knots using thin suture material or Steri-Strip™.

Staples, although popular and frequently used, are not considered first choice, if cosmetically nice-looking scars are expected. Their application is quick, but not very precise and removal must occur within a few days in order to avoid a stepladder pattern, which may cause secondary widening or dehiscence of the skin, resulting in ugly scarring.

Small, clean, simple lacerations with minimal retraction may be managed with noninvasive techniques, including suture strips (ie, Steri-Strip™, 3M™, St. Paul MN, USA), mesh and/ or cutaneous adhesives, (ie, Prineo®, Dermabond®, Johnson & Johnson Medical Ltd., New Brunswick, NY, USA).

When primary closure is not immediately possible, delayed primary closure may be considered. The wound may be conditioned for closure with a synthetic-skin substitute (eg, Epigard®, Pfizer, New York, NY, USA), which is applied to the wound initially, then removed after swelling abates and primary closure is made.

10.1.3   Secondary closure

Conditions exist, in which primary or delayed primary closure is not a viable option. Frequently, it will not be possible for fasciotomy wounds or traumatic wounds accompanied by marked swelling to be closed initially or even within 48 hours. However, several methods are available by which an acceptable, though less than perfect, closure may be obtained. Often, large surgical vessel loops fastened by staples (**Fig 10.1-12a–h**) (chapter 12.3) may be used to reapproximate wound edges that are subject to rapidly decreasing edema. When used in fasciotomy wounds, the size of a required skin graft may be markedly reduced or the skin graft may not even be needed.

Should primary closure result in wound dehiscence, and excessive tension prevent another attempt at wound closure, wound edges will be debrided and the wound may be left to heal by secondary intention, ie, by granulation tissue and reepithelialization. This may be hastened by:
- negative-pressure wound therapy
- elevation of the extremity to minimize swelling
- application of pumps such as the A-V Impulse System (Novamedix Services Limited, Andover, Hampshire, UK).

The disadvantages of secondary closure are:
- prolonged length of time for closure (up to several weeks)
- risk of infection
- much larger scar
- necessity for continued wound care while handling.

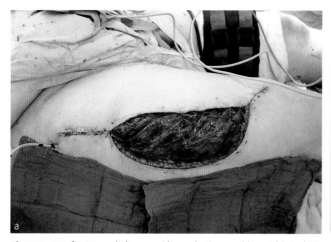 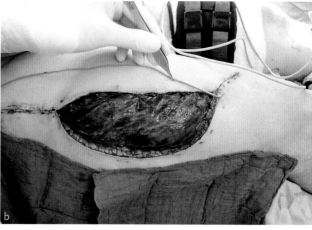

Fig 10.1-12a–h   Wound closure with an elastic vessel loop. This technique is used to reapproximate wound edges in wounds that show excessive swelling and no substantial skin loss. The large elastic vessel loop is stapled to the wound edges in a shoelace fashion. By providing gentle traction while swelling decreases, this method can help close above described wounds within a few days.
a   Surgical wound after elevation of a lateral thigh flap. Proximally and distally, the wound has been closed primarily.
b   The end of the vessel loop is knotted and stapled onto the skin.

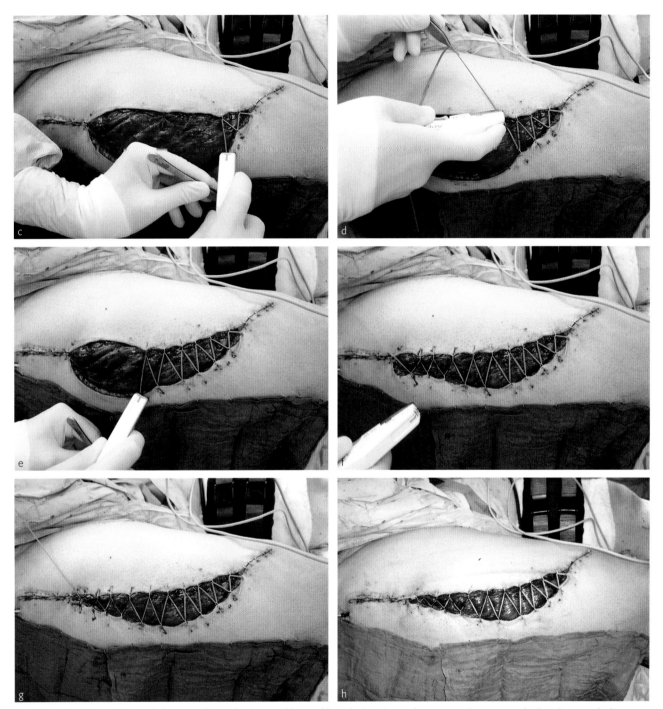

Fig 10.1-12a–h (cont) Wound closure with an elastic vessel loop. This technique is used to reapproximate wound edges in wounds that show excessive swelling and no substantial skin loss. The large elastic vessel loop is stapled to the wound edges in a shoelace fashion. By providing gentle traction while swelling decreases, this method can help close above described wounds within a few days.

c–g Alternating sides, the elastic vessel loop is now placed and stapled in a zigzag manner across the wound. Despite being held in place by staples, the elastic vessel loop can still slide through the eyelets created by the staples.

h Having applied the last staple, the elastic vessel loop is fixed by tying the end into a knot that prevents the loop from slipping through the last staple. There is the possibility of tightening these "shoelaces" every other day to further approximate the wound edges.

10.2 Skin grafts and substitutes—principles

Authors Lars Steinsträßer, Sammy Al-Benna

10.2.1 Introduction

Skin is composed of three layers: epidermis, dermis, and subcutaneous tissue (chapter 2.1, 4.1). The epidermis has a superficial layer mainly consisting of epithelial cells, ie, keratinocytes, whereas the basal or deepest epidermal cells are anchored to the underlying basal membrane. These germinal epithelial cells divide continuously and migrate toward the outermost layer to replace cells, which are lost to wear and tear. As the cells migrate, they form keratin that becomes an effective barrier to environmental hazards, such as mechanical stress, excessive water evaporation, and infection. The dermis comprises 90% of the two outermost parts of the skin and is a dynamic layer of connective tissue. The dermis is formed by the superficial papillary layer, which contains the anchoring rete pegs, and the deeper reticular layer. The fibroblast is the predominant cell type of the dermis. It produces key structural extracellular matrix proteins and collagen. The dermis contains skin appendicular structures such as sebaceous and sweat glands. Hair follicles within the dermis and lined by epithelium provide a source for epithelial cell regeneration in case of partial-thickness wounds.

Skin grafts are completely separated from their blood supply and donor-site attachments before being grafted to another area of the body, ie, to the recipient site. Skin grafted from one area of the body to another on the same individual is termed an autograft. Skin grafted between two individuals of the same species but of disparate genotypes is termed an allograft (homograft), whereas skin grafted between two different species is termed a xenograft. Skin grafting is a surgical procedure, in which skin or a skin substitute is used to reconstruct a wound defect in order to restore function of the skin (chapter 2.1). It is indicated in wounds caused by soft-tissue trauma or surgical excision, where primary closure is not an option or a flap is not necessary. Skin grafts are easy to harvest with minimal additional time for surgery and postoperative hospital stay, and, if correctly used, may offer acceptable functional and cosmetic outcome.

Skin grafts are indicated for any soft-tissue defect too large for direct closure or in case of spontaneous wound contracture that has a viable wound bed (eg, granulation tissue, muscle, fascia, peritenon, adventitia), which will generate blood supply for a graft. Granulation tissue is characterized by well-vascularized, fibrous connective tissue replacing a fibrin clot (chapter 4.1). As a general rule, any wound or defect that forms granulation tissue will support a skin graft. Wounds that will not develop granulation tissue, or show exposed bare bone and tendons, cartilage or implant material (eg, plates, nails, prosthesis) or a nylon mesh will not be able to accept a skin graft and will need an alternative surgical treatment for closure such as the transfer of vascularized tissue, ie, a flap (chapter 10.3 to 10.6).

The application of a skin graft depends on many criteria such as general and local status of the patient, site and size of the wound as well as functional and cosmetic concerns.

10.2.2 Engraftment

Skin-replacement surgery is usually performed in two steps. The first step includes the surgical excision of any grossly contaminated or necrotic tissue, resulting in a clean surgical wound. The second step consists of the application of a skin graft to the well-vascularized and clean wound bed. Engraftment or graft take is known as the integration of grafted tissue into the host's tissues. Engraftment of an autograft or allograft results in creating new vascular connections, with cellular and extracellular matrix remodeling the dermis. Only autografts can remain engrafted permanently, whereas allografts and xenografts are only temporarily accepted and will eventually be rejected. Engraftment results in healing by first intention, in which the lost skin is permanently replaced by healthy skin with normal tissue architecture of both epidermis and dermis (chapter 4.1). Skin grafts adhere and take in four distinct phases:
1. fibrin adherence
2. serum imbibition
3. inosculation
4. revascularization.

Phase of fibrin adherence

Fibrin exudation as part of the normal process of hemostasis allows initial adherence of the skin graft to its recipient bed. Within 48 hours, the fibrin starts to break down. Adhesion of the graft to the bed is then maintained by the proliferation of fibroblasts and deposition of collagen to replace the fibrin. The strength of this attachment increases rapidly, with firm anchoring within 4 days, which allows the graft to be handled safely if reasonable care is taken.

Phase of serum imbibition

Serum imbibition or fluid absorption occurs during the first 4 days after application and will be observed as swelling of the graft. The nutritive value of serum imbibition in maintaining graft viability is debated.

Phase of inosculation

The term inosculation describes the development of direct anastomosis between preexisting vessels within the graft and newly formed vessels from the granulation tissue of the recipient.

Phase of revascularization

Revascularization by vessel ingrowth into the graft starts after ~4 days. The underlying mechanism, however, is not exactly known and may comprise three different steps:

- **Inosculation:** an anastomosis between preexisting vessels within the graft and newly formed vessels within the wound bed
- **Revascularization:** ingrowth of newly formed microvessels from the recipient site into the vascular channels of the graft
- **Neovascularization:** New blood vessels develop as solid sprouts from the recipient bed across the fibrin layer and penetrate into the graft along the preexisting vascular structure of the graft. These solid sprouts of vascular endothelium are subsequently opened up, thereby initiating graft perfusion.

A pink, well-adhering graft is the most important clinical sign of successful revascularization and healing of the graft. Thereafter, the final process of graft remodeling to the histological architecture of normal skin sets in.

10.2.3 Split-thickness skin grafts

Definition

Split-thickness skin grafts (STSGs) are composed of epidermis, including the basal membrane, and a variable thickness of dermis. Split-thickness skin grafts may be subdivided into:

- thin (0.008–0.012 mm)
- medium (0.012–0.018 mm) and
- thick (0.018–0.030 mm) grafts.

Indications and advantages

Split-thickness skin grafts are most commonly used when the defect needing to be covered is of substantial size, precluding the use of a full-thickness skin graft, or whenever cosmetic concerns are not essential (chapter 12.5). Split-thickness skin grafts will tolerate less ideal conditions for survival in comparison to full-thickness skin grafts and offer a wide range of application, such as the coverage of large wounds (including lining of cavities), resurfacing of soft-tissue defects, coverage of muscle flaps (**Fig 10.2-1**), or closure of flap donor sites. The donor sites of split-thickness skin grafts heal spontaneously within 7–14 days from epithelial remnants within hair follicles and other epidermal appendices. Donor sites usually allow for reharvesting once healing is complete. However, with each increase in thickness of the graft, healing time will be prolonged.

Disadvantages

Split-thickness skin grafts are rather vulnerable, especially when applied over areas with little underlying soft-tissue bulk for support. They have a tendency to contract (chapter 11.3) during healing and they cannot grow along with the host tissues. They appear to be smoother and shinier than normal skin because the appendices of normal skin are missing. They often show inhomogeneous pigmentation, ie, hypo- or hyperpigmentation, particularly in darker-skinned individuals. The thinness, smooth texture, and lack of hair growth render these grafts rather more functional than cosmetically attractive. Accordingly, when used to cover large wounds such as after large surface abrasion, skin loss due to degloving or burns, split-thickness skin grafts may produce an undesirable mask-like appearance. Last but not least, the wound created at the donor site is often more painful than the recipient site and may result in permanent hypopigmentation (**Table 10.2-1**).

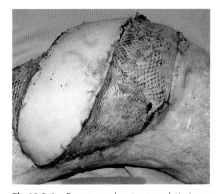

Fig 10.2-1 Free musculocutaneous latissimus dorsi flap that covers an anterior defect at the knee joint. The elliptical skin island allows better tissue match and serves for monitoring of the flap's perfusion (ie, viability, monitoring island). The rest of the latissimus dorsi muscle is covered with split-thickness skin grafts.

Parameter	Split-thickness skin graft (STSG)	Full-thickness skin graft (FTSG)
Structure	Full epidermis and variable part of the dermis	Full epidermis and dermis
Hair-growth	No	Yes
Indication	Temporarily or permanent, large surfaces	Esthetic outcome important, flap is not an option, restricted to small surfaces
Graft survival rate	↑	↓
Graft robustness	↓	↑
Contraction rate	↑	↓
Aesthetic appearance	Rather poor (color and texture mismatch)	Rather good
Common donor site	Circumference of the thigh and arm, medial aspect of the forearm, abdomen, back, buttock, scalp (especially in children)	Post- and preauricular, supraclavicular region, lateral groin crease, suprapubic area and inner surface of the arm
Availability of the donor site	Due to spontaneous healing, donor site can serve repetitively within ~14 days	Limited amount of available tissue

Table 10.2-1 Comparison of split-thickness and full-thickness skin grafts.

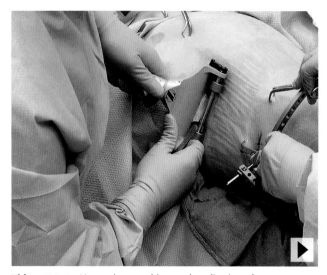

Video 10.2-1 Harvesting, meshing, and application of a split-thickness skin graft.

Contraindications

The use of split-thickness skin grafts is not indicated wherever significant wound contraction may compromise function or where mechanical resistance and cosmetic outcome are essential. Poor color and texture match as well as lack of adnexal structures contribute to the more marked "hodgepodge" appearance in comparison to full-thickness skin grafts. If the original soft-tissue defect is small, healing by secondary intention (chapter 4.1) may result in a better cosmetic outcome in comparison to reconstruction with split-thickness skin grafts. In addition, granulation tissue that develops during healing by secondary intention compensates for significant discrepancies of wound depth by "filling it up" to the level of the surrounding normal skin prior to split-thickness skin-graft application.

Technique (Video 10.2-1)

It is advisable not to prepare the donor site with Betadine®, as this tends to cause the dermatome to stick and not glide smoothly along the skin. Prior to harvesting the split-thickness skin graft, the dimensions of the recipient site are measured. A dermatome is usually used to harvest the skin graft. There are various types of dermatomes, but most involve a blade, which is mounted to the dermatome and a blade guard, which determines the width of the harvested skin. If the graft is to be meshed, the width of the graft may be adjusted by the mesh ratio. For instance, if a defect measures 3 inches (7.6 cm), a 2 inch (5.1 cm) graft may be harvested, if the mesh ratio is 1:1.5. Care should be taken to select the appropriate harvest depth. For medium thickness grafts, a #15 blade may be used to confirm the correct depth of the blade. The donor site should be selected based on several factors:

- how much graft will be required
- condition of the donor skin
- surgical convenience
- cosmetic concerns.

Skin grafts are usually harvested from areas of the body that can easily be covered by clothes such as the thigh, upper arm, back, abdomen, buttock, etc. The donor site should be free of any severe abrasions or scars.

Injecting saline solution subcutaneously at the donor site may facilitate harvesting of the graft because of the smelling of the skin. Alternatively, saline solution may be mixed with lidocaine and epinephrine in order to reduce postoperative pain respectively bleeding at the donor site. The donor site should also be prepared by applying mineral oil, ChloraPrep®

or other viscous liquid to lubricate the skin and prevent skipping of the dermatome while harvesting the graft. Tension should be applied longitudinally along the skin with a tongue blade or sharp towel clips in order to flatten the donor surface as much as possible. When properly harvested, there should be uniform punctate bleeding from the donor site (**Fig 10.2-2**).

The skin graft is then passed through a mesher to increase its surface (**Fig 10.2-3**) and then secured over the recipient site as described below (chapter 10.2.7).

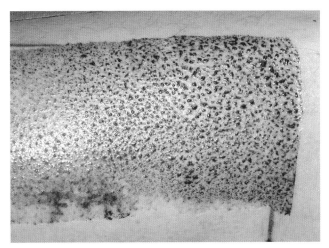

Fig 10.2-2   After correct harvesting of a split-thickness skin graft, the donor site will show evenly spread punctate bleeding, ie, decapilated papillae of the dermis.

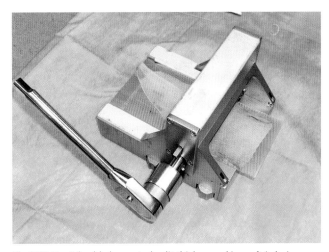

Fig 10.2-3   A freshly harvested split-thickness skin graft is being passed through a mesher in order to produce the correct-sized meshed graft necessary to fit the wound perfectly.

10.2.4   Full-thickness skin grafts

Definition
Full-thickness skin grafts (FTSGs) are composed of epidermis and the entire dermis. They are usually harvested from areas with sufficient laxity to permit direct closure of the donor site. The thicker the dermis, the better the nature of normal skin will be achieved after grafting. This is due to the increased collagen content and the higher number of dermal vascular plexuses and epidermal appendices contained within the dermis of thicker grafts.

Indications and advantages
The use of full-thickness skin grafts is indicated in defects, in which the adjacent tissues are rather immobile or scarce. Full-thickness skin grafts are ideal for exposed areas of the face that are not suitable or accessible to local flaps. Specific locations that lend themselves well to full-thickness skin grafts in the face are:
- nasal tip
- eyelids
- forehead
- ears.

This also applies to digits and toes, but less to other regions of the extremities. Full-thickness skin grafts retain more of the characteristics of normal skin including color, texture and thickness in comparison to split-thickness skin grafts. Full-thickness skin grafts also undergo less contraction while healing. This is important in the face as well as on the hand or over other mobile joint surfaces. Full-thickness skin grafts in children are more likely to grow along with the individual. Common donor sites for the reconstruction of full-thickness defects in hands or feet are the lateral groin crease, the suprapubic area or the inner surface of the arm. For the use in head and neck reconstructions, the usual donor sites are the post- and preauricular as well as the supraclavicular region.

Disadvantages
The application of full-thickness skin grafts is limited to relatively small, uncontaminated, well-vascularized wounds and, thus, they do not have as wide a range of application as split-thickness skin grafts. Full-thickness skin grafts require more favorable wound bed conditions for engraftment and survival, because of the thicker amount of tissue requiring revascularization. Donor sites must be closed primarily or, more rarely, first resurfaced with a split-thickness graft from another site (**Table 10.2-1**).

Contraindications

The major contraindication to the use of a full-thickness skin graft primarily is size. By necessity, these grafts are limited to 1–2 cm in most cases. Also, the recipient site must be highly vascularized as the entire thickness of the graft must be supported by recipient-site vessels.

Technique

A common method for harvesting a full-thickness skin graft is to perform a "pinch graft". In the forearm, a pinch of skin is elevated from the anterior forearm and a knife is used to circumscribe the base of the elevated skin. This commonly yields a 1–1.5 cm circle of full-thickness skin, which may then be used to cover a defect such as an exposed extensor tendon slip in the digit. The donor site is closed primarily. Any subcutaneous fat should be removed prior to placement of the graft on the recipient site.

10.2.5 Substitutes

Skin autografts are not always available in sufficient quantity for skin replacement surgery, while allografts and xenografts as possible alternatives only have a limited life-span. Unfortunately, skin allografts appear to carry a potential susceptibility for infections by viruses (hepatitis B and C, HIV) or prions. Prions in particular are highly resistant to conventional methods of sterilization and disinfection and have even been shown to survive in cryopreserved and glycerol-preserved tissue. The evidence of these risks is supported by case reports [3]. An engineered tissue or a combination of biomaterials could be an attractive alternative to autografts. Unlike allografts and xenografts, artificial skin replacements are not rejected by the patient's body, which is promising for the new generation of engineered tissue.

Recent progress has been observed in the development of artificial skin replacement products. Although no engineered skin product equals the patient's skin, artificial skin products can provide satisfactory options to overcome the limited availability of skin autografts and allografts in patients with large wound surfaces. Engineered skin is usually composed of a synthetic epidermis and a collagen-based dermis (ie, silicone sheet and monolayer or bilayer bovine collagen matrix: Integra®, Integra Life Sciences Technology, Plainsboro, NJ, USA). The artificial dermis consists of fibers arranged in a mesh that serves as a scaffold for the formation of new tissue. Fibroblasts, blood and lymph vessels as well as nerve fibers originating from the surrounding healthy tissue grow into the collagen scaffold, which is eventually resorbed, as these cells and structures develop a new dermis.

A silicon layer (Integra®) membrane simulating the epidermis acts as a temporary barrier and seals off the surface in order to reduce fluid loss during the process of dermal substitution. This transparent membrane allows for wound inspection and progressively loses adherence to the dermal layer as it is incorporated. After about 2–3 weeks, the silicon layer (Integra®) may be peeled off and replaced with a thin split-thickness skin graft or with a cultured epidermis. Alternative dermal substitutes and artificial skin products with their own specificities are available, including Apligraf®, TransCyte®, MATRIDERM®, and Dermagraft® (**Fig 10.2-4a–f**).

For many years, one of the goals in research has been the engineering of sheets of "skin" originating from cultured epithelial cells. These engineered autografts require skin biopsies of the patient, followed by culturing of the cells in vitro to develop confluent sheets. Presently, the adjunct of stem cells obtained from bone marrow or blood is under clinical evaluation [4]. Hopefully this approach will eventually reduce the need for autografts and decrease the complication rate of severe and large-surface injuries that are common in patients with full-thickness burns of up to 50% of the body surface in comparison to patients with orthopaedic trauma such as extensive degloving [5]. The major disadvantages of this culturing process are related to the high costs and the extreme fragility of the engineered sheets that are very susceptible to infection. However, cultured skin would overcome the delay in patient recovery due to limited availability of uninjured skin for grafting. Therefore, a lot of effort still has to be put into research including wound healing, immunology and molecular biology.

10.2.6 Degloved skin as skin graft

Degloving injuries are part of crush-avulsion trauma and are associated with severe morbidity, possibly even mortality (chapter 3.3). A primary aim, therefore, is to establish skin coverage of the degloved area. If the avulsed skin appears to show dermal bleeding at the wound edges before or after trimming, it is preserved. Sometimes, the fat beneath is also trimmed and the thinned flap repositioned immediately. The absence of dermal bleeding—resulting from disruption of perforating vessels from the degloved skin or inadequate size of the longitudinal vessels supplying the degloved flap— renders spontaneous revascularization, respectively surgical replantation, very difficult. Furthermore, if the avulsed skin flap presents with a very narrow base, survival of the degloved skin is severely jeopardized. Several authors, therefore, advocate the immediate use of obviously degloved skin as a full-thickness skin graft or a split-thickness skin graft

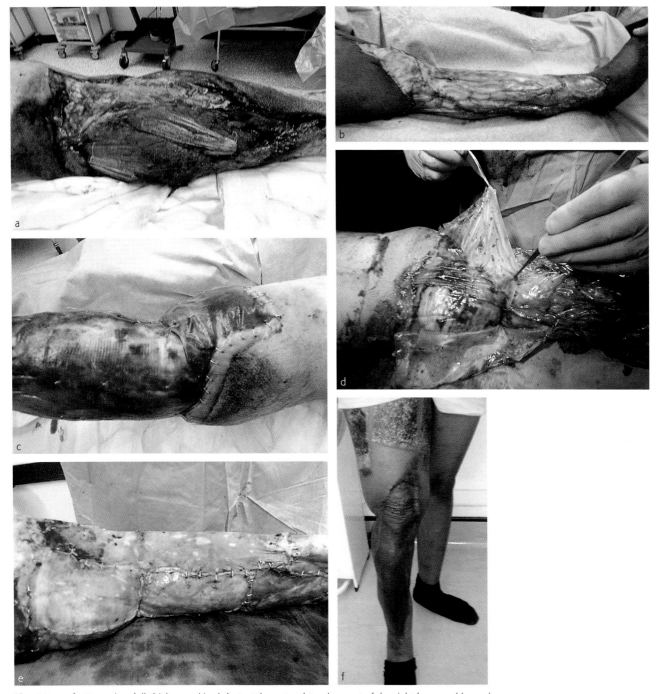

Fig 10.2-4a–f Extensive, full-thickness skin defect at the anterolateral aspect of the right knee and lower leg.
a   Viable muscles after debridement.
b   First dressing 2 days after application of a dermal substitute and a silicon sheet. Note the yellowish color of the substitute.
c   Two weeks after application of the dermal substitute. Note the patch-like appearance but red color of the substitute, indicating vessel ingrowth.
d   Peeling off of the silicon layer from the engrafted dermal substitute.
e   Immediately after application and staple fixation of the split-thickness skin graft.
f   Postoperative view at 6 months. Fully healed split-thickness skin graft. Note the rather "elastic-like" wrinkling of the skin graft over the kneecap and the hyperpigmentation of the skin graft as well as the inhomogenous pigmentation of the donor site at the thigh.

in order to guarantee the most satisfactory coverage of denuded areas (**Fig 10.2-5a–e**) [6–8]. Usually, the grafts are immediately applied as long as the wound bed is vascularized and clean. Otherwise, one option is to store the harvested skin grafts in the refrigerator, packed in sterile gauzes. Once wound conditioning has been achieved, the stored grafts may be applied after 2–5 days.

The harvesting of large, uniform skin grafts from the avulsed skin flap is technically demanding, requiring skin to be resilient. Difficulties that may arise include:

- loss of elastic skin properties due to the avulsion or degloving injury itself
- irregularity of the flap's deep surface, which hinders harvesting of a uniform skin graft due to misalignment, especially if applied tangentially to the Langer lines (chapter 1).

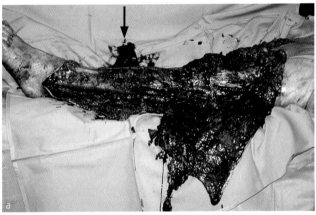
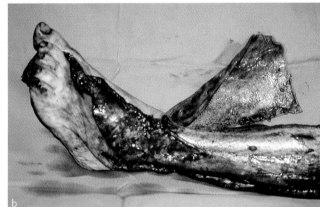
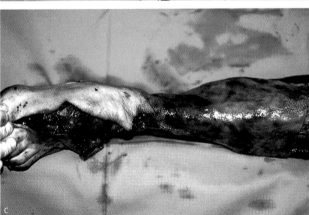
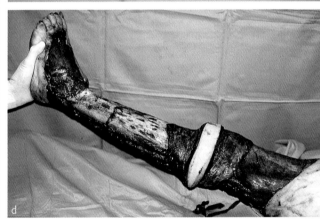
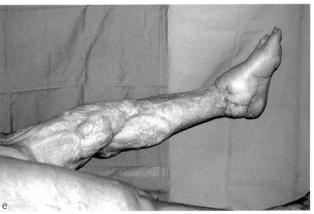

Fig 10.2-5a–e Extensive degloving injury of the left leg.

a Degloved skin of the lower leg laterally with a narrow, distally based pedicled skin flap adjacent to the medial malleolus (arrow).

b Skin flap after fat removal on the underside.

c Repositioning of the defatted skin as a pedicled flap with a disadvantageous width-to-length ratio. It will therefore function as a full-thickness skin graft to cover the medial side of the lower leg.

d Fenestrated, full-thickness skin graft, donated by a craniolateral skin flap, to cover the lateral side of the lower leg. The knee has been covered with a free musculocutaneous latissimus dorsi flap including a skin island to monitor the flap. The rest of the flap has been covered with a split-thickness skin graft.

e Fully healed leg at the 1-year follow-up.

Several methods have been described to tackle these difficulties such as having two assistants stretch the skin flap over a large abdominal pad for even distribution of pressure and using handheld, nonmechanical dermatomes, or specially adapted dermatomes, such as the Gibson-Roots dermatome [9].

Any collection of fluid beneath the degloved skin reduces close contact of the graft to the vascularized wound bed and, thus, the likelihood of its successful engraftment. The risk of hematoma formation may be minimized by meticulous hemostasis of the wound bed, the use of a meshed skin graft, and the application of a bolster dressing. If the dressing is changed within 1 day of skin grafting, any hematoma or seroma that might have accumulated beneath the graft can be drained via selective incisions through the graft above the accumulated fluid; this will permit readherence of the graft and prevent graft loss. The detection of collected fluids is much more difficult in patients with an avulsion injury without visible skin wound.

10.2.7 Graft application and dressings

Meshing of the skin graft
While planning soft-tissue reconstruction using skin grafts, the surgeon has to decide whether the graft needs to be applied onto the recipient site as a meshed or unmeshed graft. A scalpel is often used to create small slits or fenestrations, whereas a graft-meshing device is used to generate a meshed skin graft (**Fig 10.2-6**) (**Video 10.2-1**). Fenestration of the skin graft allows the drainage of serosanguineous fluid from the wound bed through the graft, which minimizes the risk of fluid accumulation beneath the graft, which would jeopardize its survival. Unless cosmetic factors predominate, fenestration is indicated in any kind of skin graft. Meshing additionally allows the graft to be expanded. This is useful in order to cover large surfaces. However, meshing the skin graft delays the ultimate epithelialization and is cosmetically less attractive, ie, it leaves a permanent diamond shaped pattern of the skin graft upon healing (**Fig 10.2-7**).

The graft-meshing device may be used if expansion of the overall surface of the graft is required (**Fig 10.2-3**). Several types of skin carriers are available. Each type is designed to produce multiple uniform slits in a skin graft, which are ~0.1 cm apart. The device allows for a skin expansion ratio of 1:1, 1.5:1, 3:1, and even up to 9:1. The use of the latter, however, is discouraged. The wider the mesh, the greater the wound area that may be covered. Yet the closure by epithelialization will take longer as the open interstices needing to be filled are larger and the margins of the mesh reticulum are farther apart. During this period there is a real risk of losing the graft. In addition, the more widely a meshed

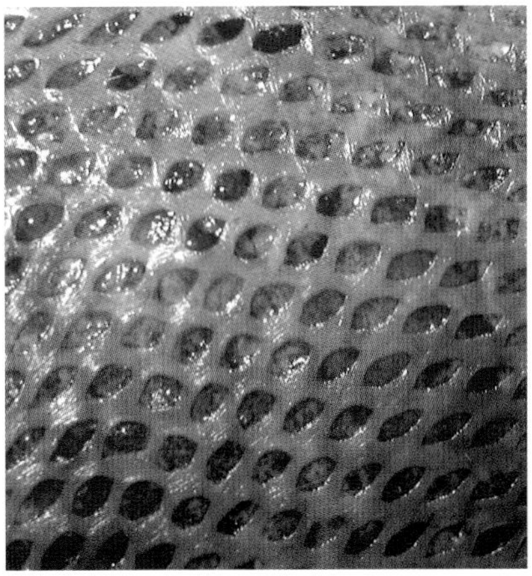

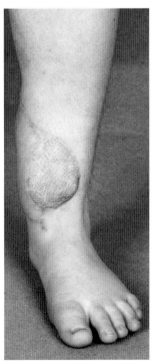

Fig 10.2-6   Diamond-shaped pattern of a meshed, split-thickness skin graft after graft placement.

Fig 10.2-7   Permanent diamond-shaped pattern of the skin graft years after healing.

graft is, the higher the potential risk of:

- hypertrophic scars
- unsatisfactory mechanical resistance
- inadequate pliability
- restricted joint mobility
- permanently poor cosmetic appearance.

Exact measurement of the skin defect allows to plan for an adequately sized split-thickness skin graft at a 1:1.5 ratio, which means that a segment of skin that is ~11 × 3 cm suffices to cover a 10 × 5 cm defect, taking into account a slight loss in length when the graft is expanded by 1.5 times to the width of the defect. Therefore, split-thickness skin grafts should be harvested ~10% longer than the actual length of the wound. The skin to be meshed is placed onto the carrier with the dermal surface facing upwards. The template and the graft are passed through the device by using a hand-crank mechanism and then covered with moist saline gauze until application onto the wound (**Video 10.2-1**).

Fixation of the skin graft

A skin graft placed on a properly prepared wound bed must remain immobilized long enough in order to allow for successful vascularization of the graft (ie, inosculation and re-vascularization). All techniques must serve to maintain fixation between the graft and the underlying wound bed in order to avoid shearing, which could disrupt the vascularization of the graft. Since 1929, when Blair and Brown stressed the importance of the application of even pressure to the graft by a carefully designed dressing [10], surgeons have been encouraged to use so-called pressure dressings on skin grafts [11]. This belief was perpetuated in 1957 by Gillies and Millard [12], who stated that by using the tie-over dressing both stretch and pressure are applied to the graft. However, the graft first has to be immobilized correctly. A variety of methods have been described for the immobilization of grafts, including sutures, staples, and tissue adhesives. The use of tissue adhesives has gained considerable momentum over the last 20 years. Biological adhesives consist of thrombin and fibrinogen as principle components. Thrombin converts fibrinogen into fibrin. Fibrin mimics the final common pathway of the coagulation cascade. To be effective, these two components are mixed with cofactors, which will form a fibrinous matrix between the wound bed and the graft. The first report of fibrin glue used as a skin-graft adhesive was published in 1944 [13]. Advantages of this technique were that sutures, staples, or bulky bolster dressings were no longer needed to fix the graft, thus changes of dressing could also be dispensed with. This had some positive impact on the general discomfort and anxiety of the patient associated with change and removal of dressings as well as on nursing time. Fibrin glue has also been reported to decrease the incidence of both hematoma and seroma formation beneath extensive skin grafts. Fibrin glue has further been associated with improved graft survival rates in infected wounds, decreased wound contraction as well as shorter immobilization time and hospital stay.

Bolstering and dressings

The bolstering of the graft to the wound, however, is achieved with dressings that provide uniform pressure over the entire graft site in order to:

- minimize dead space
- reduce hematoma and seroma formation
- decrease the risk of shear forces
- immobilize the graft.

Ideally, the dressing should be simple to apply and economical in terms of dressing material and necessary personnel. Many types of dressings have been proposed, varying from simple cotton balls, resin molds, and foam pads, to complex stent-like metals, plastic, and dental liner.

Bolster dressings are useful over joints or other areas, where motion is difficult to avoid as well as in wounds with irregular contours such as deep concave areas, where it is difficult to secure a dressing. These bolsters may be constructed from a nonadherent material such as fat gauze folded over moistened cotton balls and covered with a nonadherent, semi-occlusive, absorbent dressing material. An alternative is the tie-over dressing that results from sutures placed radially around the wound in order to tie them to each other over the bolster dressing (**Fig 10.2-8**).

Another alternative for larger, irregularly contoured wounds with difficult topography or wounds with high levels of exudate are negative-pressure wound-therapy devices (**Video 10.2-1**). This type of dressing conforms to the wound surface by suction and promotes skin-graft adherence by maximizing the contact surface while removing exudate and edema from the surrounding tissues (chapter 9.3). In such case, it is advisable to place a nonadherent interface between the skin graft and the foam in order to prevent peeling the graft off when removing the foam of the device. Negative-pressure wound-therapy devices can also immobilize an extremity and be used as a splint in order to prevent any shearing displacement of the skin graft.

Grafts placed on extremities may be managed by elevation of the limb and compression dressing applied to the entire extremity distal to the graft in order to prevent edema formation, which could cause inadequate adherence (chapter 11.4).

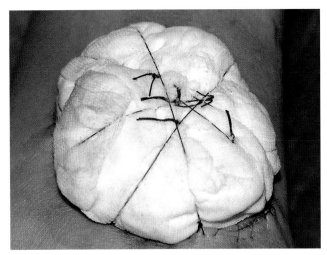

Fig 10.2-8 Tie-over dressing using sutures placed radially around the wound, which are tied to each other over a bolster dressing to cover and immobilize a split-thickness skin graft.

A cast or a splint is useful whenever grafts cover a mobile surface in order to prevent motion, to eliminate shear forces, or even to deal with a patient with poor compliance. Finally, a skin graft may also be treated without any dressing at all except for a thin layer of ointment in order to prevent desiccation. Although wounds treated in this manner are susceptible to hematoma or seroma formation beneath the graft due to the lack of pressure applied, this may be the only option in order to cover the exposed pedicle or

muscle of a transferred flap without compromising its patency, respectively vascularity.

10.2.8 Aftercare

Typically the period of immobilization ranges from 3–7 days. During the first 14 days, it is very important to take great care of the graft in order to reduce the risk of its failing. This involves the avoidance of shearing between the wound bed and graft, eg, caused by subjecting the reconstructed area to vertical forces in an upright position, which would result in an increase of hydrostatic pressure within the newly formed vessels. Patients may briefly walk with newly applied grafts, but they must wear a firm dressing or a tubular support bandage such as tubigrip™ to protect the graft. As yet, properly constructed studies in order to develop guidelines for the use of splinting and dressings have not been carried out.

Following engraftment (ie, graft take), the skin may gently be washed with soap and water. Within 2 weeks, the dressing may be left off and shoe wear may be permitted. Advise the patient on the fact that the grafted skin and the donor site are prone to hyperpigmentation if exposed to sunlight within the first 6 months after grafting. The application of sunscreen may reduce this risk. Some surgeons recommend the use of vitamin E ointment in order to lessen the likelihood of pigment mismatch.

10.3 Flaps in general—principles

Authors   Maurizio Calcagni, Pietro Giovanoli, Reto Wettstein, Yves Harder

10.3.1 Definition of the term flap

A flap is a unit of one or more tissues that maintains its own blood perfusion through a vascular pedicle, which acts as a conduit, while being transferred from a donor site of the body, where it is dispensable, to a recipient site, where it is needed. Flaps are required in order to cover tissue defects that have poor vascularity or which expose foreign bodies such as implant material. Flaps range from a simple advancement of skin and subcutaneous tissue to so-called composite units that may consist of any type of tissue including skin, subcutaneous tissue, muscle, bone, fascia or even nerve. A brief history of flaps is outlined in **Table 10.3-1**.

10.3.2 Flap classification

Categories

Decades of research, clinical and surgical experience as well as better knowledge of vascular anatomy have allowed the classification of flaps. The most commonly used categories are based on:

- type and anatomy of vascular supply (ie, source vessel)
- method of tissue transfer (ie, technique of flap elevation and movement)
- flap composition (ie, tissues that constitute the flap).

1597	Tagliacozzi	Distant arm flap
1837	Horner	Z-plasty principle
1889	Manchot	Definition of vascular patterns of cutaneous circulation by dissection
1906	Tansini	Latissimus dorsi musculocutaneous flap
1912	Blair	Osteoseptocutaneous flap
1916	Esser	Arterial (biological) flap
1919	Davis	Principles of pedicled flaps
1921	Blair	Delay phenomenon in nonpedicled flaps
1946	Limberg	Rhomboid flap
1965	Bakamjian	Deltopectoral flap
1968	Ger	Muscle flaps
1972	McGregor and Jackson	Groin flap
1973	Daniel, Taylor, O'Brien, Harii	Free flaps
1974	Reinisch	Pathophysiology of the delay phenomenon
1975	McCraw and Furlow	Dorsalis pedis flap
1977	McCraw	Description of musculocutaneous vascular territories and musculocutaneous flaps
1981	Ponten	Fasciocutaneous flaps
1987	Taylor and Palmer	Angiosomes
1988	Koshima	Perforator flap (anteromedial thigh flap)
1992	Khouri	Principles of flap prefabrication
1994	Pribaz	Principles of flap prelamination

Table 10.3-1 Summary of the milestones in the evolution of surgical flaps (with special emphasis on orthopaedic soft-tissue trauma). Table modified according to Selected Reading in Plastic Surgery, Volume 9, Number 2, 1999, page 2, The University of Texas, Southwestern Medical Center at Dallas, Baylor University Medical Center.

Classification according to the type of vascular supply

McGregor and Morgan [14] categorized flaps as random skin flap or axial pattern skin and/or muscle flap. Random pattern flaps lack a specific blood supply for their vascular pattern and are subject to restrictions in length. They must, therefore, correspond to a certain width-to-length ratio (chapter 10.4). This ratio depends on the dermal and subcutaneous vascularity (chapter 2.2). Axial pattern flaps have at least one specific, direct vascular pedicle that contains an anatomically recognizable arteriovenous system, including lymph vessels, and a nerve within the long axis of the flap (chapter 10.4, 10.5). A well-defined axial pedicle can safely perfuse a flap beyond its angiosome (chapter 2.2.3), ie, with a width-to-length ratio larger than 1:2–1:3, and is therefore more reliable in comparison to a random pattern flap. The pedicle consists of a vascular branch, originating from a source vessel, allowing it to be isolated in a specific flap. Such a vascular tree of source vessels of the lower extremity is described in (**Fig 10.3-1a–b**).

At the level of the groin, the inguinal ligament constitutes an anatomical barrier for a network of deep and superficial vessels emerging from the external iliac artery, and common femoral arteries provide a variety of source vessels more distally. The deep inferior epigastric, circumflex iliac, and external pudendal arteries emerge proximally, above the inguinal ligament, whereas their superficial counterparts branch off below the inguinal ligament with common or separate origins. These vessels supply the region of the groin, the iliac crest, and the abdominal wall offering different options for flaps. Dorsally, the superior and inferior gluteal arteries are the major vessels for gluteal muscle and skin perfusion. The inferior gluteal artery runs down the posterior aspect of the thigh, sometimes as far as 8 cm from the popliteal fossa.

While the vascularization of the thigh rarely poses a problem for wound healing in comparison to the lower leg, preservation of the medial and lateral femoral circumflex arteries, as well as branches of the deep femoral artery may be important as they may all serve as pedicles for many useful flaps. The superficial femoral artery gives off muscle branches and the superior genicular artery at the adductor hiatus. This forms a rich anastomotic network with the inferior genicular artery arising from the popliteal artery and terminating distally as the saphenous branch running with the homonymous sensitive nerve. Before bifurcating into the tibiofibular trunk and the anterior tibial artery, the popliteal artery gives off paired sural arteries, which supply the two heads of the gastrocnemius muscles, another potential source for a flap pedicle for the area of the knee. The anterior tibial artery passes over the interosseous membrane, courses distally into the anterior muscle compartment of the leg surrounded by the tibialis anterior and extensor hallucis muscles anteriorly and the interosseous membrane posteriorly to become the dorsalis pedis artery of the foot. Source arteries and their concomitant veins usually travel adjacent to—but not within—the rigid fascial envelopes, in loose connective tissue, often containing fat that helps to identify these structures. The deep fibular nerve joins the anterior tibial artery in the proximal third of the leg. Posterior to the interosseous membrane, the tibiofibular trunk divides into the fibular and posterior tibial artery. The fibular artery runs medially to the fibula between the posterior tibial and flexor hallucis longus muscles. It supplies the fibula and the overlying skin through septocutaneous vessels and forms the vascular basis for the fibula flap. Its terminal branch, the lateral calcaneal artery, may serve as an important pedicle for local flaps for soft-tissue defects in the region of the ankle. In spite of the nomenclature, neither the superficial nor the deep fibular nerve runs parallel to the

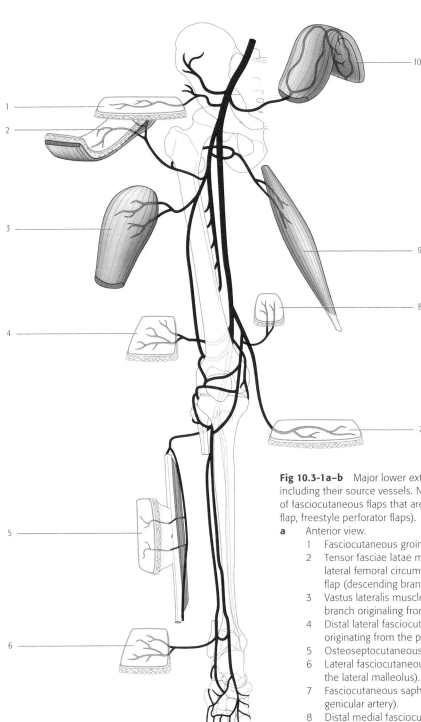

Fig 10.3-1a–b Major lower extremity vessels and sketch of respective flaps including their source vessels. Note that this sketch does not show the multitude of fasciocutaneous flaps that are based on perforating vessels (eg, lateral thigh flap, freestyle perforator flaps).

a Anterior view.
1 Fasciocutaneous groin flap (superficial iliac circumflex artery).
2 Tensor fasciae latae musculocutaneous flap (transverse branch of the lateral femoral circumflex artery); anterolateral fasciocutaneous thigh flap (descending branch of the lateral femoral circumflex artery).
3 Vastus lateralis muscle flap (perforating vessels from the descending branch originaling from the deep femoral artery).
4 Distal lateral fasciocutaneous thigh flap (lateral collateral artery originating from the popliteal artery).
5 Osteoseptocutaneous fibula flap (fibular artery).
6 Lateral fasciocutaneous supramalleolar flap (arterial arch surrounding the lateral malleolus).
7 Fasciocutaneous saphenous flap (terminal branch of the descending genicular artery).
8 Distal medial fasciocutaneous thigh flap (medial collateral artery originating from the popliteal artery).
9 Gracilis muscle flap (transverse branch of the medial femoral circumflex artery).
10 Rectus abdominis muscle flap (deep inferior epigastric artery).

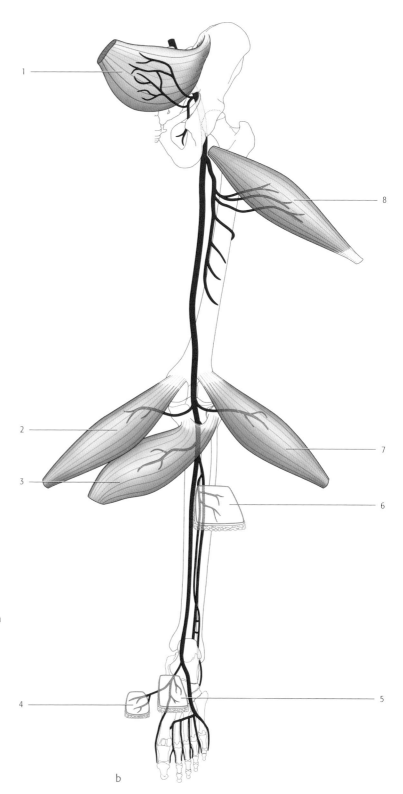

Fig 10.3-1a–b (cont) Major lower extremity vessels and sketch of respective flaps including their source vessels. Note that this sketch does not show the multitude of fasciocutaneous flaps that are based on perforating vessels (eg, lateral thigh flap, freestyle perforator flaps).

b Posterior view.

1   Gluteus maximus muscle flap (inferior and superior gluteal artery).
2   Medial gastrocnemius muscle flap (medial sural artery).
3   Soleus muscle flap (branches originating from the tibial and fibular artery).
4   Medial fasciocutaneous foot flap (cutaneous branch originating from the medial plantar artery).
5   Fasciocutaneous instep flap (medial plantar artery).
6   Sural fasciocutaneous flap (sural artery with reversed flow).
7   Lateral gastrocnemius muscle flap (lateral sural artery).
8   Biceps femoris muscle flap (branches originating from the deep femoral artery).

fibular artery. The posterior tibial artery gives off branches to supply muscles, then bifurcates into the medial and lateral plantar arteries after the distal margin of the flexor retinaculum muscle and runs parallel to the tibial nerve, which in turn is responsible for plantar sensation and intrinsic foot-muscle innervation distally. The medial plantar artery and the respective nerve supply the instep area, which provides a valuable reservoir of skin for reconstruction of the heel.

For reconstructive surgery of the upper extremity and other locations of the body, the same anatomical knowledge is required.

In addition to the knowledge of the normal anatomy of the arteries and veins and possible variations of leg perfusion, these causes for critical changes have to be taken into consideration, both, when dealing with emergency cases as well as in planning elective surgery:
- peripheral artery occlusive disease
- diabetes mellitus
- posttraumatic changes.

The exact knowledge of vascular anatomy is important, especially in regard to flap elevation, but also to surgical approaches, in view of salvage operations such as reoperations or prosthetic joint replacement, and/or tissue transfer.

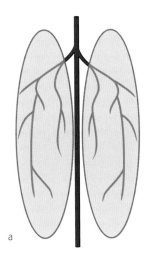
a

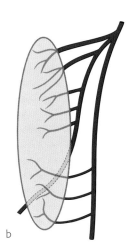
b

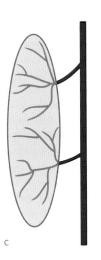
c

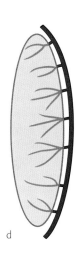
d

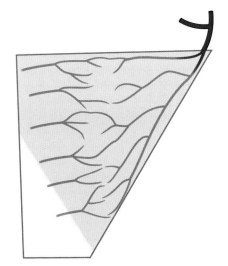
e

Fig 10.3-2a–e Classification of the vascular anatomy of muscles.
a Type 1: one single major pedicle, eg, tensor fasciae latae muscle, rectus femoris muscle, gastrocnemius muscle.
b Type 2: one major pedicle and minor pedicles, eg, gracilis muscle, vastus lateralis muscle, biceps femoris muscle, soleus muscle, semitendinosus muscle, fibular muscles, brachioradialis muscle.
c Type 3: two major pedicles, eg, serratus anterior muscle, gluteus maximus muscle, rectus abdominis muscle, semimembranosus muscle.
d Type 4: several segmental pedicles of approximately the same size, eg, sartorius muscle, tibialis anterior muscle.
e Type 5: one dominant pedicle and secondary segmental pedicles, eg, latissimus dorsi muscle, pectoralis major muscle.

For reconstructive surgery of the upper extremity and other locations of the body, the same anatomical knowledge is required. According to their blood supply, muscles have been divided into five different types (**Fig 10.3-2a–e**) [15]:

- **Type 1:** a single major pedicle
- **Type 2:** one major pedicle and minor pedicles
- **Type 3:** two major pedicles
- **Type 4:** several segmental pedicles of approximately the same size
- **Type 5:** one dominant pedicle and secondary segmental pedicles.

Classification according to the type of transfer

Local skin flaps are used to close defects immediately adjacent to the donor site and are classified according to the respective technique of transfer (chapter 10.4):

- **Advancement:** advances along the long axis of the flap, from the base towards the defect. V-Y advancement is a modification of the advancement flap.
- **Rotation:** rotation about a pivot point into the defect
- **Transposition:** rotation about a pivot point into the defect with lateral movement
- **Interpolation:** rotation about a pivot point into the defect that is nearby but not directly adjacent to the donor site, so that its pedicle must pass over or under the intervening tissues.

Regional flaps have the base of their pedicle in contiguity with the defect and the skin on the same extremity (chapter 10.5). If the pedicle consists of the vascular bundle only, without subcutaneous tissue and skin, the flaps are called island flaps.

Distant flaps are required when the recipient site or tissue defect is not in close vicinity to the donor site or because there is no healthy soft tissue adjacent to the wound. They are divided into two categories:

- attached direct distant flaps
- free flaps (ie, supplied by microvascular anastomosis) (chapter 10.6).

The expression "attached direct distant flaps" rightfully implies that flaps from a distant donor site are temporarily attached to the area of the defect. For example, the patient has an open-wound defect on the lower leg or the palmar side of a finger that requires soft-tissue coverage. The donor site for the distant flap will be chosen from the contralateral leg, respectively the dorsum of the neighboring finger. Therefore, the patient's injured lower leg or finger must initially be attached to the contralateral leg or neighboring

finger, using a cross-finger or cross-leg flap. After a period of about 2–3 weeks (cross-finger flap) or 3–4 weeks (cross-leg flap), vessels from the surrounding tissues of the recipient site grow into the flap, whereby it gradually becomes less dependent on the circulation of the donor site for survival. The flap is then separated from the donor site and, will survive in the new surrounding of the original defect. This technique not only takes several weeks to complete, it is also cumbersome and inconvenient for the patient. Today, this method will rarely be considered for the leg, only if no other options are available. For finger injuries, however, this technique should be part of the surgeon's armamentarium.

Free flaps, ie, flaps with an axial pattern-type of blood supply were developed to circumvent the disadvantages inherent to attached direct distant flaps. Free flaps along with their pedicle are completely detached from the donor site and are transferred within one procedure to the recipient site. After microsurgical anastomosis, blood flow is reestablished (chapter 10.6). Free flaps undergo a certain period of ischemia during the procedure until they are reperfused, which is, however, usually tolerated by the tissues.

Lately, techniques in flap surgery have been developed with the specific intention of optimizing reconstructive goals. Accordingly, it is possible to prefabricate, respectively prelaminate a flap prior to transfer. Prefabrication refers to the implantation of a nonnative vascular pedicle into the tissue desired for reconstruction before its actual transfer [16], whereas prelamination refers to the implantation of anything else into the future flap [17].

Classification according to tissue composition

Flaps may consist of any type and number of tissues in virtually any combination. Complexity of the defect, vascularization of the recipient site, constitution of the tissues needed, donor-site morbidity as well as patient-related factors will dictate which type of flap should be used. Composite flaps often incorporate skin, muscle, bone and the intervening subcutaneous fat and fascia, allowing single-stage reconstruction of complex defects. Specialized flaps can provide sensory skin and functional muscle to areas requiring special needs.

The three varieties of flaps (ie, type of vascular supply, technique of transfer, and tissue composition) require a proper terminology and classification that is of paramount importance not only in teaching basic knowledge about flaps, but also in daily practice. This allows the development of algorithms and treatment strategies using a large number of new flap options that are often technically demanding. Despite widespread classification systems, these often do not cover all aspects of a flap. There have been various attempts to provide a more comprehensive classification system [18, 19] (**Table 10.3-2**). One of these systems describes the circulation (vascular supply, axial pattern versus random pattern) as the core characteristic, and constituents, contiguity, construction, conformation and conditioning of the flap as further characteristics that determine flap nomenclature. These characteristics are also called the six "C"s.

Classification parameter	Subdivisions		Further subdivision/ comment
Type of vascular supply	Random (nonspecific blood supply of the dermal and subdermal plexuses)	Components: skin only	Width-to-length ratio differs according to anatomical region
	Axial (at least one specific arteriovenous system)	One or more of the following components: skin, muscle, fascia, bone	Pedicled: single-pedicled, multipedicled
			Free (microvascular)
			Perforator
Type of transfer	Local	Advancement	Pedicled: single-pedicled, bipedicled
			V-Y
			Y-V
		Rotation	About a pivot point
		Transposition	About a pivot point
		Interpolation	About a pivot point
	Regional	–	Base of the pedicle in contiguity with the defect
	Distant	Pedicled (attached)	Cross-finger, cross-leg, island
		Free (detached)	Microvascular
Type of tissue composition	Skin	–	–
	Subcutaneous tissue	–	–
	Fascia	–	–
	Bone	–	–
	Cartilage	–	–
	Nerve	–	–
	Composite	Fasciocutaneous	–
		Musculocutaneous	–
		Osteoseptocutaneous	–
		Neurocutaneous	–
Time of flap preparation	Immediate	–	–
	Delayed	Surgical delay	–
		Delay due to tissue expansion	–
		Physical delay	–
		Chemical delay	–
Type of pedicle	Skin	Single-pedicled	–
		Bipedicled	–
	Non-skin	Subcutaneous tissue	–
		Fascia	–
		Muscle	–

Table 10.3-2 Classification and nomenclature of flaps according to different characteristics. Table modified according to Selected Readings in Plastic Surgery, Volume 9, Number 2, 1999, page 2, The University of Texas, Southwestern Medical Center at Dallas, Baylor University Medical Center.

10.3.3 Zone of injury and flap surgery

Assessing the severity of a traumatic wound is very important in decision making for reconstructing soft-tissue defects (chapter 5.1, 6.2). The amount of energy imparted to the tissues during trauma determines the extent of the visible soft-tissue trauma and the so-called macroscopically invisible zone of injury, ie, inflammatory and edematous soft tissues that are characterized by disturbed microcirculation challenging the viability of flaps. Accordingly, it is often very difficult to clearly distinguish this zone of injury from the adjacent healthy tissues, especially soon after the trauma. Therefore, it is important to take into account that the ultimate extension of traumatized soft tissue almost always exceeds the area initially appreciated, especially if the trauma results from a blunt, high-energy insult. This fact is of clinical relevance because vascular pedicles originating from within the zone of injury or microvascular anastomosis performed in this area are associated with impaired healing potential as well as an increased flap loss rate [20, 21]. Today, if feasible, radical debridement followed by immediate soft-tissue coverage in order to obtain primary healing is considered the optimal approach for most if not all open injuries of the extremities (chapter 7.1). Byrd et al [20] and Godina et al [21] demonstrated the advantages of early reconstruction of complex injuries of the extremities with concomitant soft-tissue defects using pedicled or free flaps:

• reduced infection rate
• improved flap survival
• decreased length of hospital stay [22].

The authors could also show that reconstruction performed after the third day, but before the sixth week, respectively, following trauma are associated with an increased complication rate, which is the consequence of both direct and indirect trauma to the soft tissues.

Flap surgery, ie, dissecting a regional or a free flap as well as preparing its recipient vessel, should be performed using high magnification loupes. If a tourniquet is used to elevate a flap or to prepare the flap's recipient vessels, it should be released before final transfer in order to estimate the blood flow, respectively the leaking sites, once dissection has been completed. The artery should always show a clear pulsating flow without tendency to stop. If the blood flow is still inadequate and vascular spasm has been excluded, perivascular injection of papaverin at the pedicle site or shortening of the recipient vessel of a free flap can be performed until blood flow, respectively pulsation is satisfactory. In doing so, the length of the recipient vessel is accurately determined and the need for vein grafts can be reduced or even excluded.

10.3.4 Preoperative assessment of vessels and flap surgery

Before planning the elevation of a flap, and independent of its tissue composition, the surgeon in charge of the reconstructive procedure must know exactly the current condition and exact anatomical course of the vessel of interest. Assessment of blood flow—in particular in lower limb surgery—is even more important if a free tissue transfer is planned (chapter 5.1). For many years, angiography has been the gold standard for the preoperative assessment of vascular patency prior to lower-limb reconstructions [23]. Interestingly, clinical evaluation, ie, palpation of peripheral pulses and the use of duplex sonography have been shown to be of high accuracy as well [24]. The indications for angiography are manifold. They include the suspicion of an intimal lesion to the vessel as may be observed after direct or indirect trauma, with or without involvement of bone. Furthermore, the presence of concomitant diseases such as peripheral artery occlusive disease in elderly patients, diabetes, heavy smoking, or cardiovascular risk factors has to be taken into account. This investigation will inevitably determine the feasibility of a reconstruction, because inflow to the donor site (eg, pedicled flap of the calf) and recipient vessels (eg, proper site of anastomosis for free flaps) may reliably be determined. Today, computed tomographic angiography [25] and high-resolution magnetic resonance angiography [26] can accurately determine detailed vascular patterns up to the diameter of septocutaneous perforator vessels and will eventually replace conventional preoperative angiography, which exposes patients to irradiation, is more invasive, and associated with a higher rate of morbidity.

10.3.5 Surgical delay

Surgical delay consists of a stepwise elevation of the flap by repeated incisions around and below the flap. The aim of delaying surgery is to train the tissue to be transferred before separation. The goal is to reduce the extent of flap tissue that is at risk of undergoing necrosis, ie, to improve the width-to-length ratio in favor of the long axis (random pattern flap), respectively to increase the total surface of tissue supplied by the pedicle (axial pattern flap). The delay phenomenon is not yet completely understood. However, it seems to result from several orchestrated pathophysiological mechanisms. The early phase is characterized by a hypoxia-induced hyperadrenergic state, resulting in vasoconstriction at the precapillary level, lasting for 18–30 hours. During this overlapping period, a surgically induced denervation (ie, sympathectomy) of the vascular bed of the flap is performed, which causes vasodilatation. In a later phase, morphological changes are observed, including arteriogenesis (ie, an increase in the diameter of preexisting arterial vessels) as well as hypoxia and vascular endothelial growth factor-driven angiogenesis (ie, growth of new blood vessels from preexisting vessels) [27, 28]. As surgical delay needs to be invasive and time consuming in order to be effective (ie, ~2–3 weeks to prepare a flap), short-term and less invasive strategies for preconditioning of musculocutaneous tissue that appear to be effective [29] are currently under investigation in clinical studies in humans.

10.4 Local flaps—principles

Authors   Maurizio Calcagni, Pietro Giovanoli

10.4.1 Introduction

The beginning of flap surgery was challenging despite the detailed anatomical studies about vascular patterns of cutaneous circulation by Manchot [30], Spalteholz [31], and Braithwaite [32]. As the vascular supply of the skin was still poorly understood, the use of local flaps with a random type of perfusion was common. Such local flaps consisting of skin and subcutaneous tissue lack any defined alignment or axial orientation of the feeding arterioles and their respective draining veins (chapter 10.3). As the feeding vessels derive from direct musculocutaneous, fasciocutaneous, or cutaneous arterioles, the viability of the transferred tissues depends on the perfusion within dermal and subdermal plexuses (chapter 2.1), and the design and extent of the flap. In contrast to random-pattern flaps, the axial pattern flaps are based on a vascular pedicle that either runs longitudinally along the fascia or depends on perforating vessels.

10.4.2 Random-pattern flaps

Characteristics

Random-pattern flaps are not centered on a particular vessel but rather depend on a strict width-to-length ratio (chapter 10.3). In the lower extremity and the hand, width-to-length ratios of 1:1 to 1:2 are acceptable while in the face a ratio of 1:3 to 1:5 can be used safely. As an option, the ratio can be increased in favor of length by the techniques of surgical delay or tissue preconditioning (chapter 10.3.5).

More commonly, local flaps are grouped according to the technique used to move the tissue between the donor site and the immediately adjacent recipient site (chapter 10.3) (chapter 12.6 to 12.18). In practice such local flaps are often combined in order to achieve closure of the defect. In the following, the four major types of local flap transfer are described.

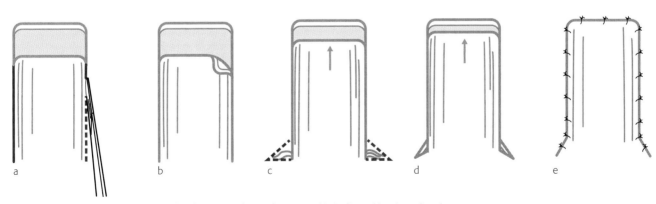

Fig 10.4-1a–e   Advancement flap. The defect needing to be covered is indicated by the colored area.

a   Incision of the flap's margins down to the muscle fascia, the paratenon, or the perineurium.

b   Elevation of the flap from the side of the defect towards the flap's base.

c   Advancement of the flap in direction of its long axis (arrow) into the defect, which may result in bulges laterally adjacent to the flap's base (waved lines). If necessary, the bulging skin can be excised in a triangular shape (Burow triangle = red dotted line).

d   Further advancement of the flap in direction of its long axis (arrow) into the defect. By doing so, the space created by excision of the Burow triangle is closed.

e   Suturing of the flap to the surrounding skin.

Advancement flaps

Advancement flaps of variable design are moved or advanced in the direction of their long axis directly into the neighboring defect by simply stretching the skin. There is no rotational or lateral movement. The best examples are:

- direct wound closure after subcutaneous mobilization
- single-pedicle advancement flap (**Fig 10.4-1a–e**)
- V-Y advancement flap (**Fig 10.4-2a–h**).

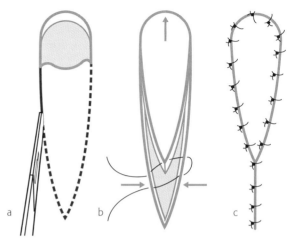

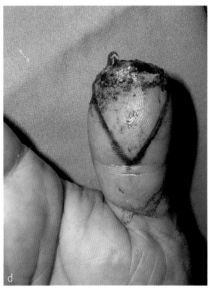

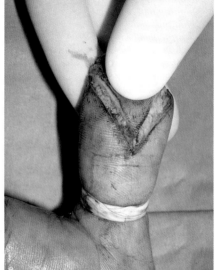

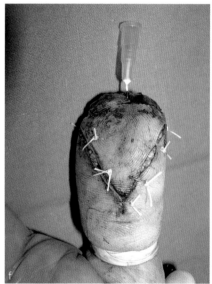

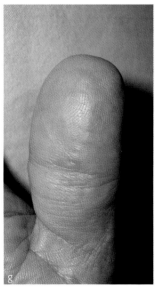

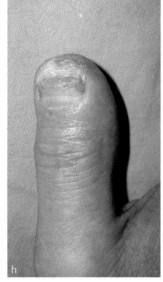

Fig 10.4-2a–h   V-Y advancement flap with clinical illustration. Defect at the tip of the right thumb.

a   Incision of the V-shaped flap.

b   The V-shaped flap is advanced in direction of its long axis (vertical arrow) into the defect, resulting in a proximal donor-site defect (horizontal arrows).

c   Primary closure of the donor-site defect by advancing the skin on each side of the V, resulting in a Y-shape.

d   Outlining of the V-shaped flap with its distal edge neighboring the defect.

e   Incision of the flap's margins and dissection of the subcutaneous pedicle.

f   Tension-free flap advancement into the defect and direct closure of the donor site. Temporary flap fixation with a cannula.

g   One year after surgery. Note the almost scar-free healing at the palmar aspect of the thumb.

h   The dorsal aspect of the thumb shows discreet malformation of the distal aspect of the nail due to shortening of the distal phalanx, respectively missing padding of the nail.

The overall distance of possible advancement mainly depends on the elasticity of the skin and the parameters of the flap's design, ie, the correct width-to-length ratio. The skin of the donor site should be rather loose and the flap's contour should be integrated within anatomical or cosmetic units in order to achieve an optimal result. Usually after advancement of the flap, extra skin (ie, dog ear) is left at its base. In order to equalize the length of the flap and the adjacent wound edge, the lateral bulges may be excised in a triangular shape (ie, Burow triangle) (**Fig 10.4-3a–e**). The excision of such extra skin is indicated whenever the bulge interferes with closure in general and/or hinders the wearing of footwear in particular, or if the patient objects from a cosmetic point of view. The vascularity of the flap will not be endangered as long as the width of the flap's base is not decreased.

Rotation flaps

Rotation flaps are semicircular in design and rotate about a pivot point into the adjacent defect needing to be closed (**Fig 10.4-4a–f**). First, the defect has to be roughly transformed into a triangle with a base shorter than its limbs. The base of the defect is then prolonged into a semicircular arch that measures at least four times the dimension of that base. After the elevation, the flap is rotated into the defect. Depending on the elasticity of the local tissues and the tension along the suture line, the need for a tension releasing back-cut has to be evaluated. This back-cut decreases the blood supply of the flap by narrowing its base and, therefore, must be planned cautiously (**Fig 10.4-4e**). In order to facilitate advancement and rotation of the flap, any extra skin appearing adjacent to the pivot point of the flap (ie, dog ear) is best excised as a Burow triangle (**Fig 10.4-4f**) (chapter 10.4.2) or the surrounding tissue can be undermined cautiously. This technique, however, is only moderately beneficial in decreasing tension along the circumference of the flap. As a general rule, attention should be paid to plan the incision line along the margin of a cosmetic unit. If performed on an extremity, the pedicle should be placed proximally and respect the long axis of the vessels in order to guarantee adequate perfusion of the flap (chapter 12.16). The donor site of the flap may either be closed by primary suture or, if needed, by a skin graft (chapter 10.2).

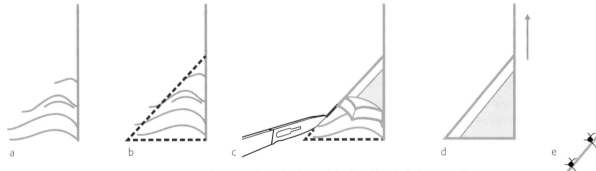

a   b   c   d   e

Fig 10.4-3a–e   Burow triangle to excise surplus tissue from the base of the flap (detail of **Fig 10.4-1d**).
a   Flap advancement results in skin bulges (ie, dog ear = waved lines) laterally at the flap's base.
b   Outlining the triangular skin excision (ie, Burow triangle = red dotted line).
c   Excision of the Burow triangle in order to balance the vertical length of the flap to the surrounding wound edges.
d   The excision is made outside the flap's base in order not to endanger its vascularity by narrowing the flap's base.
        Closing of the defect by advancing the flap in direction of its long axis (arrow).
e   After primary closure of the Burow triangle.

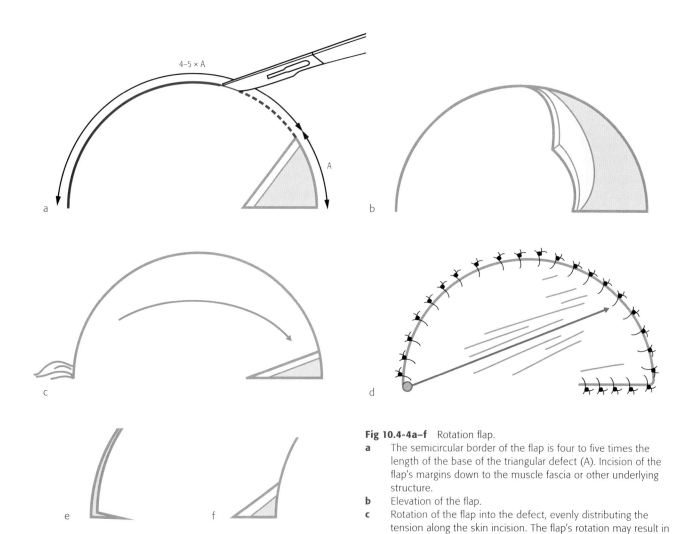

Fig 10.4-4a–f Rotation flap.

a   The semicircular border of the flap is four to five times the length of the base of the triangular defect (A). Incision of the flap's margins down to the muscle fascia or other underlying structure.

b   Elevation of the flap.

c   Rotation of the flap into the defect, evenly distributing the tension along the skin incision. The flap's rotation may result in a bulge laterally adjacent to the flap's base (waved lines).

d   Note the position of the pivot point (blue dot) and the line of greatest tension (blue line).

e   In case of excessive tension, a back-cut is performed at the base of the flap in order to release the tension and to allow for an easier rotation into the defect. However, the back-cut narrows the flap's base and may compromise its perfusion.

f   Alternatively, an eccentric Burow triangle may be excised at the flap's base. Direction of the tension lines of the skin determines the position of the Burow triangle and the type of flap movement (details see **Fig 10.4-3a–e**).

Transposition flaps

A transposition flap is transferred about a pivot point in a lateral direction into the adjacent defect (**Fig 10.4-5a–f**). Depending on the shape of the defect, the vascularization of the local tissues and the region of the body, these flaps exist in a broad variety of geometrical designs (chapter 12.6, 12.7). The flap must be planned larger and longer than the defect needing to be covered, because the more the flap needs to be moved laterally into the defect, the more its length is shortened (**Fig 10.4-6a–f**). Sometimes a back-cut may still be necessary. The resulting tissue defect at the donor site may be closed by direct suture. In case of extensive tension, this defect may also be covered by a secondary flap (eg, bilobed flap) or a skin graft.

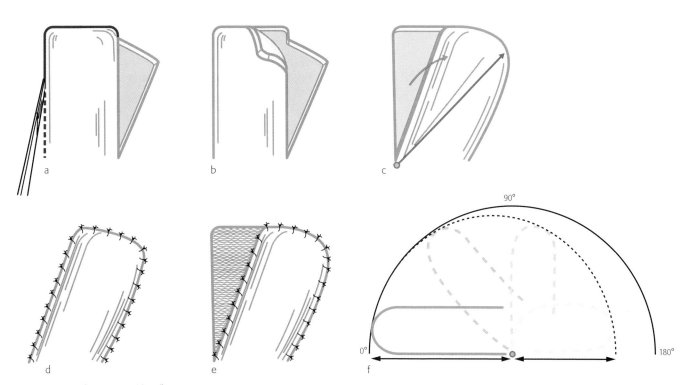

Fig 10.4-5a–f   Transposition flap.
a   Incision of the flap's margins down to the muscle fascia or other underlying structure.
b   Elevation of the flap.
c   Transposition of the flap into the defect (green arrow). Line of greatest tension (blue line) corresponds to the diagonal of the rectangular flap and originated at the level of the pivot point (blue dot).
d   Following flap transposition, tension free closure to the surrounding skin.
e   If the secondary defect resulting from flap elevation cannot be closed primarily because of undue tension, a skin graft (gray) or a secondary flap is applied.
f   A skin flap transposed about a pivot point (blue dot) is always shortened in length the farther it is transposed. This must be considered when planning such a flap, especially with regard to the width-to-length ratio.

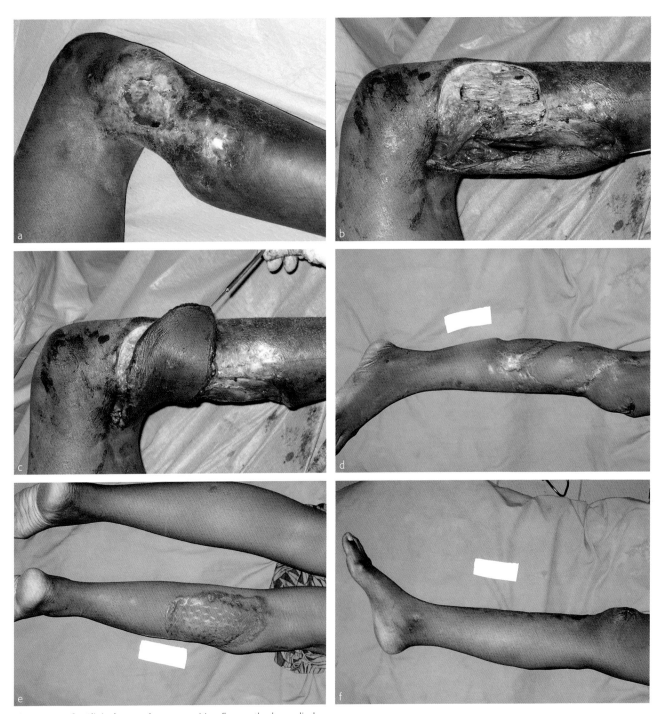

Fig 10.4-6a–f Clinical case of a transposition flap on the lower limb.
a   Chronic, nonhealing wound after semicircular deep skin abrasion at the lateral aspect of the right lower leg proximally.
b   After excision of the granulation tissue and unstable scar as well as elevation of a randomly perfused flap that was planned almost as wide but longer than the defect.
c   After transposition of the flap. Note the excess of length with regard to the defect.
d   After uneventful healing, soft flap tissue covers the region of the proximal fibula.
e   Donor site of the flap covered with split-thickness skin graft.
f   Medial aspect of the lower leg.

A variation of the transposition flap is the Z-plasty, in which two identical triangular flaps are outlined and exchanged between each other. The three limbs of the Z must be of equal length, while the amount of length gained relates to the degree of the angles of the Z. The classic Z-plasty is based on angles of 60°, which allows obtaining maximal length at the central limb of the Z (**Fig 10.4-7a–h**). On closure, the Z is reversed and rotated by 90°. A single large Z-plasty is more effective for lengthening of the skin than multiple smaller ones, although the latter may well be used to correct and conceal a scar, make it less conspicuous, or to release and break up a contracture following scarring. Accordingly, the Z-plasty is mostly used to prevent or correct scar contracture.

The Limberg flap (ie, rhomboid flap) is another transposition flap and, like the Z-plasty or the bilobed flap, depends on the looseness of surrounding skin. Therefore, this type of flap is better suited for the face, the back, the forearm, or the hand than the leg. The Limberg flap is ideal for rhomboid defects with angles from 60–120° [33]. The limbs should have the same length as the transverse axis of the rhomboid (**Fig 10.4-8a–b**). Dufourmentel modified this technique to close defects with any acute angle [34].

Interpolation flaps

Interpolation flaps are dislocated about a pivot point by a lateral movement into a defect that is in close vicinity but not directly adjacent to the donor site. Its pedicle must pass beneath (or above) the interposed intact tissue. Strictly speaking, these flaps may be regarded as regional flaps (chapter 10.5).

Pearls and pitfalls

As the name suggests, the vascular supply of the flap is assumed to be somewhere within the flap. The presence of these vessels in the skin, the subcutaneous tissue and the fascia allows planning random-pattern flaps almost everywhere on the body's surface. However, exact planning that takes width-to-length ratio, angles, and the donor site into consideration, is necessary in order to successfully elevate and move these types of flaps into the defect. Otherwise, wound dehiscence and partial flap necrosis might occur. Technically, dissection of these local flaps is rather easy.

10.4.3 Axial pattern flaps

Characteristics

Axial pattern flaps are characterized by a well-defined pedicle consisting of one artery and usually two concomitant veins as well as lymph vessels (chapter 10.3) that are some-

times accompanied by a nerve (eg, latissimus dorsi flap, lateral arm flap). This vascular bundle runs in the subcutaneous fat immediately above the muscle and its fascia and parallel to the skin surface (**Fig 10.4-9**) or within the muscle. The longitudinal course of the arteries allows elevation of a circumscribed unit of skin and subcutaneous tissue or a muscle with or without overlying skin. Taylor [35] defined the concept of angiosomes, ie, composite anatomical vascular territories of the skin that are supplied by vessels originating from segmental cutaneous (eg, superficial circumflex iliac artery) or muscle arteries (eg, fibular artery) that are interconnected (chapter 2.2.3). From these, ~400 perpendicular vessels feed the surface of the body [36]. Basically, all these vessels are able to supply a skin flap with blood. Although their nomenclature is still heterogeneous, they can be grouped into vessels perforating muscles (ie, true musculocutaneous perforators) or vessels running along septa (ie, septocutaneous perforators). Even though the exact position of a perforating vessel may vary between individuals, the basic anatomy in humans most often is quite constant and predictable.

Perforator flaps

Based on the above knowledge, perforator flaps supplied by a single perforating vessel may be transferred locally to cover small to medium-sized soft-tissue defects on an extremity (**Fig 10.4-10a–f**). These flaps are also called free-style perforator flaps, because they are based on a perforating vessel adjacent to the defect that acts as pivot point for the flap. Although sometimes delicate to dissect at the site of the perforating vessel, these flaps are versatile and quite reliable. The perforators can be precisely identified preoperatively using a handheld Doppler device. The intensity of the signal grossly indicates the diameter of the vessel. Duplex sonography may provide further information about the diameter and the course (ie, intramuscular versus intraseptal) of the vessels. Once the perforating vessel is selected as the basis of the flap's pedicle, the flap is carefully planned to fit the defect. The measurement of the flap must include the exact distance from the perforating vessel to the most distal wound edge. Any misjudgment may render the flap too short and the subsequent advancement of the flap will be more difficult because of too much tension on the pedicle, which in turn will compromise the flap's perfusion. After planning, the flap is gradually elevated with or without fascia, depending on the reconstructive needs, starting distally from the defect and trying to safely visualize the pedicle as early as possible. To adequately judge the blood flow within the pedicle and the flap, the preparation and elevation of the flap should be done with loupe magnification and bipolar cautery or vascular clips but without application

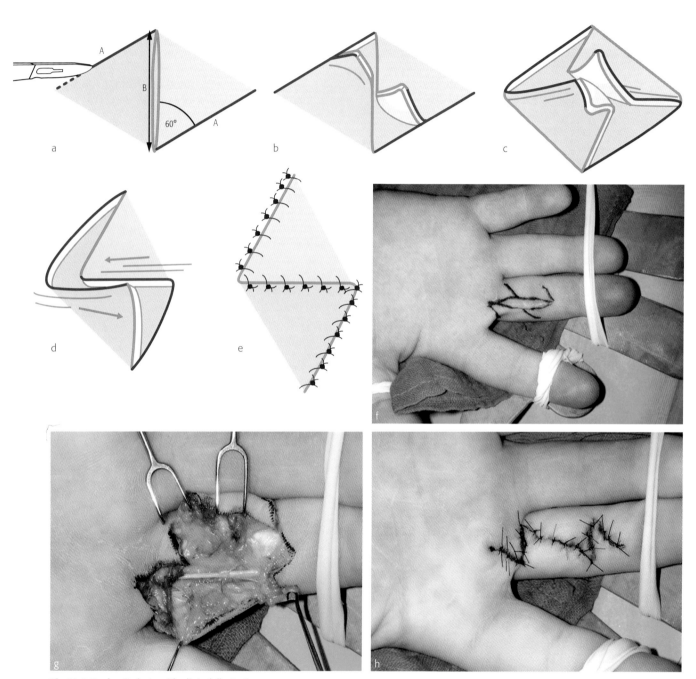

Fig 10.4-7a–h Z-plasty with clinical illustration.
a Classic 60°-angle Z-plasty. The limbs (A) of the Z are all of equal length to the central member (B), which may be a laceration, a defect, or a scar. Incision of the three sides (Z) of the flap down to the fascia.
b Elevation of the resulting two triangular flaps.
c–d The position of the flaps is then exchanged and they are transposed into the defect (arrows).
e After primary closure, the resulting central limb has been rotated by 90° in comparison to the original central limb. The Z-plasty allows a lengthening of the scar in one direction by recruiting surrounding skin (eg, the 60°-angle Z-plasty gains 73% in length).
f Scar contracture after palmar cut of the middle finger radially. Planning of a double Z-plasty to correct the contracture.
g After incision, excision of all scar tissue and freeing of the radial digital nerve.
h After transposition of the flaps and tension-free suture.

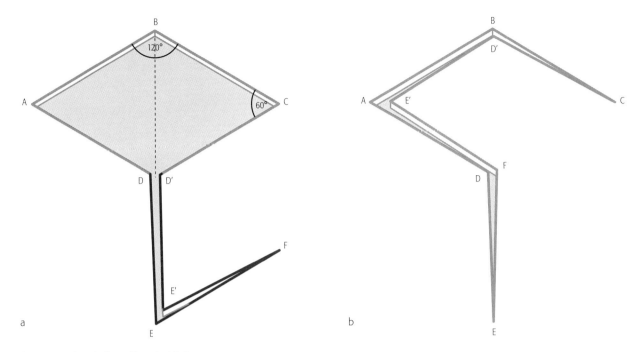

Fig 10.4-8a–b Limberg (rhomboid) flap.

a When planning a Limberg flap, the rhomboid defect (indicated by color) must have angles of ~60–120°. The short line between B and D (dotted line), which equals the length of each side of the defect, is extended by its own length to point E. The line between E and F is drawn parallel to the line between C and D and is of equal length.

b After elevation, the flap is transposed into the rhomboid defect and the skin closed by primary suture. Note the new position of the points D', E', and F.

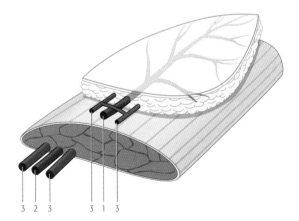

Fig 10.4-9 Blood supply to skin and muscle.
1   Direct cutaneous artery.
2   Direct muscle artery.
3   Accompanying veins.

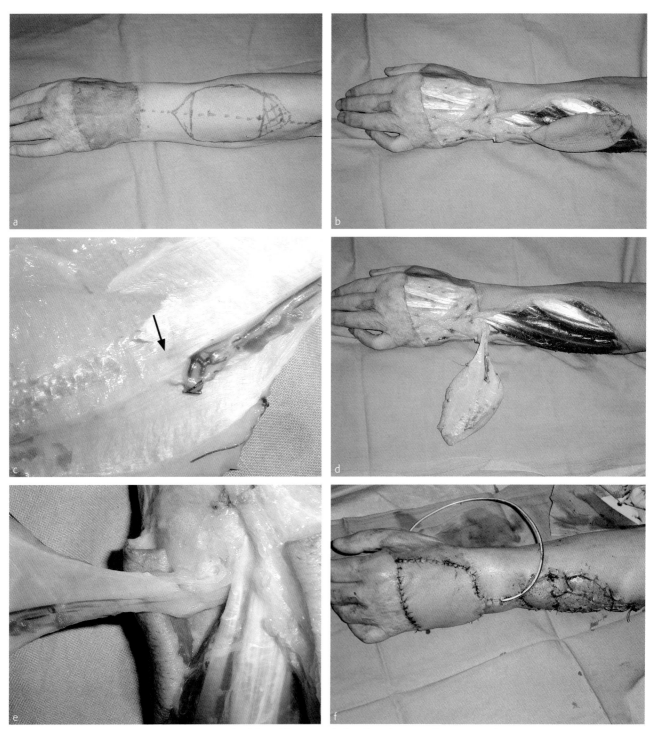

Fig 10.4-10a–f Clinical case of an interosseous island flap with retrograde flow based on a perforating vessel.
a Outlining of the flap within the middle third of the forearm.
b Identification of the pedicle (septocutaneous perforating vessels) passing through the intermuscular septum and dissection of the flap.
c Close-up of the perforating vessel feeding the flap (arrow).
d The pedicle is freed distally to gain additional length.
e The intermuscular septum and the artery follow the tendons of the extensor carpi ulnaris and extensor digiti minimi muscles.
f Insertion of the flap and closure of the donor site with a split-thickness skin graft.

of a tourniquet. The surgeon must ensure that the position of the perforating vessel correlates with the preoperative markings and has a good pulsatile flow. However, there are no exact criteria in order to decide before or during surgery whether the perforating vessel is large enough to adequately feed the flap. As a rule of thumb, a minimal diameter of 0.5 mm is necessary to reliably perfuse such a flap. The skin incision around the flap is then completed and the perforating vessel is dissected through the fascia and even deeper, if necessary. Such a flap cannot be advanced over a long distance but should rather be transposed into the defect by gently redirecting the pedicle. Especially in obese patients, such a flap transposition usually does not allow primary closure of the donor site. Initially after flap transfer, its reperfusion generally appears to be delayed, particularly if the flap had to be rotated along the rather short pedicle by 180°.

Modified perforator flaps

A very useful alternative to the described single perforator flap is the so-called propeller flap (chapter 12.15). This flap is planned around an eccentrically located perforating vessel as pivot point, which lies somewhere along the long axis between the pedicle and the defect. The total flap length A equals the distance B (from the perforating vessel to the proximal wound edge) plus the axial length of the defect C (**Fig 10.4-11**). The flap then resembles an eccentrically mounted propeller. After flap elevation and dissection of the pedicle, the propeller flap is gently rotated by 180° into the defect. The careful freeing of the pedicle is particularly important because it has to be long enough in order to tolerate the twisting but avoiding the occlusion of the delicate accompanying veins, which would induce venous stasis of the flap. If elevated in the direction of arterial blood flow, the proximal area of the propeller flap lies within the donor site, reducing tension during primary closure, which should be achieved in the majority of the cases. In case a dead space needs to be plugged, muscle tissue from beneath the fascia may be included (**Fig 10.4-12a–j**).

Pearls and pitfalls

In contrast to the random-pattern flap, the axial pattern flap is supplied by one well-defined vascular pedicle. Accordingly, this flap is very reliable if well dissected, even beyond its anatomical border that is formed by the corresponding angiosome. However, the dissection of this flap depends on the exact localization of the vascular pedicle, which will somewhat limit its availability. Vessel branches originating from these vascular pedicles, often true perforators, will increase the availability of axially perfused flaps due to their abundant occurrence in almost any area of the body.

Despite a rather constant anatomy of the general vascular architecture, the anatomy of perforators is subject to a high degree of individual variability. Although the dissection of a flap based on such a perforating vessel avoids the need to sacrifice any major vessel, gentle preparation of the perforating vessel is critical in order to guarantee viability. Preparation of the pedicle should be continued for 2–4 cm through the muscle fascia and, if needed, into the muscle itself. Any extra length of pedicle will allow for some limited advancement and, in particular, will compensate for twisting or rotating of the pedicle that should never exceed 180°. A high degree of flexibility is required in planning and executing these flaps, which must include a back-up option in case of inadequate perfusion or intraoperative injury to the perforating vessel.

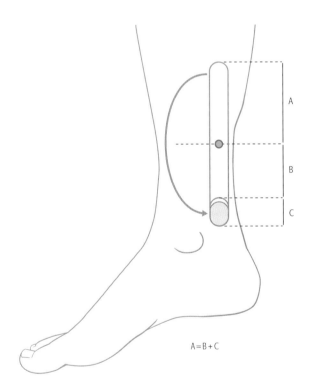

Fig 10.4-11 Principle of the propeller flap. The total flap length A (ie, distance from the perforating vessel (ie, pivot point = blue dot) to the distal end of the flap) equals the distance from the perforating vessel to the proximal wound edge B plus the axial length of the defect C.

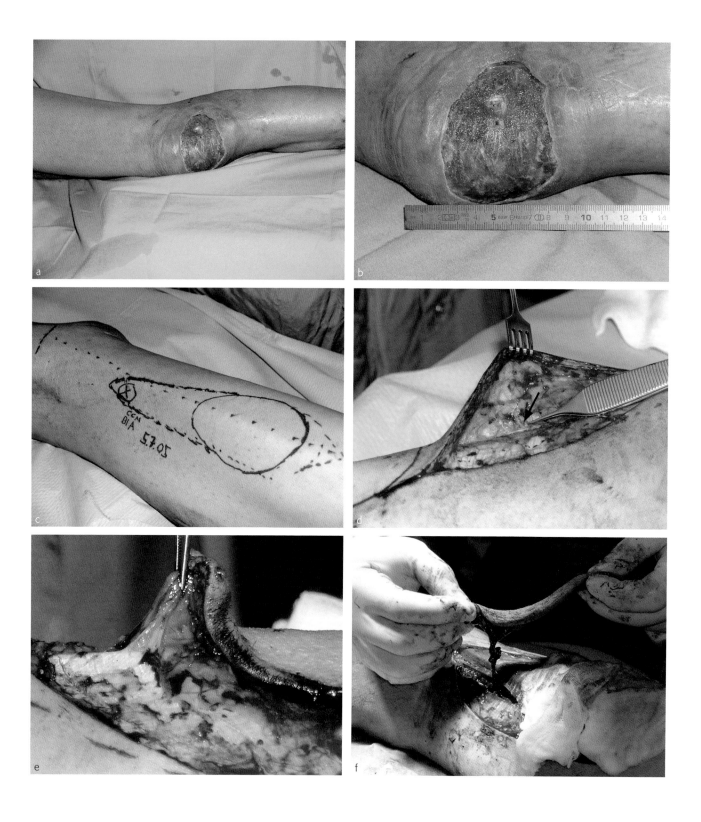

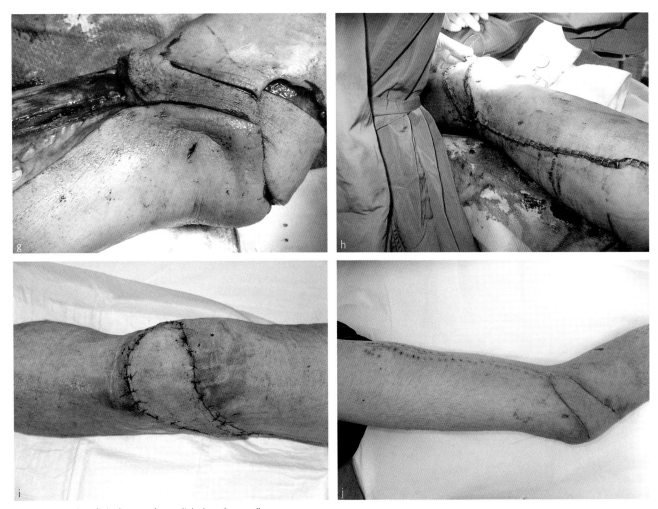

Fig 10.4-12a–j Clinical case of a pedicled perforator flap.
a   Soft-tissue defect over the patella that needs coverage with well-vascularized tissue in order to permanently pad this exposed region.
b   Close-up of the defect showing a thin layer of granulation tissue and exposed bone.
c   Marking of the perforating vessel at the anterolateral aspect of the thigh (x) and outlining of the flap to fit the defect.
d   Medial approach and incision of the skin down to the muscle fascia in order to identify the perforating vessel (arrow).
e   Completion of the incision from lateral and elevation of the flap.
f   After elevation of the flap and complete dissection of the perforating vessel. Note the incision of the muscle fascia and iliotibial band and the further dissection of the pedicle within the muscle in order to increase the length of the pedicle.
g   After transfer of the flap into the defect. Note the rather tension-free course of the pedicle.
h   After tension-free primary closure of the donor site and insertion of the flap.
i   Postoperative view at day 2 with uneventful healing.
j   One month after surgery: uneventful healing with good color, texture, and thickness match of the flap with the surrounding tissues.

Finally, these flaps may individually be tailored to the defect and possess soft-tissue characteristics, which are similar to the lost skin in order to replace like with like. Since the amount of available soft tissue is rather limited in the lower extremities, these flaps only represent an excellent option for small to medium-sized defects. Nevertheless, their use should be assessed carefully in acute trauma with extensive bruising, because increased pressure due to interstitial edema of the skin could induce venous stasis of the flap, endangering its viability (**Fig 10.4-13a–b**).

Nevertheless, two points of debate persist:
- What is the role of these flaps in patients suffering from peripheral occlusive arterial disease or diabetes mellitus or in smokers?
- Should perforator flaps be considered as first choice for soft tissue defects of the extremities or rather considered as a back-up option for failed free flaps?

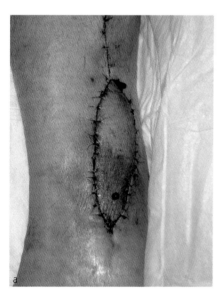 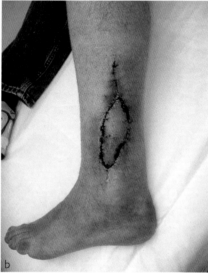

Fig 10.4-13a–b Clinical case of a pedicled perforator flap.
a Pedicled perforator flaps, particularly propeller flaps that are rotated by 180° may often develop venous congestion of the distal area (dark blue bleeding after scarification of the flap) due to twisting of the often short pedicle.
b Most often, however, the venous congestion resolves spontaneously.

10.5 Regional flaps—principles and specific flaps

Authors   Maurizio Calcagni, Pietro Giovanoli, John S Early, Yves Harder

10.5.1 Introduction

Regional flaps are characterized by a pedicle that remains in continuity with the tissue defect while the transferred tissue (eg, skin, muscle, bone) originates from the same extremity. If the pedicle consists of the vascular bundle, and sometimes an accompanying nerve and more or less of the surrounding adipose tissue (ie, pedicle without skin), the flap is called an island flap. Accordingly, these flaps have a longer arc of rotation in comparison to local flaps (chapter 10.4). A selection of techniques for the transfer of regional flaps must be part of the surgeon's armamentarium in order to reliably treat soft-tissue defects following trauma. More-

over, the following factors will strongly influence the outcome of the flap:
- the general condition of the patient (age, health risks, comorbidities, etc)
- the local vascular status of the patient (comorbidities, etc)
- the mechanism and energy of the trauma, ie, the visible extent of the injury as well as the invisible zone of injury, which is usually less evident or even hidden (chapter 10.3.3)
- a careful clinical evaluation of the regional vascular perfusion in the area of interest using different imaging techniques (chapter 10.3.4).

It order for a pedicled flap to become an option, these factors must be checked first. In case the patient's general condition is bad, comorbidities are present, or the extremity is severely injured, it has been proven that the outcome of the flap will be inferior compared to that in healthy patients and nontraumatized donor sites.

This chapter illustrates the most commonly used pedicled flaps: fasciocutaneous and muscle flaps as well as their surgical variations with regard to supplying pedicles, direction of blood flow, and tissue composition. The choice and details concerning flap dissection reflect the authors' personal preferences. The proposed positions during surgery usually allow simultaneous and easy access to both the donor and the recipient site.

10.5.2 Fasciocutaneous flaps

Radial forearm flap

Anatomy and blood supply
The radial forearm flap is a fasciocutaneous flap that is supplied by multiple, vertically directed septocutaneous perforating vessels arising along the entire course of the radial artery, which run within the radial intermuscular septum. Proximally the radial artery courses between the supinator muscle and the fibrous origin of the flexor digitorum superficialis muscle. In the medial third of the forearm, the artery runs between the pronator teres and brachioradialis muscles, and further distally anterior to the flexor pollicis longus muscle. At the wrist, the artery may be palpated between the radius and the tendon of the flexor carpi radialis muscle. From there, the superficial palmar branch passes anteriorly or through the thenar muscles to join the superficial branch of the ulnar artery forming the superficial palmar arch. At the snuff box, the first dorsal metacarpal artery gives off the princeps pollicis artery to the thumb and terminates in the deep palmar arch. The venous drainage is provided by the basilic and cephalic vein, respectively (superficial system), and by paired concomitant veins (deep venous system) that travel with the arteries and terminate in the cubital vein.

Indication and landmarks
For tissue defects of the upper extremity, the radial forearm flap having a long, wide and reliable pedicle is a very good option. It may be used in different compositions of tissues including fascia, tendons, nerve, and bone. It may also be used as a flow-through flap (eg, defect coverage proximally and revascularization of the fingers distally) or a sensitive flap, including the antebrachial cutaneous nerve [37]. The

distally based pedicled radial forearm flap with retrograde flow is versatile and suitable for reconstructions of the hand, the fingers and the forearm. With a proximally based pedicle and antegrade blood flow the radial forearm flap is usually used for reconstructions around the elbow (**Fig 10.5-1a–b**). It has been challenged by pedicled perforator flaps (chapter 10.4), other fasciocutaneous or free muscle flaps. When planning a radial forearm flap, the patency of the ulnar artery with sufficient blood supply to all fingers must be assessed by the Allen test. This test is used to check the collateral circulation of the hand by alternating evaluation of the patency of the radial and ulnar arteries. It involves the following:
1. The patient is asked to make a fist for ~30 seconds with the hand elevated.
2. Pressure is applied in order to temporarily occlude both the radial land ulnar arteries.
3. The elevated hand is opened and should appear blanched (pallor can be observed at the fingernails).
4. Pressure is released, and the color should return within ~7 seconds, demonstrating adequate recapillarization due to a patent radial/ulnar artery.

In doubtful cases (eg, after direct trauma to the arm or in elderly patients), Duplex sonography or angiography may be indicated in order to demonstrate an adequate perfusion of the palmar arches. The size and position of the skin island for the flap are chosen so that they will fit the defect. The flap usually measures 5–8 cm in width and 8–10 cm in length. Its widest extension may reach from ~3 cm proximal to the cubital fossa to the distal crease of the wrist (ie, 10–12 cm in width and 20–30 cm in length) (**Fig 10.5-1c**). The landmarks consist of the cubital fossa, the palmaris longus muscle and the flexor carpi radialis muscle as well as the snuff box and, if visible or palpable, the cephalic vein.

Surgical technique

General procedure
The patient lies in supine position with the abducted arm on a hand table. Use of a tourniquet is optional, yet most often very useful for flap preparation. Complete exsanguination using an Esmarch bandage is not advisable in order to allow better visual access to the small septal branches.

Distally based pedicled flap with retrograde blood flow
After outlining the island flap on the skin, the dissection begins proximally on the ulnar margin (**Fig 10.5-1d**). The deep fascia of the forearm is included and temporarily fixed to the skin (**Fig 10.5-1e**). The incision is continued distally, identifying and exposing the radial artery and its associated veins. Dissection continues from ulnar to radial beneath the

deep fascia preserving the paratenon of the flexor carpi radialis muscle as far as the ulnar aspect of the intermuscular septum. Next, the skin is incised on the radial side, again including the deep fascia, but taking care not to injure the superficial branch of the radial nerve. The brachioradialis muscle is retracted exposing the radial artery and its accompanying veins within the intermuscular septum radially (**Fig 10.5-1f**). The vascular pedicle can now be isolated as far distally as defined by the pivot point. All small periosteal and muscle branches are coagulated or clipped and transected. Proximal clamping of the vascular pedicle and

releasing the tourniquet allows observing whether distal reperfusion and capillary filling of the flap's septum and skin island and the fingers is adequate. If this is the case, the pedicle is divided proximally and the flap may now be elevated completely and transposed into the defect needing to be covered (**Fig 10.5-1g–h**). The donor site is usually covered with a split-thickness skin graft, possibly supplemented by dermal substitutes (eg, Matriderm® or Integra®) (chapter 10.2). If small-sized flaps are used, donor-site closure may be achieved by primary intention, possibly supplemented by a local advancement and/or a rotation flap,

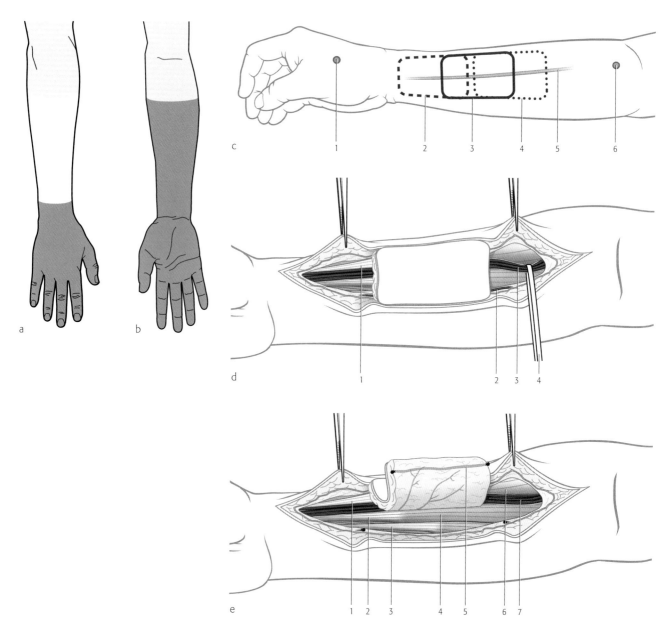

Fig 10.5-1a–h   Radial forearm flap.

a–b Schematic view of the areas which can be covered by the radial forearm flap. Proximally based flap = light blue; distally based flap = dark blue.

a Posterior view.

b Anterior view.

c Planning of a radial forearm flap to be prepared at the middle third of the forearm.
1 Pivot point of the distally based flap pedicle at the first web space.
2 Idealized skin island preparation of a proximally based flap.
3 Outline of the standard skin island that may be used for distally or proximally based flaps.
4 Idealized skin island preparation of a distally based flap.
5 Course of the radial artery.
6 Pivot point of the proximally based flap pedicle between the flexor muscles of the forearm.

d Visual access to the pedicle by skin incisions distally and proximally to the flap (skin island).
1 Tendon of the brachioradialis muscle.
2 Cephalic vein (superficial venous system).
3 Radial artery with concomitant veins.
4 Vessel loop.

e Flap dissection begins at the ulnar side of the skin island until the vascular pedicle can be inspected laterally.
1 Tendon of the brachioradialis muscle.
2 Tendon of the flexor carpi radialis muscle.
3 Tendon of the palmaris longus muscle.
4 Flexor carpi radialis muscle.
5 Cephalic vein.
6 Brachioradialis muscle.
7 Radial artery with concomitant veins.

f The flap is elevated radially from the brachioradialis muscle (red line) and the superficial branch of the radial nerve is separated from the flap's skin island. The pedicle can be identified in the depth.
1 Tendon of the flexor carpi radialis muscle.
2 Superficial branch of the radial nerve.
3 Brachioradialis muscle.

g Transection of the pedicle proximally.
1 Flexor digitorum superficialis muscle.
2 Flexor carpi radialis muscle.
3 Brachioradialis muscle.

h If the pedicle has to be prolonged, a skin incision across the snuff box may be performed (red dotted line).

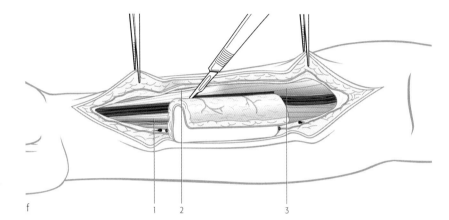

f   1   2   3

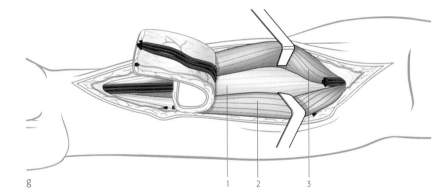

g   1   2   3

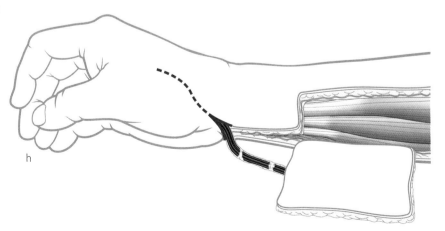

h

pedicled on the ulnar artery. The following modifications of the flap are useful:

Proximally based pedicled flap with antegrade blood flow

Elevation of the flap is performed in analogy to the distally based flap with retrograde blood flow. However, the pedicle is transected distally. The cephalic vein should be routinely included in the dissection of the vascular pedicle and followed as far as the cubital fossa, where a communicating branch to the concomitant veins of the radial vein is encountered. The concomitant veins can be ligated proximally to guarantee venous drainage along the superficial and deep venous system.

Osteofasciocutaneous flap

If a bone segment has to be included within the flap, the skin island should be planned between the insertion of the pronator teres muscle proximally and the tendon of the brachioradialis muscle distally. Dissection of the skin paddle is performed in analogy to the proximally based flap with antegrade blood flow, followed by an incision of the pronator quadratus and the flexor pollicis muscles on the ulnar side of the intermuscular septum. Then a longitudinal osteotomy is performed through the ulnar and radial cortices of the radius. The distal and proximal osteotomies are conducted in an oblique manner in order to reduce the risk of stress fractures. If periosteal and musculoperiosteal attachments are preserved, a bone segment of 10–12 cm by 1.5 cm may now be harvested.

Sensate radial forearm flap

To use the flap as a sensate one, dissection may include the medial or lateral antebrachial cutaneous nerve that is sutured to a recipient nerve using neurography for monitoring.

Further specific variants of the radial forearm flap

It is further possible to divide the skin island longitudinally or transversally into subunits of skin vascularized by independent branches of the radial artery running within the intermuscular septum. Another possibility is to integrate the palmaris longus tendon within the flap as a vascularized tendon, which is a useful option for reconstructions of tendons in the hand. The superficial branch of the radial nerve may be transferred as a vascularized nerve accompanying the radial artery and concomitant veins. The adipofascial flap, ie, a skin island without epidermis and dermis, may be used to replace missing gliding tissue around tendons and nerves in the distal forearm or wrist. Appearance and function of the donor site are better with an adipofascial flap than with a fasciocutaneous flap, because normal skin will still cover the donor site once the adipofascial flap has been elevated. Finally, it is possible to elevate the flap in a suprafascial plane in order to increase the rate of skin-graft take at the donor site, in particular over exposed tendons [38, 39]. Finally, the radial forearm flap is even more versatile, if it is used as a free flap. Its versatility even increases if it is used as a composite free flap.

Outcome

Most complications develop at the donor site including delayed wound healing and/or skin-graft loss with reduced function of the hand as well as hypo- or hyperesthesia along the dorsal aspect of the thumb and index (superficial branch of the radial nerve) (chapter 12.12).

Pearls and pitfalls

- The flap is versatile in its use and one of the best flaps for the hand.
- The flap has a wide, safe, and reliable pedicle.
- Venous drainage may be provided by the superficial and/or deep venous system.
- Gentle dissection of the skin island is advised in order to preserve the paratenon of the flexor tendons and thus ensure skin-graft take.
- Careful flap elevation is recommended in order to preserve septal branches for vascularization of the skin island.
- In situ preservation of the superficial branch of the radial nerve is advised.
- Poor donor-site appearance may result if large skin islands are raised and the donor site is covered with a split-thickness skin graft.

Distally based sural flap (Video 10.5-1)

Anatomy and blood supply

The distally based sural flap is a fasciocutaneous flap with retrograde blood flow based on a dense arterial network surrounding the sural nerve, which arises from the superficial sural artery and the fibular artery. The former originates either from the popliteal artery or from the sural artery [40]. After perforating the fascia that separates the two heads of the gastrocnemius muscles, the superficial sural artery follows the lesser saphenous vein and sural nerve distally to the lateral malleolus. This artery is connected to a consistent network of musculocutaneous perforators from the fibular artery. The most distal one, which may be localized about 4 cm proximal to the lateral malleolus with a handheld Doppler device, is also the most distal pivot point for the flap.

Indication and landmarks

The distally based sural flap has a wide arc of rotation that

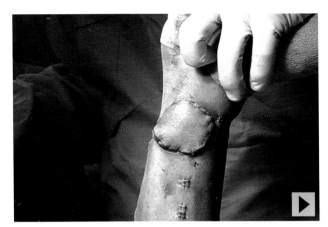

Video 10.5-1   Distally based sural flap.

easily reaches:

- the distal third of the lower leg (chapter 12.13) [41]
- both malleoli
- the posterior aspect and the weight-bearing area of the heel [42]
- the dorsum of the foot (**Fig 10.5-2a–c**).

The skin island may be elevated anywhere along the oblique course of the sural nerve and artery within the distal two thirds of the lower leg and it is designed to fit the defect. As a rule of thumb, the size of the skin island should not exceed the muscle bellies of the gastrocnemius muscle laterally, respectively medially, and it should be centered onto the pedicle (**Fig 10.5-2d**). Landmarks are the popliteal fossa, the crease between both heads of the gastrocnemius muscle and the posterior aspect of the lateral malleolus. Sometimes the lesser saphenous vein is visible.

Surgical technique

General procedure

With the patient in prone or lateral position, the island is outlined and the skin incised along the course of the pedicle in a straight, curved, or zigzag pattern. The distal pedicle is dissected—leaving ample subcutaneous tissue around the sural nerve, the adjacent superficial sural artery, and the lesser saphenous vein—resulting in a 2–4 cm wide adipofascial pedicle (**Fig 10.5-2e**). Next, the skin island is incised including the muscle fascia followed by ligation and transection of the pedicle proximally at the proximal end of the skin island (**Fig 10.5-2f**). Finally, the flap is elevated from proximal to distal as far as the defined musculocutaneous perforator, ie, the pivot point of the flap, and gently rotated into the defect. A donor-site defect of up to 4–6 cm in width may usually be closed primarily, otherwise a split-thickness

skin graft is necessary for coverage (**Fig 10.5-2g**) (chapter 10.2). Following modifications of the flap are useful:

Distally based sural flap with fasciocutaneous pedicle
Some authors advocate elevating the pedicle of a wide flap together with the overlying skin or use a tear drop shaped skin island in order to prevent tension when transferring the flap into its recipient site [43].

Adipofascial sural flap
If a very thin and pliable flap is needed, the flap may be elevated without overlying skin. The donor site may easily be closed by primary closure of the skin. However, the flap needs split-thickness skin-graft coverage that may not take completely [44].

Outcome
While the functional outcome is often good, the reported morbidity may be considerable with rates of partial flap failure of up to 27%, which mostly depends on the patency of the fibular artery. In case of peripheral artery occlusive disease, the sural artery network may be unreliable, possibly contributing to ischemic complications [43]. Fasciocutaneous flaps are more reliable than adipofascial flaps. Cosmetic outcome depends on the need of a skin graft at the donor site. Accordingly, the use of large fasciocutaneous flaps should be thoroughly discussed, especially in case of female patients.

Pearls and pitfalls
- It is a straightforward one-stage operation without microsurgery and few technical pitfalls.
- No major limb vessel is sacrificed.
- Identification of the most distal musculocutaneous perforators (ie, pivot point) and the course of the pedicle is necessary using a handheld Doppler device.
- It has a large arc of rotation.
- A tear-drop shape of the skin island can reduce tension over the pedicle.
- Primary closure of the donor site is required if the skin island is < 4–6 cm.
- It is less reliable than muscle flaps of the leg.

Lateral supramalleolar flap

Anatomy and blood supply
The lateral supramalleolar flap is one of the types of flaps with blood flow, which depend on a dense arterial network that originates from the fibular and the anterior tibial artery. If the fibular artery is divided, the flap (ie, an extended Masquelet flaps) is supplied by a reversed blood flow.

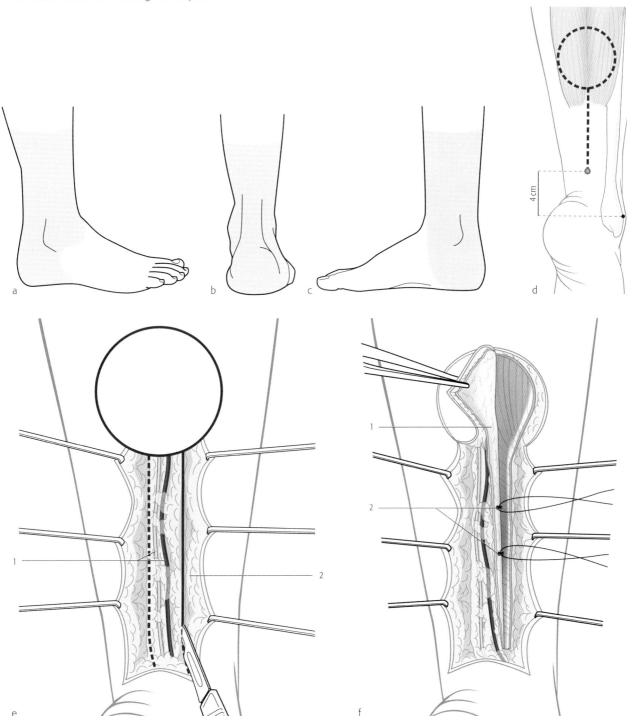

Fig 10.5-2a–g   Distally based sural flap.

a–c   Schematic view of the areas which can be covered by the distally based sural flap.

a   Lateral view.

b   Posterior view.

c   Medial view.

d   Planning of an idealized skin island approximately at the middle to distal third of the gastrocnemius muscle. The planned skin incision follows the course of the flap's pedicle (red dotted line) with its pivot point (blue dot) ~4 cm proximal to the lateral malleolus (black dot).

e   Separation of the skin from the wide flap's pedicle surrounded by subcutaneous tissue (red line).

   1 Sural nerve and lesser saphenous vein.

   2 Subdermal dissection of the flap's pedicle.

f   Flap elevation.

   1 The crural fascia of the muscle is included.

   2 Ligation or cauterization and transection of the perforating vessels originating from the fibular artery laterally is indicated.

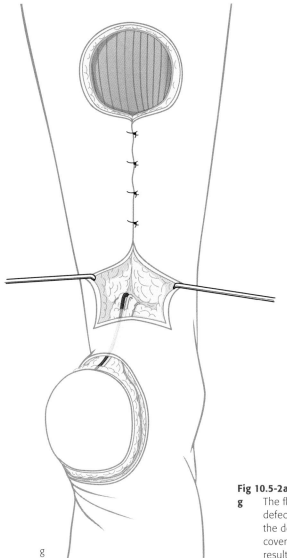

The main vessel that perforates the interosseous membrane is located within the tibiofibular angle—lying ~5 cm proximal to the lateral malleolus and palpable as a depression—and anastomoses with the lateral tarsal artery distally. Proximally, this vascular network is interconnected with the vessels accompanying the superficial fibular nerve. Drainage is provided by a dense superficial venous network that accompanies the arteries.

Fig 10.5-2a–g (cont)   Distally based sural flap.

g   The flap is passed through a tunnel proximally to the traumatic defect. The pedicle now lies subcutaneously. After flap insertion, the donor site and the area of the pedicle at the pivot point is covered with a split-thickness skin graft if primary closure would result in undue tension.

g

Indication and landmarks

Indications for this type of flap depend on the configuration needed. The reach of the flap includes the anteromedial aspect of the lower leg and the medial malleolus (transposition flap), the dorsum, the medial and the lateral aspect of the foot as well as the area of the Achilles tendon and the heel (island flap) (**10.5-3a–d**). The flap is not indicated for defects in the weight-bearing area of the foot, because of its thin and delicate skin. The limits of the flap are the middle third of the lower leg proximally, the tibial crest medially and the posterior margin of the fibula posteriorly. Distally, the flap should always extend beyond the perforating vessels for 2–3 cm (**Fig 10.5-3e**).

Surgical technique

General procedure

With the patient in supine position, the leg is internally rotated and the knee slightly flexed. The common approach to the distally based island flap consists of a lateral incision, which is started anteriorly and prolonged distally to identify the pedicle that lies beneath the superior extensor retinaculum. The retinaculum is also incised in order to identify the tibiofibular ligament (**Fig 10.5-3f**). The flap is usually elevated including the muscle fascia. At this point, it is important to identify the following vessels: the perforating vessel, the cutaneous branch to the flap and the anastomosis with the anterolateral malleolar artery, which is usually ligated. In order to have a proper view, the interosseous membrane needs to be opened (**Fig 10.5-3g**). Now, skin incision is completed proximally and dorsally to identify the fibular muscles. In the next step, the pedicle and the superficial fibular nerve are divided proximally and included within the flap in order not to endanger the vascular structures. The intermuscular septum separating the anterior from the lateral muscle compartment is incised (**Fig 10.5-3h**) and detached from the fibula towards the tarsal sinus (**Fig 10.5-3i**). In order to avoid compression at the pedicle's site distally, it is important to transect the fascia of the extensor digitorum brevis muscle. Donor-site closure includes attachment of the fibular muscle to the extensors and coverage of the defect with a split-thickness skin graft (chapter 10.2). Following modifications of the flap are useful:

Distally based island flap with subcutaneous pedicle

Another variant is the island flap with a subcutaneous pedicle detached from the overlying skin. In this manner, elevation of a reliably perfused skin island is possible, which can be tailored to a distal defect (eg, toes). However, a long subcutaneous pedicle will only supply a small skin island, resulting in very limited defect coverage if the flap is used

at the limits of the arc of rotation (**Fig 10.5-3j**). The perforating vessel is defined as the pivot point of the flap.

Distally based flap with cutaneous pedicle

This variant is easy and quick to elevate as the pedicle is not dissected. Moreover, the skin paddle does not need to be extended down to the exit point of the perforating branch. However, the arc of rotation is limited.

Outcome

The lateral supramalleolar flap—especially the distally based variant without subcutaneous pedicle— is reliable as long as the perforating vessel has been identified prior to surgery [45]. The accompanying functional loss is minimal in daily activities. Cosmetic outcome at the donor site is the main drawback, because primary closure is hardly ever possible and a skin graft applied to the distal lower leg has an unpleasant appearance. Accordingly, the possible use of this flap should be thoroughly discussed with the patient in advance.

Pearls and pitfalls

- It is a reliable flap for small defects of the distal third of the lower leg and proximal half of the foot.
- It is an unreliable flap for injuries at the lateral perimalleolar region (ie, point of emergence of the feeder artery).
- It is a straightforward, one-stage operation without need for microsurgery and few technical pitfalls.
- No major limb vessel needs to be sacrificed.
- In order to plan the exact localization of the flap, identification of the perforating vessel branch between tibia and fibula using a handheld Doppler device is essential.
- If a distally based flap is elevated, the opening of the interosseous membrane is mandatory in order to have a complete and safe view of the perforating vessel branch.
- Long and adaptable arc of rotation allows the flap to be tailored to the needs of the defect by including the descending vessel branch or by placing the skin island more proximally on the leg.
- Postoperative elevation of the limb is often mandatory, particularly in the distally based variant of the flap (ie, retrograde blood flow).

Medial plantar flap (instep flap)

Anatomy and blood supply

The medial plantar flap consists of glabrous skin that accounts for only 4% of the total body surface. This specialized skin resists tangential stress because of its dermal-epidermal junctions and fibrous septa, offers adequate padding over bony prominences, and permits perception of the environ-

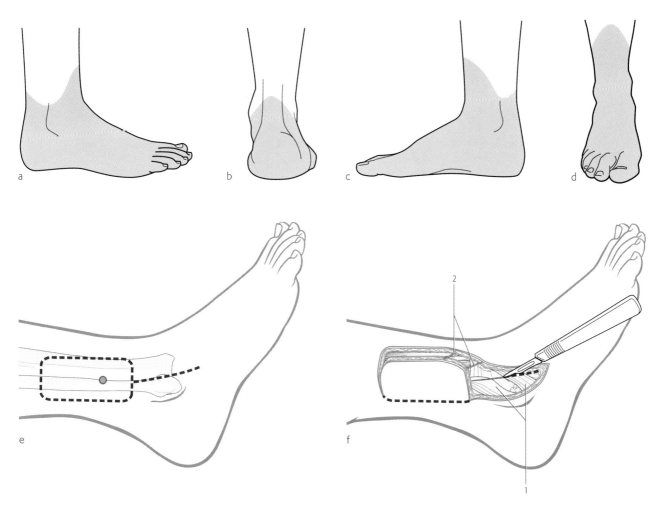

Fig 10.5-3a–j Lateral supramalleolar flap.
a–d Schematic view of the areas that can be covered by the lateral supramalleolar flap.
a Lateral view.
b Posterior view.
c Medial view.
d Anterior view.
e Planning of the flap to fit a defect (eg, distally based flap = red dotted line) with a skin island based on the perforating vessel branch (pivot point = blue dot) ~2–3 cm proximal to the flap's distal end.
f Proximal and anterior skin incision that is prolonged distally to identify the pedicle. Division of the superior extensor retinaculum.
  1 Superior extensor retinaculum of the foot.
  2 Branches of the superficial fibular nerve.

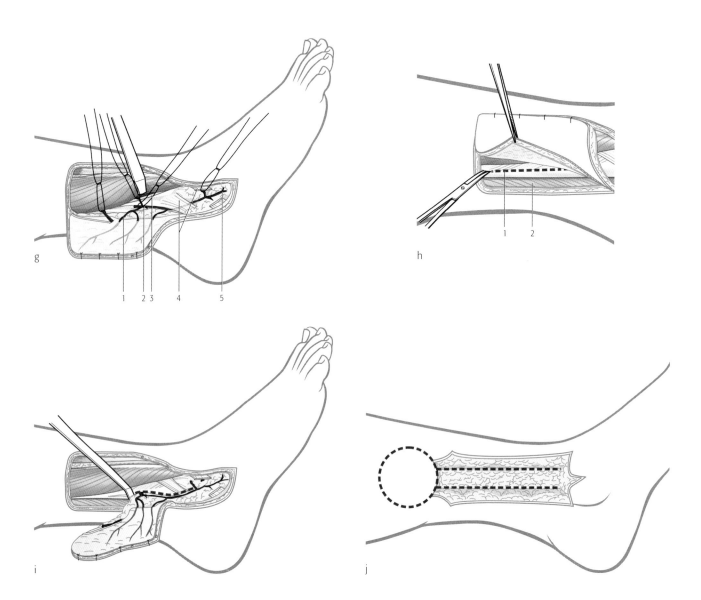

Fig 10.5-3a–j (cont)   Lateral supramalleolar flap.
g   Dissection of the pedicle distally. Division of the superficial fibular nerve proximally and the arteriovenous branches laterally.
   1 Branches of the anterolateral malleolar artery.
   2 Anterior tibial artery.
   3 Deep fibular nerve.
   4 Superior extensor retinaculum.
   5 Vascular anastomosis of the pedicle with lateral tarsal artery.
h   Completion of the skin incision dorsally to identify the fibular muscles.
   1 Incision of the intermuscular septum (red dotted line) separating the anterior from the lateral muscle compartment at the level of the fibula.
   2 Fibularis longus muscle.
i   Freeing of the flap (red dotted line) by detachment from the intermuscular septum, separating the anterior from the lateral compartment.
j   Alternatively, the flap (idealized skin island) may be dissected as an axially perfused island flap with a wide subcutaneous pedicle (red dotted line).

ment due to the high concentration of mechanoreceptors. Therefore, plantar glabrous skin is particularly suited for zones involved in weight bearing and walking.

Behind the medial malleolus, the posterior tibial artery is accompanied by the concomitant veins and the tibial nerve and is located between the flexor digitorum longus muscle anteriorly and the flexor hallucis longus muscle posteriorly. More distally, the artery bifurcates into two terminal branches—the medial plantar artery anteromedially and the lateral plantar artery more posterolaterally. These arteries, which are also accompanied by concomitant veins and a nerve, pass deep to the abductor hallucis muscle and enter the plantar surface of the foot. More distally, in the mid sole, the artery, and nerve lie in a plane beneath the plantar fascia (plantar aponeurosis) and the flexor digitorum muscle. The medial plantar artery is 3–5 cm long and has an external diameter of 1–2 mm. It is possible to prolong the pedicle of the flap by including a portion of the posterior tibial artery proximal to the bifurcation of the medial and lateral plantar artery. In this context, it is noteworthy that the lateral plantar artery is much larger in diameter than the medial plantar artery, representing the continuation of the posterior tibial artery. The medial plantar nerve provides sensation to the medial three and one-half toes as well as the medial sole. Sensation to the plantar mid sole skin is provided by cutaneous branches arising along the course of the medial and lateral plantar nerves coursing distally in their respective sulci.

Indication and landmarks

The most common indication for this flap is to resurface weight-bearing areas on the plantar surface of the foot, especially over the metatarsal heads and the heel. The reach of the flap further includes the posterior aspect of the heel (**Fig 10.5-4a–b**) (chapter 12.14). If care is taken to avoid injury to the lateral surface of the mid sole, the insult to the donor site of the non-weight-bearing surface is minimal. The fasciocutaneous flap preserves the underlying muscles and is usually elevated as a true neurosensory flap. In adults, the average dimensions of the flap from the mid sole (avoiding the heel, metatarsal heads and lateral mid sole) are 5–7 cm in length and 3–4 cm in width (**Fig 10.5-4c**).

Surgical technique

The patency of the anterior and posterior tibial artery has to be demonstrated preoperatively. Normal blood supply is sufficient to supply the entire mid sole plantar fasciocutaneous flap. With the patient in supine position, the extremity is elevated, exsanguinated, and the tourniquet inflated.

Usually the flap is marked out centered on the medial plantar artery, preserving the deep plantar arch. The mid sole flap is outlined 2–3 cm proximally to the metatarsal heads, distal to the heel, sparing the lateral mid sole weight-bearing area.

The flap is incised distally and medially towards the posterior aspect of the medial malleolus, exposing the medial plantar artery and accompanying nerves and the posterior tibial artery (**Fig 10.5-4d**). Following ligation of the medial plantar artery distal to the flap, dissection continues proximally beneath the plantar aponeurosis, including the medial plantar artery and the neurovascular bundles to the overlying fascia and skin (**Fig 10.5-4e-f**). This requires the intraneural dissection of the mid sole cutaneous branches from those fascicles supplying three and one-half toes. Often the second common digital nerve is included within the branches to the flap in order to avoid the difficulties that would otherwise be encountered in separation. The flap is elevated in a distal to proximal direction in the plane between the plantar fascia and the first layer of muscles. Fascial communications to the clefts between the underlying muscles (abductor hallucis and flexor digitorum brevis muscles and abductor digiti minimi and flexor digitorum brevis muscles) are cut.

Fascicles from the lateral plantar nerve may also be included within the flap following intraneural dissection. The length of these fascicles is kept as long as possible when they are cut proximally. The flexor digitorum brevis muscle may require sectioning proximally in order to expose these fascicles. The medial plantar artery and associated fascicles of the medial plantar nerve are traced proximally to the abductor hallucis muscle. Depending on the length of the neurovascular pedicle required, the abductor hallucis muscle may be cut and dissection continued on the ankle.

Once an adequate pedicle length is achieved, the flap is monitored for perfusion while dissection continues at the recipient site (**Fig 10.5-4g**).

Outcome

The medial plantar flap is reliable, especially the variant without subcutaneous pedicle as long as the perforating vessel has been identified prior to surgery. Only minimal functional loss in daily activities results. The cosmetic outcome of the donor site, however, is a major drawback, because primary closure is almost never possible. Fortunately, the skin graft is applied to the non-weight-bearing area of the mid foot.

Pearls and pitfalls

- It is a reliable flap for small defects of the weight-bearing areas of the foot and posterior aspect of the heel, especially if elevated as a neurosensory flap.
- No major limb vessel needs to be sacrificed.
- Increase of pedicle length is possible by including a portion of the posterior tibial artery proximal to the bifurcation.
- There is firm adhesion to the underlying osseous-tendinous structures minimizing tangential stress.

- Hyperkeratosis may appear at the junction of the plantar flap and adjacent skin.
- Separation of the cutaneous fascicles from the medial plantar nerve may be difficult, often requiring sacrifice of the common digital nerve of the second web space.
- If used as a free flap, this flap only has limited advantages for replacement of glabrous defects of the hand due to its bulk.

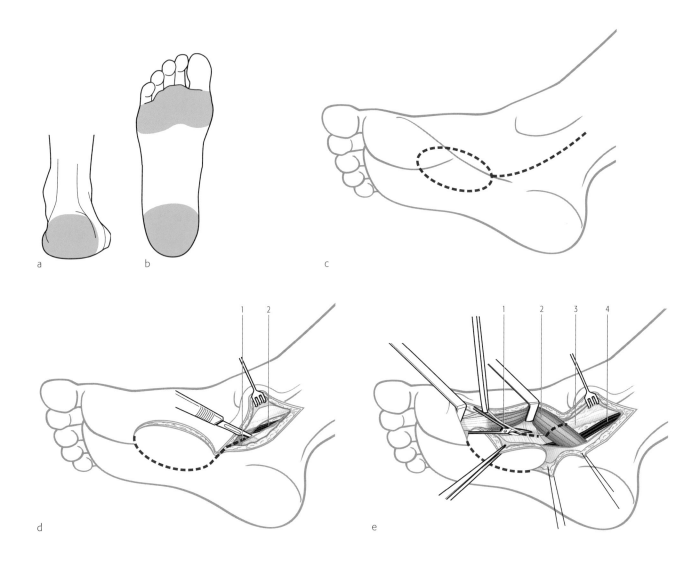

a   b   c

d   e

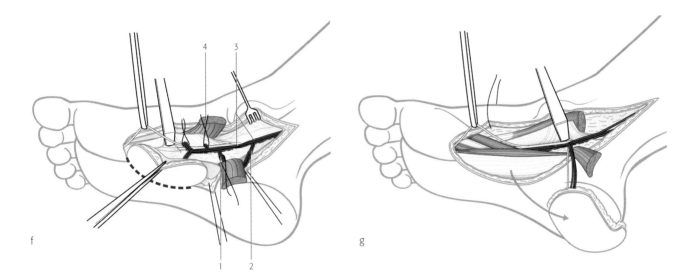

Fig 10.5-4a–g   Medial plantar flap.
a–b   Schematic view of the areas that can be covered by the medial plantar flap.
a   Posterior view.
b   Plantar view.
c   Planning of an idealized skin island of the flap that includes the non-weight-bearing area of the sole of the foot.
d   Medial skin incision and freeing of the fascia covering the abductor hallucis muscle. Dorsal to the medial malleolus an incision of the flexor retinaculum (1) is made to free the posterior tibial artery and its concomitant veins (2).
e   After freeing of the abductor hallucis muscle, both the plantar fascia and the muscle are transected (red dotted line). Care is taken to identify the medial plantar artery and the medial branch of the plantar nerve.
   1   Medial branch of the plantar nerve.
   2   Abductor hallucis muscle.
   3   Tendon of flexor hallucis longus muscle.
   4   Posterior tibial artery and concomitant veins.
f   Step-by-step freeing of the medial branch of the plantar nerve, from distal to proximal, in order to separate it from the superficial branch of the medial plantar artery that supplies the flap.
   1   Ligation of the pedicle supplying the abductor hallucis muscle.
   2   Lateral plantar artery and concomitant veins.
   3   Medial plantar artery and concomitant veins.
   4   Transected abductor hallucis muscle.
g   After complete freeing of the pedicle, the flap's arc of rotation may reach defects including the weight-bearing area and the dorsal aspect of the heel. Donor-site closure includes approximation of the abductor hallucis muscle to the flexor digitorum brevis muscle and split-thickness skin-graft coverage. Exposed plantar fascia may be excised.

10.5.3 Muscle flaps

Gastrocnemius flap—medial head (Video 10.5-2)

Anatomy and blood supply

The gastrocnemius muscle forms the superficial part of the triceps muscle of the lower leg. The medial head originates at the posterior surface of the femoral condyle and inserts together with the lateral head into a common tendon of 10–15 cm in length. The medial head is longer and, thus, more often used as a flap than the lateral head. The corresponding skin territory covering the muscles is ~23 cm long and 10 cm wide [46]. The medial head is about 15–20 cm long, 8 cm wide and 2–3 cm thick. The medial sural artery (4–5 cm long; 2–2.5 mm in diameter) arises from the popliteal artery 1–2 cm proximal to the knee joint and enters the muscle 4–5 cm distal to the popliteal crease, slightly lateral to the mid line of the muscle belly (Mathes and Nahai [15]: type I blood supply). In the majority of cases, the intramuscular pedicle divides into two or more branches, allowing for a longitudinal splitting of the distal half of the muscle into two separate units (**Fig 10.5-5a**). Venous drainage is provided by paired concomitant veins that travel with the artery and drain into the popliteal vein.

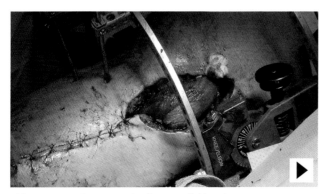

Video 10.5-2 Gastrocnemius flap—medial head.

Indication and landmarks

The arc of rotation of the muscle flap allows for safe coverage of defects of the anterior and medial aspect of the knee, the proximal third of the lower leg, and the popliteal fossa (**Fig 10.5-5b–c**). The landmarks are the knee-joint line, the posteromedial border of the tibia, the medial malleolus and the posterior mid line of the lower leg. With the foot held in forced dorsal flexion, the medial gastrocnemius muscle may easily be outlined 2–3 cm dorsal to the posteromedial border of the tibia.

Surgical technique

General procedure

With the patient in supine position and the contralateral buttock elevated, the affected lower leg is externally rotated and the knee slightly flexed. The usual approach consists of a straight incision parallel and ~2–3 cm dorsal to the posteromedial border of the tibia, curving slightly to join the popliteal fossa (**Fig 10.5-5d**). The greater saphenous vein and its accompanying nerve are gently retracted under the medial skin flap (**Fig 10.5-5e**), whereas the sural nerve that runs from proximal to distal between the two heads of the gastrocnemius muscle before perforating the fascia at the junction of the proximal and middle third of the leg is visible. Next, the junction between the medial head and soleus muscles is identified and the muscle fascia (ie, crural fascia) is incised. Further dissection within this avascular plane should be blunt until the insertion of the Achilles tendon becomes visible. If present, the tendon of the plantaris muscle is identified and preserved as it lies on the soleus muscle. The medial head is transected distally at the musculotendinous junction and subsequently detached from the lateral head until enough length has been gained while the vascular pedicle emerging from the depth of the popliteal fossa is carefully spared (**Fig 10.5-5f**). Longitudinal, respectively transverse, mesh-like incisions of the muscle fascia at the undersurface of the flap and transection of the proximal tendon allow for increases in the width and the length of the flap as well as its arc of rotation by 3–4 cm. Denervation of the muscle, if indicated or in order to exclude postoperative pain, may be performed proximally in the popliteal fossa in order to avoid injury to muscle branches. The flap may now be rotated directly into the defect or passed through a subcutaneous tunnel and fixed to the adjacent tissues (**Fig 10.5-5g**). The muscle belly is covered with a split-thickness skin graft (chapter 10.2) and the donor site may be closed primarily. The following modifications of the flap are useful:

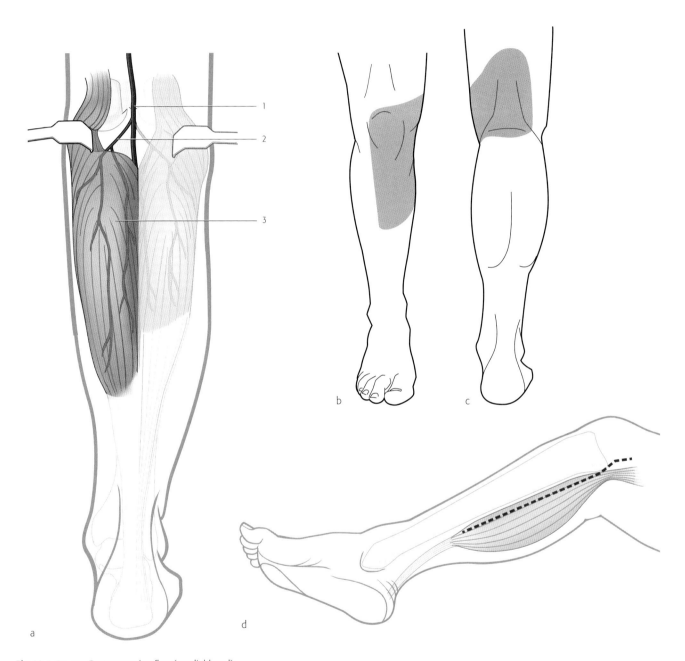

Fig 10.5-5a–g Gastrocnemius flap (medial head).

a Two-headed gastrocnemius muscle supplied by sural arteries proximally originating from the popliteal artery. The arteries are accompanied by concomitant veins and a nerve. Each head may be elevated individually. Note that the lateral head is ~25% shorter than the medial head.

    1 Popliteal artery.
    2 Medial sural artery.
    3 Medial muscle head.

b–c Schematic view of the areas that can be covered by the medial gastrocnemius muscle flap.

b Anterior view.

c Posterior view.

d Anteromedial skin incision with the affected leg externally rotated and the knee slightly flexed. The incision parallels the tibia at its middle third ~2–3 cm dorsal to the posteromedial border and is curvilinear more proximally to join the popliteal fossa (red dotted line).

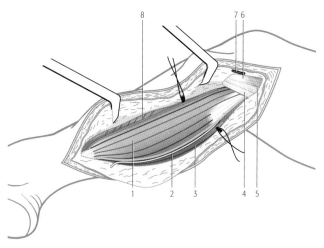

e

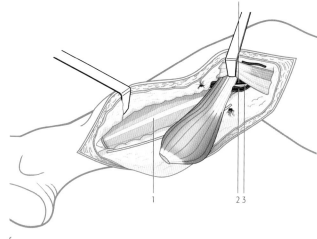

f

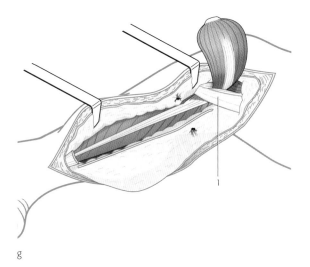

g

Fig 10.5-5a–g (cont)   Gastrocnemius flap (medial head).

e   Visual access to the intermuscular area (dark blue line) separating the soleus muscle and the medial head of the gastrocnemius muscle. As well as to the intermuscular area (light blue line) separating the two gastrocnemius muscles.
   1 Gastrocnemius muscle (medial head).
   2 Sural nerve.
   3 Gastrocnemius muscle (lateral head).
   4 Tendon of the semitendinosus muscle.
   5 Tendon of the gracilis muscle.
   6 Tendon of the sartorius muscle.
   4–6 Pes anserinus.
   7 Greater saphenous vein.
   8 Soleus muscle.

f   Distal transection of the muscle (usually within the tendinous part) and step-wise elevation from distally to proximally. If present, the tendon of the plantaris longus muscle is identified beneath the elevated muscle belly.
   1 Tendon of the plantaris longus muscle.
   2 Neurovascular bundle entering the proximal segment of the gastrocnemius muscle (medial head).
   3 Tibial nerve.
   4 Popliteal artery and concomitant veins.

g   The flap's arc of rotation may be increased to easily reach the anterior side of the knee joint if the flap is detached from its origin at the femur. However, the flap has to be passed beneath the pes anserinus (tendons of the semitendinosus, gracilis and sartorius muscles) (1).

Musculocutaneous flap

The medial gastrocnemius muscle may also be elevated with a pliable and sensitive skin island measuring at most 23 cm in length and 10 cm in width, extending from the popliteal fossa to ~5 cm proximal to the medial malleolus and from 1 cm posterior to the posteromedial border of the tibia to the mid line of the calf. The skin island is vascularized through fascial vessel branches and musculocutaneous perforators of the sural artery. The skin is first incised and then fixed to the gastrocnemius muscle in order to avoid a shearing injury to the perforators. The donor site can only be covered by a skin graft, which results in a cosmetically poor outcome. The musculocutaneous flap variation has a smaller arc of rotation medially than the muscle flap due to the variable size of the skin island. However, it may reach from the lower thigh to the middle third of the lower leg.

Musculocutaneous flap with vascularized tendon

If the skin island overlaps the musculotendinous junction and remains attached to the tendon, the distal part of the medial gastrocnemius muscle may be elevated as a vascularized tendon, which is an option for reconstructions of the patellar or quadriceps tendon [47].

Outcome

The medial gastrocnemius muscle flap is very reliable as cover for defects around the knee and proximal tibia medially. The loss of function is minimal for daily activities because this is well compensated by the remaining lateral head and the soleus muscle. Athletes or climbers may experience some loss of strength with movements such as stair climbing [48]. Cosmetically the outcome at the donor site is quite acceptable if primary skin closure can be performed. Any skin graft applied to the calf will have an unsightly appearance. Accordingly, the use of musculocutaneous flaps should thoroughly be discussed with the patient.

Pearls and pitfalls

- It is a straightforward procedure with few technical pitfalls.
- There is a wide and consistent pedicle that does not require microsurgical dissection.
- Branching of the vascular pedicle within the muscle allows for longitudinal splitting of the distal half.
- Transverse mesh-like incisions of the muscle fascia and transection of the proximal tendon allow for increasing the size and the arc of rotation of the flap.
- The musculocutaneous variation allows the transfer of a large island of pliable and sensitive skin.
- For simultaneous elevation of both medial and lateral heads, a mid-line incision in prone position is recommended.
- Contour deformity is acceptable when using only one head of the muscle.

Gastrocnemius flap—lateral head

Anatomy and blood supply

The lateral head of the gastrocnemius muscle originates at the lateral condyle of the femur. It is 12–17 cm long, 6 cm wide, and 2–3 cm thick. The lateral sural artery (4–5 cm in length; 2–2.5 mm in diameter) arises from the popliteal artery 1–2 cm proximal to the knee joint (Mathes and Nahai [15]: type I blood supply). It enters the lateral muscle head 4–5 cm distal to the popliteal crease (**Fig 10.5-6a**). Venous drainage is provided by paired concomitant veins that run with the artery and drain into the popliteal vein.

Indication and landmarks

The lateral gastrocnemius muscle is used less frequently than the medial head not only because it is shorter but because the fibula hinders an easy transfer to the anterior aspect of the knee including the tibial crest. Nevertheless, this flap is essential to safely cover defects in the area of the popliteal fossa and the anterolateral aspect of the proximal third of the lower leg (**Fig 10.5-6b–c**). The musculocutaneous variation of the flap has a smaller arc of rotation laterally, reaching from the lower thigh to the middle third of the lower leg.

The landmarks consist of the knee joint, the anterior margin of the lateral head of the gastrocnemius, the lateral malleolus, and the posterior mid line of the lower leg. With the foot held in forced dorsal flexion, the lateral gastrocnemius muscle is easily outlined 2–3 cm dorsal to the intermuscular septum.

Surgical technique

With the patient in supine position and the ipsilateral buttock elevated, the affected lower leg is internally rotated and the knee slightly flexed. The anterolateral incision parallels the posterior border of the fibula (**Fig 10.5-6d**). At the level of the fibular neck, the common fibular nerve that courses between the posterior border of the biceps femoris muscle and the lateral head of the gastrocnemius muscle must carefully be identified and preserved. After incision of the muscle fascia laterally, blunt dissection is performed within the avascular plane between the gastrocnemius and soleus muscles as far the tendinous junction forming the Achilles tendon. Transection is performed at the musculotendinous junction distally, followed by subsequent separation from the medial head until enough length is obtained. Care must be taken to spare the vascular pedicle of the sural artery emerging from the popliteal fossa. If denervation of the muscle is indicated, it should be performed proximally in the popliteal fossa in order to avoid injury to the muscular branches. The technique of flap transposition

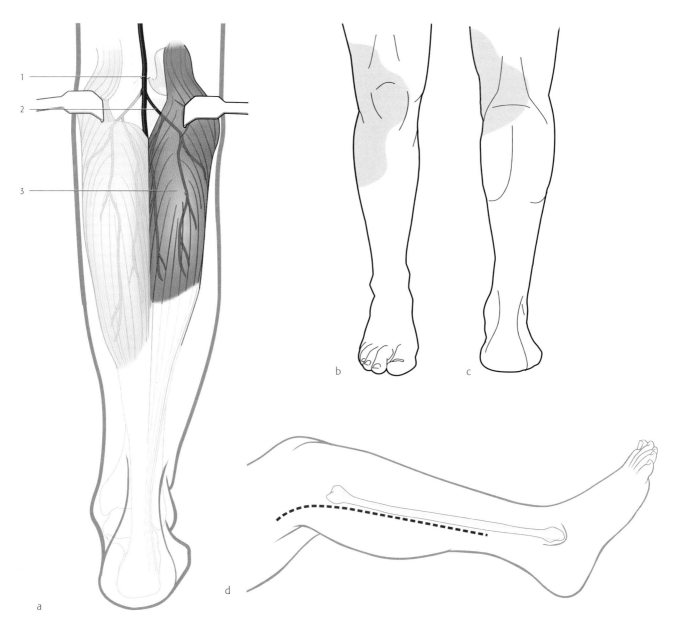

Fig 10.5-6a–d Gastrocnemius flap (lateral head).

a Two-headed gastrocnemius muscle supplied by sural arteries proximally originating from the popliteal artery. The arteries are accompanied by concomitant veins and a nerve. Each head may be elevated individually. Note that the lateral head is ~25% shorter than the medial head.

    1 Popliteal artery.
    2 Lateral sural artery.
    3 Lateral muscle head.

b–c Schematic view of the areas that can be covered by the lateral gastrocnemius muscle.

b Anterior view.

c Posterior view.

d Anterolateral skin incision with the affected leg internally rotated and the knee slightly flexed. The incision parallels the posterior border of the fibula and is curvilinear more proximally to join the popliteal fossa (red dotted line).

into the defect, muscle coverage and donor site closure is performed in the same way as for the medial gastrocnemius flap.

The same variations as for the medial calf region are also possible for the lateral gastrocnemius flap, with the outcome being similar. However, the arc of rotation is considerably shorter in comparison to the flap at the medial aspect of the calf.

Outcome

The lateral gastrocnemius muscle flap is very reliable as cover for defects around the knee and the fibula. The loss of function is minimal for daily activities because it is well compensated by the remaining stronger and bigger medial head and the soleus muscle.

Pearls and pitfalls

In comparison to the medial gastrocnemius flap, the dissection of the lateral flap is more demanding (common fibular nerve), while it has a smaller volume and a smaller arc of rotation.

Soleus flap (Video 10.5-3)

Anatomy and blood supply

The soleus muscle has a tapered shape from proximal to distal. It is positioned in the deep part of the triceps muscle of the lower leg. The two-headed muscle (ie, tibial and fibular head) originates medially on the posterior aspect of the tibial head and laterally on the posterior and medial aspect of the fibular head. Distally it joins the tendinous parts of the gastrocnemius muscles to form the Achilles ten-

don. The soleus receives its blood supply proximally from major pedicles originating from the posterior tibial artery 3–4 cm distal to the soleus arcade, respectively from the fibular artery. Distally, the most reliable minor pedicles are located between 6–7 cm [49] and 11–13 cm [50] proximal to the medial malleolus (Mathes and Nahai [15]: type II blood supply) (**Fig 10.5-7a**). Venous drainage is provided by paired concomitant veins that course with the arteries and drain into the tibial or fibular vein. The soleus muscle belly is wider than the gastrocnemius heads. Its width may be increased by longitudinal, mesh-like incisions of the posterior muscle fascia.

Indication and landmarks

The soleus muscle may be elevated as an entire flap or, more commonly, as a medial hemisoleus flap based on the proximal major pedicles as cover for defects in the middle third of the tibia. A distally pedicled hemisoleus flap that depends on minor pedicles may also be elevated. The reach may go as far distally as the lower leg and almost to the proximal foot (**Fig 10.5-7b**). The landmarks consist of the medial malleolus, the Achilles tendon and the posterior border of the tibia.

Surgical technique

General procedure

With the patient in supine position, the contralateral buttock slightly elevated and the lower leg externally rotated, the anteromedial skin incision parallels the palpable crease between the medial head of the gastrocnemius muscle and the soleus muscle, which may be identified better by passive dorsal flexion of the foot. In case the skin-bridge between the surgical incision and the defect appears to be too narrow, the incision may include the defect—often close to the tibial crest—and may be extended posteriorly towards the lateral crease between the two muscles mentioned above (**Fig 10.5-7c**). Both the greater saphenous vein and the saphenous nerve should be preserved. After incision of the thin muscle fascia medially, blunt dissection is performed between the medial gastrocnemius and soleus muscle posteriorly and between the soleus and flexor digitorum longus muscle anteriorly, taking care to spare the posterior tibial artery and veins (**Fig 10.5-7d–f**). At this point the decision has to be made about the final composition of the flap, ie, hemisoleus or full muscle; proximal or distal pedicle. Proximally, the dissection is continued until the desired arc of rotation is reached. Distally, the flap is sharply separated from the Achilles tendon (**Fig 10.5-7g**). The muscle is then transposed into the defect, fixed and covered with a split-thickness skin graft (chapter 10.2) and the donor site

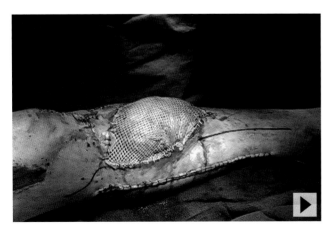

Video 10.5-3   Proximally based soleus flap.

closed primarily. The following modifications of the flap are useful:

Hemisoleus flap with proximal pedicle

The muscle belly has to be split longitudinally along the mid line. All secondary branches have to be transected for the medial hemisoleus flap whereas the vascular branches to the lateral head should be spared. This flap is well suited for narrow defects within the middle third of the lower leg, where less bulk is needed and functional loss is limited (**Fig 10.5-7h**).

Hemisoleus flap (reversed flap) with distal pedicle

The muscle is split proximally and rotated about the two most distal minor pedicles originating from the posterior tibial artery. This technique allows the transfer of one half or up to two thirds of the muscle (**Fig 10.5-7i**) [49].

Musculocutaneous flap

A skin component may be marked as a peninsula or as a circumscribed island. The musculocutaneous hemisoleus flap may either be transposed on the medial or on the lateral side. Distally it can reach to the ankle or even further if surgical delay or preconditioning is applied (chapter 10.3).

Outcome

The proximally based soleus flap is very reliable. Only major injury to the proximal pedicles resulting from direct trauma or peripheral artery occlusive disease may cause partial or total flap necrosis (chapter 11.3). The distally based flap is less reliable with a failure rate of ~20% [49]. Flap morbidity may be reduced substantially, if two distal minor pedicles perfuse the flap and if only the medial part is used after discarding its proximal third (chapter 12.11) [51].

Pearls and pitfalls

- It is a straightforward procedure with few technical pitfalls.
- There is a wide and consistent pedicle that does not require microsurgical dissection.
- The incision to approach the flap may include the defect in order to avoid a narrow skin bridge between the defect and the surgical approach.
- Musculocutaneous variation transfers a large island of pliable and sensitive skin.
- Preservation of two distal minor pedicles is necessary for the less reliable distally based hemisoleus flap.
- Little functional donor site morbidity for daily living activities.
- There is substantial loss of strength if both soleus and gastrocnemius muscles are used, therefore, contraindicated in athletes and climbers.

- Poor appearance results if the donor site has to be covered with a skin graft.

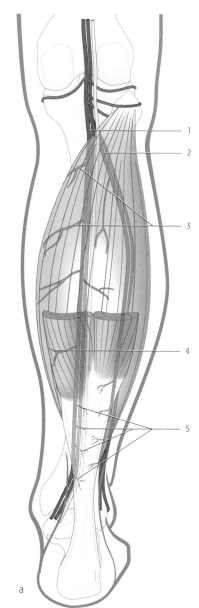

a

Fig 10.5-7a–i Soleus flap.

a   The muscle is supplied by various pedicles originating from the posterior tibial artery and the fibular artery. The arteries are accompanied by concomitant veins and a nerve.
1 Posterior tibial artery.
2 Fibular artery.
3 Two to three major pedicles proximally.
4 Secondary pedicle.
5 Variable number of minor pedicles distally.

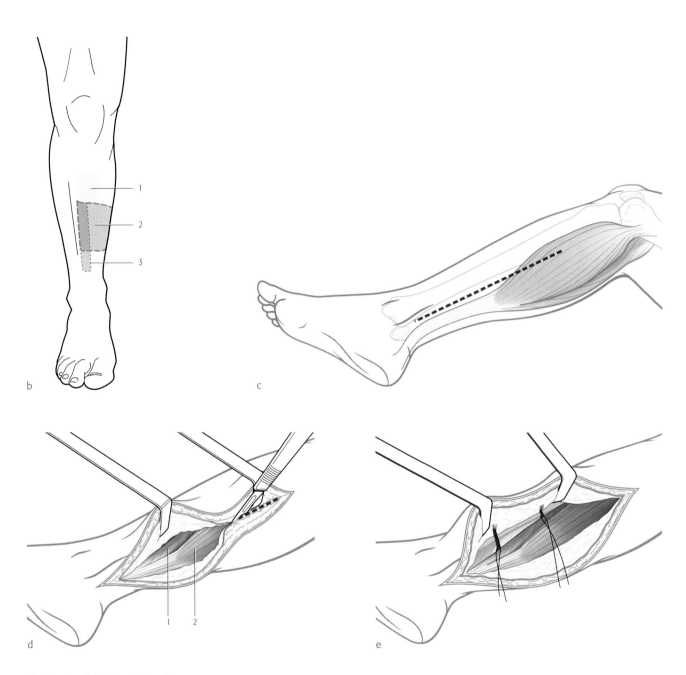

b

c

d

e

Fig 10.5-7a–i (cont)   Soleus flap.
b   Schematic view of the areas that can be covered by the soleus muscle showing the flap's arc of rotation in its different variations.
  1 Proximally based hemisoleus muscle.
  2 Soleus muscle.
  3 Distally based hemisoleus muscle.
c   Anteromedial skin incision with the affected leg externally rotated and the knee slightly flexed. The planned incision (red dotted line) parallels the crease between medial gastrocnemius muscle and soleus muscle that is identified by active contraction of the calf muscles or by passive dorsal flexion of the foot ~ 1 cm dorsal to the posterior border of the tibia.
d   Preservation of the greater saphenous vein and its accompanying nerve within the subcutaneous tissue is indicated. Incision of the crural fascia (red dotted line) and bilateral skin flap elevation.
  1 Soleus muscle.
  2 Gastrocnemius muscle (medial head).
e   Visual access to the intermuscular area (dark blue line) separating the soleus muscle and the medial head of the gastrocnemius muscle.

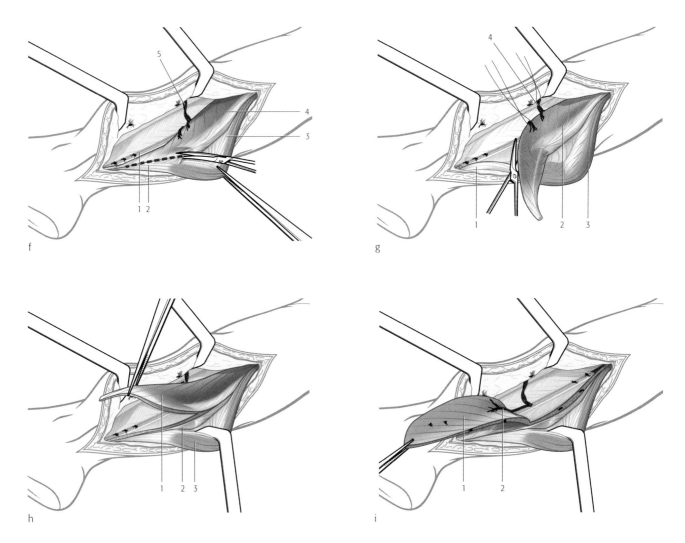

Fig 10.5-7a–i (cont)   Soleus flap.

f   Incision of the fragile muscle fascia and blunt dissection separating the bellies of the soleus muscle and the medial head of the gastrocnemius muscle (red dotted line).
1 Posterior tibial artery, concomitant veins, and tibial nerve.
2 Achilles tendon.
3 Gastrocnemius muscle (medial head).
4 Soleus muscle.
5 Secondary vascular pedicle within the middle third of the muscle.

g   After distal transection of the tendon, sharp dissection of the soleus muscle from the tendinous part of the gastrocnemius muscle distally where both muscles form the Achilles tendon. Gentle freeing of the muscle fascia fixed to the fibula.
1 Achilles tendon.
2 Soleus muscle.
3 Gastrocnemius muscle (medial head).
4 If the required length of the flap mandates it, secondary pedicles originating from the fibular artery are ligated or cauterized.

h   Narrow defects at the anterior and proximal aspect of the tibia may be covered with the proximally based hemisoleus flap.
1 Medial hemisoleus flap.
2 Lateral hemisoleus flap.
3 Gastrocnemius muscle (medial head).

i   Narrow defects at the anterior and distal aspect of the tibia may be covered with the distally based hemisoleus flap. Its elevation starts proximally and continues to the level of the secondary pedicle. The latter is approximately located in the middle of the tibial mid third.
1 Medial hemisoleus flap.
2 Vascular pedicle.

10.6 Free flaps—principles

Authors   Stefan Langer, Hans-Ulrich Steinau, Christoph Andree, Lars Steinsträßer

10.6.1 History

Since the 1980s, the microvascular technique has become a standard procedure particularly in plastic surgery. It is of great help for reconstructive surgery because almost any defect at any site of the body has become "repairable" using autologous tissue transplantation. The range of flaps has increased dramatically during the last decades, as a result of various anatomical works describing meticulously the anatomy of muscle pedicles (chapter 10.3). By now, almost every muscle can be raised as a free flap (**Fig 10.6-1a–d**). With increasing interest in the vascular distribution within muscles, the contribution of blood circulation in muscles for the

overlying skin was finally recognized, ie, each superficial muscle provides vascular connections via musculocutaneous and/or septocutaneous perforating vessels to the overlying skin (chapter 2). Accordingly, it became possible to include a segment of skin with the muscle flap, thus creating the musculocutaneous flap [52]. Based on Taylor's concept of skin circulation [35], fasciocutaneous [53] or perforator flaps [54] have been described that are widely used today (chapter 10.3). Refinements in free-flap surgery are made with regard to donor-site morbidity (ie, functional loss, extensive scaring, and contour deformity) and the choice of the most suitable flap for a specific defect including tissue composition, volume, texture, and color.

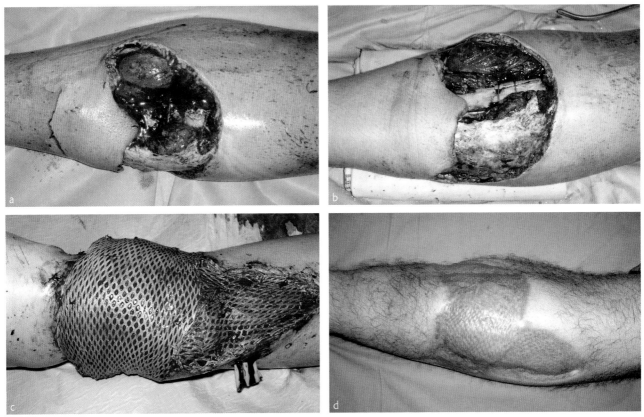

Fig 10.6-1a–d   Free gracilis muscle flap.
a   Open fracture of the middle third of the left lower leg with subsequent soft-tissue loss and exposed tibial bone following two debridement procedures after initial open reduction and internal fixation (ORIF).
b   Resulting soft-tissue defect and bare tibial bone after radical debridement.
c   Immediately after defect coverage using a free gracilis muscle flap and meshed split-thickness skin graft from the ipsilateral leg.
d   Fourteen months after soft-tissue reconstruction. The muscle has atrophied, the split-thickness skin graft remains hyperpigmented and shiny with a permanent diamond-shaped pattern.

10.6.2   Basic considerations in free flap surgery

Surgical skills

Any surgeon can be trained in microsurgery. He or she requires similar technical skills, good eye-hand coordination, great care in handling tissues in general and soft tissues in particular, as well as much patience and practice. Given proper instruction and training in a microsurgical laboratory course of 1–4 weeks, the necessary skills needed to pass into the clinical setting can be acquired. Before actually performing an anastomosis, several preconditions should be met as defined by Acland [55]:
- careful preoperative planning
- enjoyable working environment
- appropriate equipment (surgical loupes, microscope, micro instruments, and sutures) adapted to these vascular calibers
- comfortable sitting position and hand support
- anatomical knowledge of access and exposure
- proper choice of vessels
- hemostasis.

Equipment for microsurgery

The microsurgeon sees his operative field magnified through two instruments: the surgical loupes and the operating microscope. The operating microscope traditionally provides the necessary magnification (~12-fold) and illumination for microsurgery in order to adequately perform the anastomosis of vessels of ~1–4 mm in diameter, respectively sutures of nerves. The microscope should be double headed in order to allow both surgeon and assistant to see the same operative field, which is transmitted by beam splitters. In addition, individual control of focus and zoom mechanisms through separate optical systems and remote control by foot are advisable. Finally, coaxial illumination is a necessity in order to guarantee a clear, bright, and sharp visual field without shadows. Video and photographic attachments compliment the entire system. Disadvantages include the cost, size, maintenance, setup time and adequate storage of the equipment.

The use of high-power and customized surgical loupes (magnification 2.5–4-fold) has been advocated for the crucial steps during dissection of the flaps and their vascular pedicles at the donor site as well as the preparation of the recipient vessels. Furthermore, refinements of the loupes concern the variability of the working distance (~25–50 cm), the width of the visual field ranging from a normal to an extended field, the integrated light source and the weight. Altogether this generates more freedom of movement than a microscope. Microscopes mounted on a head set may eventually combine the advantages of the operating microscope and the surgical loupes, though the wearing comfort is limited due to weight and a tensed and stable fixation onto the head, possibly inducing head and neck pain. Although the microscope on a foot rest may be cumbersome, it is still the ideal magnifier because it allows the assistant to see what the surgeon sees.

The list of instruments necessary to perform microsurgical procedures includes (**Fig 10.6-2**):
- jeweler's forceps (straight and angled)
- micro-scissors (round-tipped for dissection and sharp-tipped for vessel cutting)
- needle holder (round-tipped for easier passing of the needle through the vessel)
- vessel-dilating forceps
- micro-toothed forceps
- microsurgical clamps (approximating or double clamp and single clamp) of different sizes. Do not use "bulldog" clamps because of the traumatizing "imprints" to the vessel wall.
- clamp-applying forceps.

All of these instruments are extremely delicate and, therefore, highly prone to damage.

Nonresorbable polypropylene or polyamide 8-0 to 9-0 sutures are usually used for vascular anastomosis in free-flap surgery and 10-0 sutures for digital arteries and veins. The appropriate needle is nontraumatic and round in shape.

In search for faster "no-suture" methods for anastomosis, a variety of devices is currently in use or under clinical investigation, such as staples, ring clips, coupling devices, magnets, and laser welding. However, except for the venous coupling device, none of the "faster" methods has yet proven to be superior to a diligent and meticulous microsurgical technique, especially in the reconstruction of defects in the lower extremities.

Anastomoses

Atraumatic tissue handling refers to minimizing damage inflicted on the vessel, both in dissection and anastomosis and directly correlates with patency of the anastomosis. The following factors may influence anastomotic patency [56]:
- atraumatic surgical handling of the vessel
- diameter of the vessel
- flushing of the flap
- absence of tension and kinking of the anastomosis
- mean arterial pressure and blood flow especially during freeing of blood flow after completion of the anastomosis and during reperfusion of the flap
- use of anticoagulant and antithrombotic molecules (dextran, unfractionated heparin, low-molecular-weight heparin, acetylsalicylic acid, etc).

An anastomosis may be carried out in an end-to-end or an end-to-side fashion, using the interrupted single-stitch technique with the surgeon's knot lying on the outside of the vessel's lumen (**Fig 10.6-3a–b**). Alternatively, a venous anastomosis can be performed with uninterrupted or interrupted sutures according to the preference of the surgeon.

Since compression and kinking of vascular pedicles are associated with disturbed inflow and/or outflow, some advocate the local application of ~2 ml fibrin glue once the anastomosis is completed, even though fibrin glue is not seen as an alternative to suturing [57]. Fibrin glue seals small holes within the vessel wall and gives the pedicle some rigidity

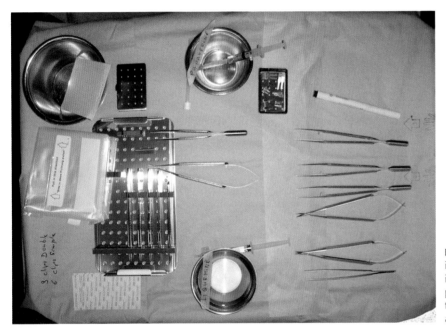

Fig 10.6-2 Microsurgical instruments. They include microvascular clamps, heparin diluted in saline solution to flush the flap before performing the anastomosis and papaverine to inject into adventitial tissue of the artery after completion of the anastomosis.

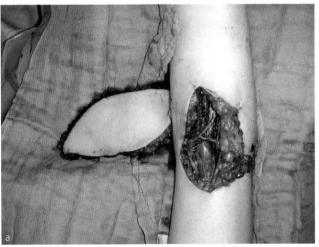
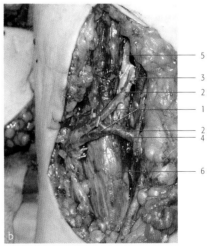

Fig 10.6-3a–b Intraoperative status showing microsurgical reconstruction of a soft-tissue defect of the posterior and anterior (not shown) elbow region with a free latissimus dorsi musculocutaneous flap. The flap has been elevated with two skin islands to cover each defect.

a Intraoperative view of the groove of the right elbow after completion of arterial and venous end-to-end anastomosis.

b The magnified cutout shows adequate caliber of the thoracodorsal vessels of the flap (1) anastomosed (2) onto the inferior ulnar collateral artery (3) and median cubital vein (4). Brachial artery (5); brachioradialis muscle (6).

and adherence to the adjacent tissues, protecting it from shear stress-induced movements, while tailoring the flap during its placement.

10.6.3 Indications and composition of free flaps

As a free flap is transferred with intact circulation, its use is indicated whenever the simple skin graft would be out of place and whenever a flap is preferable or even necessary in order to cover exposed, vital or nonvascularized structures (ie, tendons, bare bone, joints, or implant material) (**Fig 10.6-4a–f**). Other indications are the restoration of function (muscle = functional motor unit) or cosmetic units. Free flaps are also used to pad bone prominences (ie, sacrum, ischium, trochanter, or heel) and to cover traumatized areas for which secondary operations are planned in order to repair underlying structures (eg, implant exchange and bone

grafting for nonunion, knee prosthesis for post traumatic osteoarthritis). Customized free flaps are more versatile and can be optimally adapted to a defect in comparison to local or regional pedicled flaps if available at all. Whether it is preferable to use fasciocutaneous tissue instead of muscular tissue, particularly in regard to contaminated or infected traumatic wounds, is still a matter of debate. Mathes et al were the first to experimentally compare in vivo musculocutaneous flaps with randomly perfused skin flaps in order to determine the bacterial clearance and oxygen tension of each [58]. Bacterial challenge of the flaps resulted in total necrosis of the skin flap, whereas the musculocutaneous flaps demonstrated long-term survival. These results correlated well with a low bacterial count and a high oxygen tension measured beneath the musculocutaneous flap. Although microvascular tissue transfer has become the gold standard for complex defects in the lower extremities, no prospective study comparing fasciocutaneous flaps

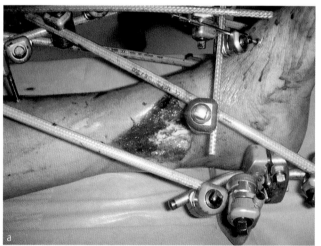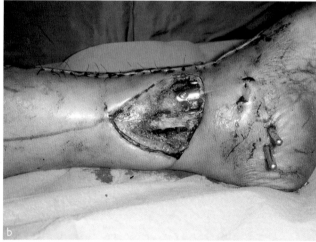

Fig 10.6-4a–f Free fasciocutaneous radial forearm flap.
a Open bimalleolar fracture initially treated by external fixation. Subsequent skin necrosis developed, exposing the medial malleolus.
b After debridement and switching from external fixator to open reduction and internal fixation. Exposed implant material and bare tibial bone.

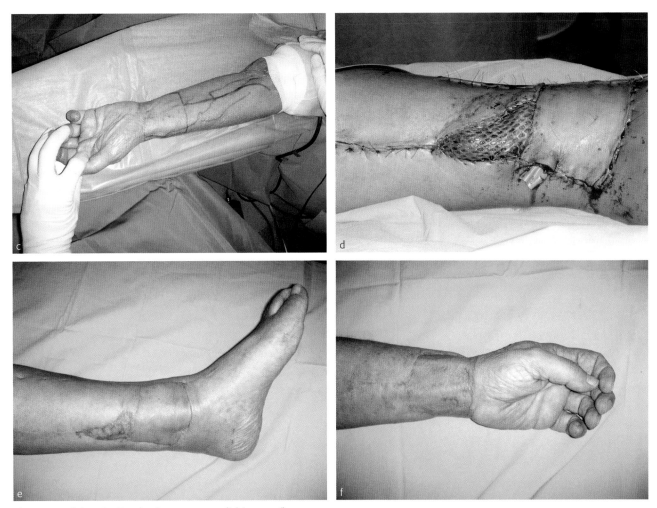

Fig 10.6-4a–f (cont) Free fasciocutaneous radial forearm flap.

c Marking of the rectangular skin island proximally to the wrist's crease. Superficial veins are also marked to be included within the vascular pedicle.

d Immediately after defect coverage using a free fasciocutaneous radial forearm flap and a small meshed split-thickness skin graft to cover the pedicle proximally and to prevent it from coming under too much tension.

e Six months after soft-tissue reconstruction. The forearm skin is well integrated within the surrounding skin of the ankle; the appearance of the split-thickness skin graft remains slightly hyperpigmented and shiny, with a permanent diamond-shaped pattern.

f Six months after flap harvesting. Soft-tissue padding is missing after split-thickness skin grafting of the donor site. The flexor carpi radialis and palmaris longus tendons are well covered.

(**Fig 10.6-5a–b**) with muscle flaps (**Fig 10.6-6**) has been carried out to date. Nevertheless, the good results obtained with fasciocutaneous flaps have seriously challenged the dictum of only reconstructing soft-tissue defects with muscle flaps, particularly in the presence of infection (**Fig 10.6-7a–f**) [59]. From an antiinfection point of view, fasciocutaneous flaps seem to be of equal value in comparison to muscle flaps. Moreover, fasciocutaneous flaps are more pliable and often result in a better match with the cutaneous environment than muscle flaps. Angiogenesis allows a faster and safer integration of the flap into surrounding tissues, thus rendering these flaps less dependent on the pedicle in comparison to muscle flaps. Accordingly, fasciocutaneous flaps will tolerate secondary surgical procedures earlier and better [60]. However, defects with considerable, deep tissue loss including bone might still benefit from large muscle flaps acting as a plug.

Special subgroups of free flaps comprise:
- **The composite flap** (eg, osteoseptocutaneous fibula flap (chapter 12.20), musculocutaneous latissimus dorsi flap): a flap consisting of various tissues (eg, skin, fascia, muscle, bone, cartilage).
- **The chimeric flap** (eg, latissimus dorsi and serratus flap) (chapter 12.19): a versatile tissue construct combining regional flaps, the pedicles of which all derive from a single main vessel [61] (**Fig 10.6-8**).

- **The prelaminated flap:** Additional tissue is added to an existing flap (without manipulation of its axial blood supply) in order to produce a multilayered, composite flap [62].
- **The prefabricated flap:** It involves the introduction of a new blood supply by means of transferring a vascular pedicle into a volume of tissue. After a period of neovascularization, this flap may be transferred, based only on its implanted vascular pedicle [62].
- **The flow-through flap:** Both the proximal and the distal ends of the vascular pedicle acting as a conduit are anastamosed to provide blood flow to distal tissues, eg radial forearm flow-through flap. Flow-through flaps may be considered if segmental revascularization and coverage of a defect is indicated, because these flaps provide dual functionality in one operation, ie one native vascular conduit and at the same time tissue for defect coverage. Accordingly, two separate operations including reconstruction of the vascular conduit by means of a vein graft subsequently followed by flap coverage of the defect can be avoided, as can the morbidity of both procedures [63, 64].

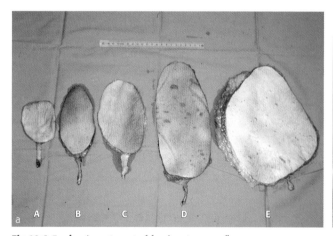 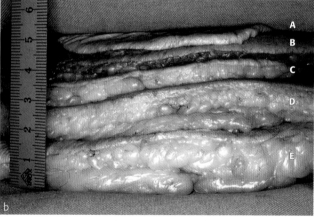

Fig 10.6-5a–b Assortment of fasciocutaneous flaps.
a   Cadaveric preparation showing the variability in available skin and thickness. The ratio of skin island to pertaining pedicle is important, thus, the difference in relative pedicle length is the following: A > C > B > D > E.
    A Dorsalis pedis flap.
    B Lateral arm flap.
    C Radial forearm flap (pedicle length depends on the size of the skin island).
    D Scapular flap.
    E Groin flap.
b   Note the difference in flap thickness: A < B < C < D < E.

Classification of free flaps according to their perfusion demand:

- **High-flow flaps:** high perfusion demand such as muscle flaps
- **Low-flow flaps:** low perfusion demand such as fasciocutaneous or osseous flaps

High-flow flaps are composed of tissues that consume a lot of oxygen, which is not synonymous with partial oxygen tension of the tissue (pO_2). In contrast, low-flow flaps are composed of tissues that consume little oxygen. Skeletal muscles and skin show pO_2-values of 20 mmHg and 45 mmHg, respectively.

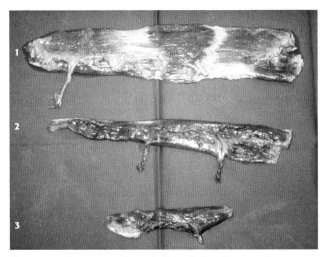

Fig 10.6-6   Assortment of muscle flaps. Cadaveric preparation showing the variability in available muscle and thickness.

1   Rectus abdominis muscle. Type III muscle according to Mathes and Nahai (chapter 10.3) [15].
2   Gracilis muscle. Type II muscle according to Mathes and Nahai (chapter 10.3) [15].
3   Pectoralis minor muscle. Type V muscle according to Mathes and Nahai (chapter 10.3) [15].

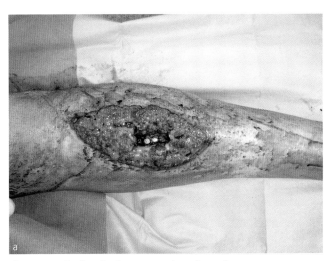
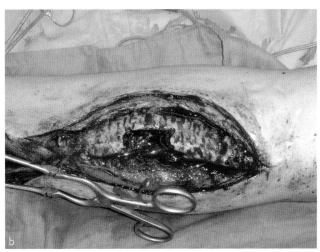

Fig 10.6-7a–f   Free fasciocutaneous lateral arm flap.
a   Soft-tissue defect with osteomyelitis at the anterior aspect of the lower leg after open fracture. Antibiotic beads implanted into the medullary canal. Infected granulation tissue.
b   After debridement and decortication of the tibial bone. 50% of the bone circumference remains.

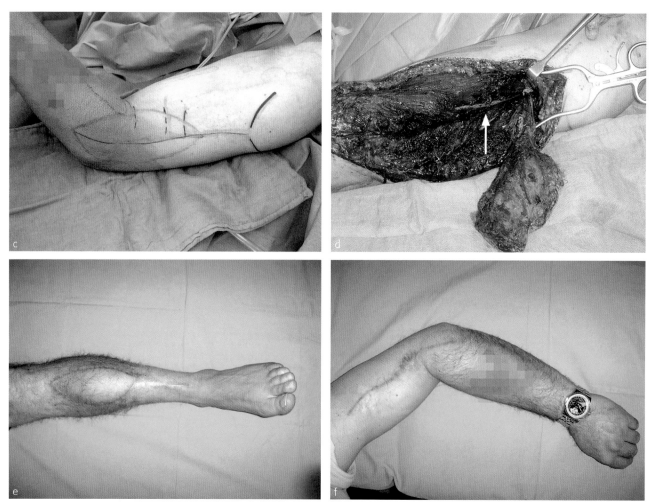

Fig 10.6-7a–f (cont)   Free fasciocutaneous lateral arm flap.

c   Marking of the spindle-shaped skin island at the level of the lateral epicondyle of the humerus.

d   During flap elevation. The pedicle lies within the lateral septum. Freeing of the radial nerve (arrow).

e   Twelve months after soft-tissue reconstruction. The skin is well integrated within the surrounding tissues with rather good matching of tissue and color.

f   Twelve months after flap harvesting and primary closure. Almost no donor-site morbidity on the arm.

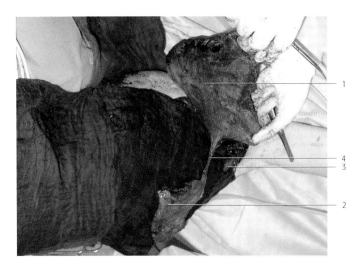

Fig 10.6-8 Elevation of a a chimeric flap in a patient in supine position having his left arm abducted by 90°. The flap consists of a latissimus dorsi muscle flap (1) and a serratus muscle flap (2) nourished by the subclavia, respectively thoracodorsal artery. Lateral border of the pectoralis muscle (3). Branch to the serratus anterior muscle almost always arising from the thoracodorsal artery (4).

10.6.4 Donor-site morbidity of free flaps

Flap harvesting should take care to limit donor-site morbidity to a minimum and to guarantee a good functional and cosmetic result. Therefore, following points should be taken into consideration when choosing a free flap for soft-tissue reconstructions of the extremities:

- If the defect is located on an extremity, the donor site should whenever possible be planned and chosen on the affected limb (in order not to harm another region of the body).
- Avoid raising a flap from the dominant arm (**Fig 10.6-9a**).
- Fasciocutaneous flaps are ideal for skin defects however limited in size (width of the skin paddle) if the donor site is to be closed primarily (eg, lateral arm flap (chapter 12.17), scapular/parascapular flap, anterolateral thigh flap (chapter 12.18)) (**Fig 10.6-9b**).

- Closure of the donor site using skin grafts should be avoided (**Fig 10.6-9a**).
- Muscle flaps may be associated with functional loss, especially in athletes (eg, latissimus dorsi, gracilis, rectus abdominis or rectus femoris muscle).
- The resulting scar and contour deformity caused by flap elevation (eg, lateral arm flap (chapter 12.17), anterolateral thigh flap (chapter 12.18), latissimus dorsi flap) must be taken into consideration (**Fig 10.6-9c**).

Despite specific surgical infrastructure, technical skills and experience that is needed, selected patients may benefit from microsurgical reconstruction because the customized flap will be adapted specifically to the local situation and to the defect in comparison to pedicled flaps originating from the neighborhood. This may also avoid the need for repeated surgery, long hospital stay or recovery time.

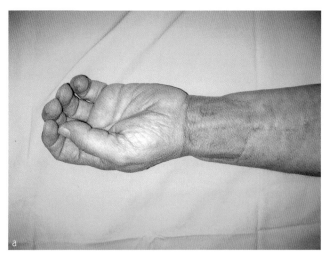
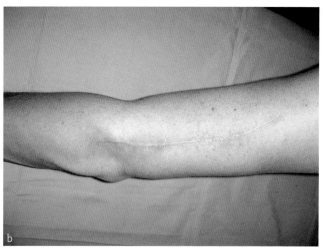
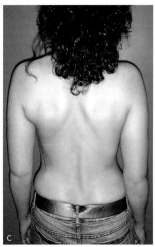

Fig 10.6-9a–c Donor-site morbidity.
a Donor site of a nondominant forearm after having harvested a quadrangular fasciocutaneous radial forearm flap and coverage of the donor-site defect with a meshed split-thickness skin graft. Note the visible depression and the almost invisible mesh-like structure of the skin graft.
b Donor site of a nondominant arm after having harvested a fasciocutaneous lateral arm flap. Note the straight scar after primary closure.
c Donor site after having harvested a musculocutaneous latissimus dorsi flap on the left. Note the straight scar along the posterior axillary line and the contour deformity along the lateral border of the scapula.

10.7 Postoperative management

Authors   Jörn A Lohmeyer, Yves Harder, Reto Wettstein

10.7.1   Introduction

Postoperative management after any type of surgical wound closure begins in the operating room. It includes dressing, splinting, immobilization of the involved extremity, and bedding of the patient as well as thromboprophylaxis, perioperative antibiotic prophylaxis and postoperative antibiotic therapy. This chapter highlights general aspects of postoperative management after primary or delayed primary closure, secondary closure, skin graft, and flap reconstructions, and also discusses personal views of the authors. As a general rule, the overall postoperative management should be simple to apply and economical in terms of dressing ma-

terial and manpower, yet safe for the patient in order to keep morbidity low.

10.7.2   Immediate aftercare of wounds

Dressing and bedding
Basically, every surgical wound must be handled with care, no matter whether it is a primary closure (chapter 10.1), a skin graft (chapter 10.2), or a complex flap reconstruction (chapter 10.3 to 10.6). Dressings (chapter 9.1) are intended to protect the wound, absorb exudates, and may also add stability to the suture (Steri-Strip™, Mefix®, OpSite®, Vari-

hesive®, etc), depending on the location, suture technique, tension, underlying pathology and presence of drainage.

In complex reconstructions, a part of the flap should be easily accessible for inspection and surveillance (color, capillary refill, swelling, and temperature). In addition, a reference point is marked with a marking pen or a stitch (in free flaps) for machine-based monitoring (temperature, Doppler, etc) (chapter 5.1). Hematoma, seroma and edema formation as well as external pressure exerted by the dressing, especially over the pedicle of the flap, and patient positioning may cause flap failure secondary to compromised flap perfusion. Therefore, circumferential dressings increase the risk of compression and should be used cautiously and applied loosely, especially if inelastic gauzes are used. Stretchable soft cotton dressings that will yield are ideal for coverage and padding of complex reconstructions.

The extremity, particularly if reconstructed with a flap, must be embedded and maintained in position softly (eg, pad, pillow, foam splint) in order to avoid any external pressure and shearing. It is also advisable to prevent direct pressure by the sheets or blankets. This may be ensured by using a special frame for the bed. Very rarely, the transitory application of an external fixator is indicated in order to suspend the extremity and prevent flap compression.

The timing of when to change the first dressing depends on various factors. In general, the dressing applied in the operation room is the cleanest and the first dressing change should only be performed as necessary (eg, soiling, bleeding, severe pain). Frequently the first dressing change is scheduled on the second postoperative day since most infections become manifest after this period of time. Thereafter, dressings should be applied and changed as required individually. The surgeon and the nursing staff must be aware of possible blisters (ie, epidermolysis) or signs of intolerance that may develop with the use of self-adhesive dressings. They may be painful for the patient and very cumbersome to handle in case of considerable exudation or lack of suitable alternative dressings.

Removal of sutures, respectively staples, mainly depends on the suture technique and location. Bear in mind that both sutures and staples will leave hypopigmented, scarred marks (rope ladder) that may be minimized by the use of thin sutures and early removal, or even be completely prevented by an intradermal suture technique (chapter 10.1). Generally, sutures are removed about 14 days after the procedure. However, on the face they should be removed earlier (5–7 days) and be left longer on the heel (21 days). A wound that has not healed within 2–3 weeks and is only held together by the suture material will probably not heal. After analysis of the reasons for failed wound healing, removal of the stitches and revisional surgery or change to open wound care and secondary wound healing should follow.

Systemic monitoring and flap monitoring

In flap surgery in general, but in free flaps in particular, normotensive values should preferably be obtained with volume management rather than vasoactive agents that may induce arterial constriction and potentially compromise flap perfusion. Also, postoperative hypertension may cause bleeding and hematoma formation, which may affect flap perfusion. The hematocrit for optimal flap perfusion is about 30% [65]. This should be kept in mind since transfusion of red blood cells will increase blood viscosity and thus affect blood rheology which in turn jeopardizes microvascular perfusion.

Flap monitoring should detect any signs of compromised perfusion. Pedicled flaps usually do not require any specific surveillance of their vascularity except for 1–2 clinical examinations per day to exclude tension and perfusion failure secondary to hematoma, swelling or external compression. Free flaps, on the other hand, must be monitored intensively during the first few days for vascular patency. Occlusion of an anastomosis requires immediate surgical revision since only rapid intervention with reestablishment of perfusion is able to save the flap. Any delay in revision would be detrimental and inevitably threaten flap survival. Many different monitoring devices and protocols exist [66], but most include a clinical examination (except for buried flaps) and a Doppler probe check for venous and arterial signals every 1–2 hours during the first 24–48 hours (chapter 5.1).

Thromboprophylaxis

Another problem in posttraumatic, often temporarily immobilized patients is the risk of hypercoagulability and thromboembolic events. Therefore, thromboprophylaxis is mandatory. It consists of different measures such as compression stockings or elastic bandages, and so-called calf pumps applied with intermittent pressure. Medical thromboprophylaxis generally consists of the administration of subcutaneous low-molecular-weight heparin (LMWH) once per day, unless the patient presents with an increased risk of thromboembolic complications or with a contraindication to LMWH. The daily dose is usually administered according to the patient's risk for developing thrombosis, or—less frequently—according to the patient's weight. Thromboprophylaxis is also administered to prevent thrombosis within the pedicle of a flap. Usually arterial occlusion develops more rapidly in comparison to venous occlusion [67]. The risk of occlusion is highest within the first 48–72 hours and occurs in about 4% of lower extremities undergoing free flap reconstruction [68]. In general after flap surgery, low-molecular-weight heparin is preferred to unfractionated heparin, because it offers the same antithrombotic potency in comparison to unfractionated heparin, yet it is associated with an almost 10-fold decreased risk of developing a heparin-induced thrombocytopenia (HIT) [69] as well as a considerably decreased risk of postoperative bleeding [70, 71]. Plasma expanders such as low-molecular-weight dextran lead to intravascular volume expansion and, therefore, enhance microrheology. However, they considerably increase the risk of pulmonary edema, pleural effusion, congestive heart failure, and bleeding [72]. They may even induce a hypercoagulable state [73–75].

It must be understood that soft-tissue reconstructions of the lower extremities go along with an increased risk of thromboembolic complications in comparison to other regions of the body, particularly if flaps are used [68]. Therefore, alternative schemes of thromboprophylaxis administering unfractionated heparin at a thromboprophylactic dose (eg, 10000 IU heparin/24 hours) associated with a plasma expander such as low-molecular-weight dextran during the first 1–2 days after surgery have to be discussed on a case-specific basis. Criteria that might favor an initial intravenous or combined thromboprophylaxis in comparison to subcutaneous administration of low-molecular-weight heparin are the following:
- known and symptomatic peripheral artery occlusive disease
- marginal perfusion of the flap during surgery
- difficult microsurgery or revision of the anastomosis
- delayed filling of the flap after freeing blood flow.

Given the fact that currently there is no consensus about postoperative thromboprophylaxis, the surgeon, therefore, has to balance the antithrombotic effects of the administered drugs to the increased risk of postoperative complications. This also includes postoperative anti-platelet-aggregation and anticoagulation [76].

Antibiotic prophylaxis and therapy
Perioperative administration of a single-shot prophylaxis is almost universally accepted (eg, sultamicillin 3 g intravenous, cefuroxime 1.5 g intravenous), particularly for open soft-tissue injuries and for surgical procedures exceeding 4 hours. While the initial prophylaxis is empiric, ongoing treatment should be based on cultures resulting from swabs and/or tissue biopsies [77]. The perioperative and postoperative use

of antibiotics may vary considerably from institution to institution despite the presence of guidelines. This might also be based on the fact that, currently, the guidelines are not based on randomized controlled trials but rather on clinical experience and consecutive studies that are often retrospective [78]. The regimen of antibiotic prophylaxis seems evident in uncomplicated and closed fractures. However, in fractures that are neither classified as clean, nor clearly contaminated, perioperative administration of antibiotics and particularly postoperative administration of antibiotics is still debatable and, therefore, may vary considerably.

10.7.3 Mobilization and weight bearing of the patient

Patients with uncomplicated wounds that are well bandaged in order to prevent edema may be mobilized immediately after surgery. In case of a combined trauma including soft tissue and bone, mobilization and weight bearing are dictated by the stability of the fracture. Basically, any soft-tissue reconstruction without bone, tendon, vessel, or nerve involvement may be fully loaded, depending on the level of pain the patient can tolerate.

For skin grafts, the ultimate goal is to have maximum adherence between graft and wound bed in order to permit vascular ingrowth. Any mobilization causing shear forces at the skin-graft-wound interface must be prevented. Vertical positioning of the reconstructed area and vertical forces have to be avoided in order to prevent damage to the newly formed, yet immature, microvessels. Ideally, high intravascular pressure should, therefore, be postponed for 4–5 days until the skin graft has taken and is stable (chapter 10.2). Thereafter, cautious mobilization is allowed, using a circular bandage or a compression stocking.

Postoperative immobilization of the patient will usually take 2 days for pedicled flaps, respectively 5 days for free flaps. This depends on several factors:
- flap type and localization
- patient comorbidities
- patient compliance.

A flap spanning a joint or located in a pressure zone will have to be treated differently from a flap used for reconstruction of a pretibial defect. Obviously, any movement between the flap and the wound bed is suboptimal for adherence of the flap and increases the probability for seroma formation. Moreover, tension created on the sutures may lead to delayed wound healing and partial flap necrosis. In any case, the affected limb should be wrapped with an elastic bandage or a compression stocking. If a free flap has been transfered from the upper to the lower extremity, a training phase of progressively increasing intervals of dependent position is recommended. Thereby, the flap tissue, which is disconnected from any functional lymph vessels, will adjust to its new environment with a different orthostatic pressure (flap training). Generally, mobilization or verticalization, ie, having the patient sit up or stand up, is increased by ~30 minutes per day. Although this is rather arbitrary, flap training is continued until the patient is able to tolerate 3 consecutive hours of limb verticalization. If the flap tolerates this time of mobilization well, flap training may be regarded as completed. Of course, mobilization can be repeated many times per day as long as the lower extremity is bandaged or the patient is wearing a custom-made stocking. As a matter of fact, these principles also hold true for the upper extremity. Since verticalization and loading can often be easily avoided in the upper extremity, flap training as described is rarely necessary.

Once the postoperative edema has regressed (fasciocutaneous flap: ~2–3 weeks) and skin grafts covering muscle flaps are stable, compression bandages may be substituted for custom-made compression garments that should be worn during daytime. Atrophy of muscular and musculocutaneous flaps approximately takes 3 months. Fasciocutaneous flaps flatten secondary to decreased or improved lymphatic drainage and not secondary to atrophy. Therefore, volume decrease takes longer than in muscle flaps.

Sometimes, soft-tissue reconstructions are performed even despite unstable fracture fixation. In addition, reconstructions may comprise tendons, vessels or nerves that require some type of temporary immobilization (eg, splint, plaster, external fixator). In general, splints and casts bear the risk of compressing the skin overlying a bony protuberance, a flap pedicle, or a skin graft. Such conditions may induce pressure sores and might compromise flap perfusion.

10.7.4 Secondary surgery after flap coverage

In case revision or secondary surgery is needed for bone, tendon, or nerve reconstruction, complete wound healing should be achieved before surgical refinement. Ideally, a period of ~3 months has to elapse in order to provide safe conditions for corrective surgery. Bear in mind that fasciocutaneous flaps will be integrated better within the surrounding tissues in comparison to muscle flaps, which usually remain dependent upon their pedicle (chapter 11.4).

Whenever a flap remains too bulky, presents with considerable contour irregularities or skin excess, different surgical options exist to remodel the flap. Especially small fasciocutaneous flaps are prone to develop the so-called trap-door phenomenon that describes a stepwise contour irregularity with the flap being elevated from the surrounding healthy tissue resulting in an uneven and bulky aspect secondary to lymphedema of the flap.

References and further reading

[1] **Rajasekaran S, Dheenadhayalan J, Babu JN, et al** (2009) Immediate primary skin closure in type-III A and B open fractures: results after a minimum of five years. *J Bone Joint Surg Br*; 91(2):217–224.

[2] **Hohmann E, Tetsworth K, Radziejowski MJ, et al** (2007) Comparison of delayed and primary wound closure in the treatment of open tibial fractures. *Arch Orthop Trauma Surg*; 127(2):131–136.

[3] **Gottesdiener KM** (1989) Transplanted infections: donor-to-host transmission with the allograft. *Ann Intern Med*; 110(12):1001–1016.

[4] **Mavilio F, Pellegrini G, Ferrari S, et al** (2006) Correction of junctional epidermolysis bullosa by transplantation of genetically modified epidermal stem cells. *Nat Med*; 12(12):1397–1402.

[5] **Pellegrini G, Ranno R, Stracuzzi G, et al** (1999) The control of epidermal stem cells (holoclones) in the treatment of massive full-thickness burns with autologous keratinocytes cultured on fibrin. *Transplantation*; 68(6):868–879.

[6] **Kudsk KA, Sheldon GF, Walton RL** (1981) Degloving injuries of the extremities and torso. *J Trauma*; 21(10):835–839.

[7] **Widgerow AD, Chait LA** (1993) Degloving injuries and flap viability assessment. *S Afr Med J*; 83(2):97–99.

[8] **McGrouther DA, Sully L** (1980) Degloving injuries of the limbs: long-term review and management based on whole-body fluorescence. *Br J Plast Surg*; 33(1):9–24.

[9] **Gibson T, Ross DS** (1965) Dermatome for preparing large skin-grafts from detached skin and fat. *Lancet*; 1(7379):252–253.

[10] **Blair VP, Brown JP** (1929) The use and uses of large split skin grafts of intermediate thickness. *Surg Gynecol Obstet*; 49:82-97.

[11] **Wolf Y, Kalish E, Badani E** (1998) Rubber foam and staples: do they secure skin grafts? A model analysis and proposal of pressure enhancement techniques. *Ann Plast Surg*; 40(2):149–155.

[12] **Gillies H, Millard DR** (1953) *Principles and art of plastic surgery, Vol. 1.* 1st ed. London: Butterworth, 98.

[13] **Tidrick RT, Warner ED** (1944) Fibrin fixation of skin transplants. *Surgery;* 15:90–95.

[14] **McGregor IA, Morgan G** (1973) Axial and random pattern flaps. *Br J Plast Surg;* 26(3):202–213.

[15] **Mathes SJ, Nahai F** (1981) Classification of the vascular anatomy of muscles: experimental and clinical correlation. *Plast Reconstr Surg;* 67(2):177–187.

[16] **Khouri RK, Upton J, Shaw WW** (1992) Principles of flap prefabrication. *Clin Plast Surg;* 19(4):763–771.

[17] **Pribaz JJ, Fine NA** (1994) Prelamination: defining the prefabricated flap—a case report and review. *Microsurgery;* 15(9):618–623.

[18] **Tolhurst DE** (1987) A comprehensive classification of flaps: the atomic system. *Plast Reconstr Surg;* 80(4):608–609.

[19] **Hallock GG** (2004) The complete classification of flaps. *Microsurgery;* 24(3):157–161.

[20] **Cierny G 3rd, Byrd HS, Jones RE** (1983) Primary versus delayed soft tissue coverage for severe open tibial fractures. A comparison of results. *Clin Orthop Relat Res;* 178:54–63.

[21] **Godina M** (1986) Early microsurgical reconstruction of complex trauma of the upper extremities. *Plast Reconstr Surg;* 78(3):285–292.

[22] **Yaremchuk MJ, Brumback RJ, Manson PN, et al** (1987) Acute and definitive management of traumatic osteocutaneous defects of the lower extremity. *Plast Reconstr Surg;* 80(1):1-14.

[23] **Isenberg JS, Sherman R** (1996) The limited value of preoperative angiography in microsurgical reconstruction of the lower limb. *J Reconstr Microsurg;* 12(5):303–306.

[24] **Boström A, Ljungman C, Hellberg A, et al** (2002) Duplex scanning as the sole preoperative imaging method for infrainguinal arterial surgery. *Eur J Vasc Endovasc Surg;* 23(2):140–145.

[25] **Jin KN, Lee W, Yin YH, et al** (2007) Preoperative evaluation of lower extremity arteries for free fibula transfer using MDCT angiography. *J Comput Assist Tomogr;* 31(5):820–825.

[26] **Fukaya E, Saloner D, Leon P, et al** (2010) Magnetic resonance angiography to evaluate septocutaneous perforators in free fibula flap transfer. *J Plast Reconstr Aesthet Surg;* 63(7): 1099–1104.

[27] **McFarlane RM, Heagy FC, Radin S, et al** (1965) A study of the delay phenomenon in experimental pedicle flaps. *Plast Reconstr Surg;* 35:245–262.

[28] **Reinisch JF** (1974) The pathophysiology of skin flap circulation. *The delay phenomenon. Plast Reconstr Surg;* 54(5):585–598.

[29] **Harder Y, Amon M, Schramm R, et al** (2005) Heat shock preconditioning reduces ischemic tissue necrosis by heat shock protein (HSP)-32-mediated improvement of the microcirculation rather than induction of ischemic tolerance. *Ann Surg;* 242(6):869–879.

[30] **Manchot C** (1889) *[The skin arteries of the human body].* Leipzig: F.C.W. Vogel. German.

[31] **Spalteholz W** (1893) [The distribution of blood vessels in the skin]. *Arch Anat Physiol;* 19:1–54. German.

[32] **Braithwaite F** (1951) Some observations in the vascular channels in tubed pedicles. II. *Br J Plast Surg;* 4(1): 28–37.

[33] **Lister GD, Gibson T** (1972) Closure of rhomboid skin defects: the flaps of Limberg and Dufourmentel. *Br J Plast Surg;* 25(3):300–314.

[34] **Dufourmentel C** (1962) [Closure of limited loss of cutaneous substance. So-called "LLL" diamond-shaped L rotation-flap]. *Ann Chir Plast;* 7:60–66. French.

[35] **Taylor GI, Palmer JH** (1987) The vascular territories (angiosomes) of the body: experimental study and clinical applications. *Br J Plast Surg;* 40(2):113–141.

[36] **Taylor GI** (2003) The angiosomes of the body and their supply to perforator flaps. *Clin Plast Surg;* 30(3):331–342.

[37] **Serafin D** (1996) The radial forearm flap. *Serafin D (ed), Atlas of microsurgical composite tissue transplantation.* 1st ed. Philadelphia: W.B. Saunders, 389–401.

[38] **Chang SC, Miller G, Halbert CF, et al** (1996) Limiting donor site morbidity by suprafascial dissection of the radial forearm flap. *Microsurgery;* 17(3):136–140.

[39] **Avery C** (2007) Prospective study of the septocutaneous radial free flap and suprafascial donor site. *Br J Oral Maxillofac Surg;* 45(8):611–616.

[40] **Masquelet AC, Romana MC, Wolf G** (1992) Skin island flaps supplied by the vascular axis of the sensitive superficial nerves: anatomic study and clinical experience in the leg. *Plastic Reconstr Surg;* 89(6):1115–1121.

[41] **Rajacic N, Darweesh M, Jayakrishnan K, et al** (1996) The distally based superficial sural flap for reconstruction of the lower leg and foot. *Br J Plast Surg;* 49(6):383–389.

[42] **Hasegawa M, Torii S, Katoh H, et al** (1994) The distally based superficial sural artery flap. *Plast Reconstr Surg;* 93(5):1012–1020.

[43] **Huisinga RL, Houpt P, Dijkstra R, et al** (1998) The distally based sural artery flap. *Ann Plast Surg;* 41(1):58–65.

[44] **Suliman MT** (2007) Distally based adipofascial flaps for dorsal foot and ankle soft tissue defects. *J Foot Ankle Surg;* 46(6):464–469.

[45] **Valenti P, Masquelet AC, Romana C, et al** (1991) Technical refinement of the lateral supramalleolar flap. *Br J Plast Surg;* 44(6):459–462.

[46] **Serafin D** (1996) The gastrocnemius flap. *Serafin D (ed) Atlas of microsurgical composite tissue transplantation.* Philadelphia: W.B. Saunders, 303–310.

[47] **Babu NV, Chittaranjan S, Abraham G, et al** (1994) Reconstruction of the quadriceps apparatus following open injuries to the knee joint using pedicled gastrocnemius musculotendinous unit as a bridge graft. *Br J Plast Surg;* 47(3):190–193.

[48] **Kramers-De Quervain IA, Läuffer JM, Käch K, et al** (2001) Functional donor-site morbidity during level and uphill gait after a gastrocnemius or soleus muscle-flap procedure. *J Bone Joint Surg Am;* 83(2):239–246.

[49] **Magee WP Jr, Gilbert DA, McInnis WD** (1980) Extended muscle and musculocutaneous flaps. *Clin Plast Surg;* 7(1):57–70.

[50] **Ginouves P, Baron JL, Bermudez J, et al** (1988) [Use of a distal pedicle hemisoleus muscle in the treatment of residual osteitis of the lower quarter of the leg]. *Ann Chir Plast Esthet;* 33(4):350–354. French.

[51] **Tobin GR** (1985) Hemisoleus and reversed hemisoleus flaps. *Plast Reconstr Surg;* 76(1):87–96.

[52] **McCraw JB, Dibbell DG, Carraway JH** (1977) Clinical definition of independent myocutaneous vascular territories. *Plast Reconstr Surg;* 60(3):341–352.

[53] **Pontén B** (1981) The fasciocutaneous flap: its use in soft tissue defects of the lower leg. *Br J Plast Surg;* 34(2):215–220.

[54] **Koshima I, Soeda S, Yamasaki M, et al** (1988) The free or pedicled anteromedial thigh flap. *Ann Plast Surg;* 21(5):480–485.

[55] **Acland RD** (1979) Factors that influence success in microvascular surgery. *Serafin D, Buncke HJ Jr (eds). Microsurgical composite tissue transplantation.* 1st ed. St. Louis, MO: C.V. Mosby, 216–229.

[56] **Acland RD** (1980) *Microsurgery practice manual.* 1st ed. St. Louis, MO: C.V. Mosby.

[57] **Andree C, Munder BI, Behrendt P, et al** (2008) Improved safety of autologous breast reconstruction surgery by stabilisation of microsurgical vessel anastomoses using fibrin sealant in 349 free DIEP or fascia-muscle-sparing (fms)-TRAM flaps: A two-centre study. *Breast;* 17(5):492–498.

[58] **Mathes SJ, Alpert BS, Chang N** (1982) Use of the muscle flap in chronic osteomyelitis: experimental and clinical correlation. *Plast Reconstr Surg;* 69(5):815–829.

[59] **Zweifel-Schlatter M, Haug M, Schaefer DJ, et al** (2006) Free fasciocutaneous flaps in the treatment of chronic osteomyelitis of the tibia: a retrospective study. *J Reconstr Microsurg;* 22(1):41–47.

[60] **Yazar S, Lin CH, Lin YT, et al** (2006) Outcome comparison between free muscle and free fasciocutaneous flaps for reconstruction of distal third and ankle traumatic open tibial fractures. *Plast Reconstr Surg;* 117(7):2468–2477.

[61] **Hallock GG** (1991) Simultaneous transposition of anterior thigh muscle and fascia flaps: an introduction to the chimera flap principle. *Ann Plast Surg;* 27(2):126–131.

[62] **Pribaz JJ, Fine NA** (2001) Prefabricated and prelaminated flaps for head and neck reconstruction. *Clin Plast Surg;* 28(2):261–72.

[63] **Soutar DS, Scheker LR, Tanner NS, et al** (1983) The radial forearm flap: a versatile method for intra-oral reconstruction. *Br J Plast Surg;* 36(1):1–8

[64] **Foucher G, van Genechten F, Merle N, et al** (1984) A compound radial artery forearm flap in hand surgery: an original modification of the Chinese forearm flap. *Br J Plast Surg;* 37(2)139–148.

[65] **Erni D, Wettstein R, Schramm S, et al** (2003) Normovolemic hemodilution with Hb vesicle solution attenuates hypoxia in ischemic hamster flap tissue. *Am J Physiol Heart Circ Physiol;* 284(5):H1702–1709.

[66] **Tenorio X, Mahajan AL, Wettstein R, et al** (2009) Early detection of flap failure using a new thermographic device. *J Surg Res;* 151(1):15–21.

[67] **Yu P, Chang DW, Miller MJ, et al** (2009) Analysis of 49 cases of flap compromise in 1310 free flaps for head and neck reconstruction. *Head Neck;* 31(1):45–51.

[68] **Wettstein R, Schürch R, Banic A, et al** (2008) Review of 197 consecutive free flap reconstructions in the lower extremity. *J Plast Reconstr Aesthet Surg;* 61(7):772–776.

[69] **Martel N, Lee J, Wells PS** (2005) Risk for heparin-induced thrombocytopenia with unfractionated and low-molecular-weight heparin thromboprophylaxis: a meta-analysis. *Blood;* 106(8):2710–2715.

[70] **Ritter EF, Cronan JC, Rudner AM, et al** (1998) Improved microsurgical anastomotic patency with low molecular weight heparin. *J Reconstr Microsurg;* 14(5): 331–336.

[71] **Khouri RK, Cooley BC, Kunselman AR, et al** (1998) A prospective study of microvascular free-flap surgery and outcome. *Plast Reconstr Surg;* 102(3):711–721.

[72] **Disa JJ, Polvora VP, Pusic AL, et al** (2003) Dextran-related complications in head and neck microsurgery: do the benefits outweigh the risks? A prospective randomized analysis. *Plast Reconstr Surg;* 112(6):1534–1539.

[73] **Namdar T, Bartscher T, Stollwerck PL, et al** (2010) Complete free flap loss due to extensive hemodilution. *Microsurgery;* 30(3):214–217.

[74] **Ng KF, Lam CC, Chan LC** (2002) In vivo effect of haemodilution with saline on coagulation: a randomized controlled trial. *Br J Anaesth;* 88(4):475–480.

[75] **Treib J, Haass A, Pindur G** (1997) Coagulation disorders caused by hydroxyethyl starch. *Thromb Haemost;* 78(3):974–983.

[76] **Hanasono MM, Butler CE** (2008) Prevention and treatment of thrombosis in microvascular surgery. *J Reconstr Microsurg;* 24(5):305–314.

[77] **Hoffman RD, Adams BD** (1998) The role of antibiotics in the management of elective and post-traumatic hand surgery. *Hand Clin;* 14(4):657–66.

[78] **Slobogean GP, Kennedy SA, Davidson D, et al** (2008) Single- versus multiple-dose antibiotic prophylaxis in the surgical treatment of closed fractures: a meta-analysis. *J Orthop Trauma;* 22(4):264–269.

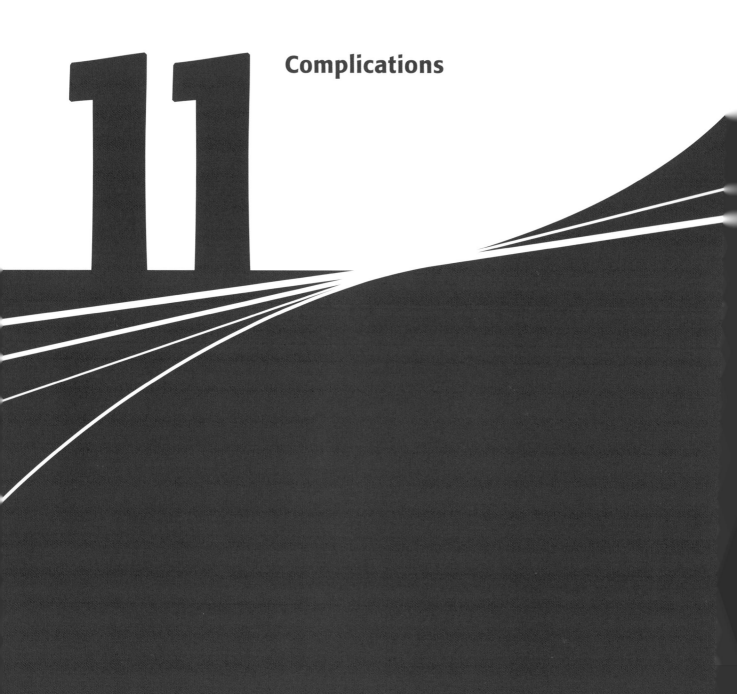

11 Complications

11.1 Complications related to the injury

Author   David A Volgas

11.1.1   Introduction

The surgeon should be vigilant for complications related to the injury. In many cases, the force that caused the orthopaedic injury also caused damage to vital organs. For instance, a fracture of the scapula should alert the surgeon to the possibility of a lung contusion or rupture of the thoracic aorta. Pelvic fractures are often associated with significant vascular lesions within the pelvis, ureteral tears, and ruptures to hollow and/or solid organs. Furthermore, soft-tissue injuries such as crush, burns, or electrical injuries may have a profound systemic effect.

11.1.2   Compartment syndrome

Compartment syndrome occurs when the pressure within a muscle compartment exceeds the end arteriolar pressure (**Animation 11.1-1**). While sustained pressures above capillary pressure may lead to chronic problems, pressures above ~30 mmHg (end arteriolar pressure) may lead to the death of muscle, nerve and other soft tissues. Permanent damage may occur in as short a time as 6 hours after onset, thus, early diagnosis and emergent treatment is essential.

The most common location for compartment syndrome to occur is the lower leg, specifically in the anterior and deep posterior compartments. It is also commonly seen in the forearm. Less common and therefore frequently overlooked

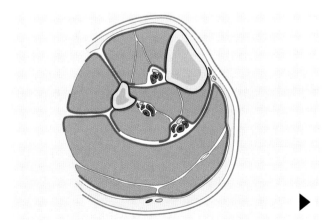

Animation 11.1-1 Compartment syndrome. Excessive pressure is released by extensive fasciotomy.

locations include the foot, hand, thigh, and buttocks. Compartment syndrome may occur after blunt trauma or crush injury with or without a fracture. When associated with fractures, the presence of an open wound does not exclude compartment syndrome.

The five "P"s remain the cornerstone of diagnosis:
- pain out of proportion to the injury or with passive stretching
- pallor
- pulselessness
- paresthesia
- paralysis.

Of these signs, the cardinal sign is pain in excess of what one would expect due to the injury, or severe pain with passive stretching. Furthermore, pain that is not responding adequately to pain medication (ie, opiates) may also indicate compartment syndrome. Often, there are no other signs until much later in the course of the injury. These symptoms may be difficult to elicit in an unconscious patient, therefore, invasive monitoring with a pressure transducer may be required.

Several techniques for the measurement of compartment pressures are available. They should not substitute a clinical exam (pain out of proportion to the injury, nonresponse to pain medication) if possible. Standard fracture textbooks describe these techniques well and, therefore, they are not presented here. When compartment measurements are taken [1] as an adjunct to clinical examination and in order to decide whether the muscle compartment should be released ot not, the surgeon may use either an absolute value of > 30 mmHg or a δ P value of < 30 mmHg, which represents the difference between the diastolic blood pressure and the measured compartment pressure. Surgeons should note that pressures within a compartment may vary inversely to distance from the fracture, and, therefore, should attempt to measure at the area associated with peak pressures, ie, near the fracture site.

The treatment for compartment syndrome consists in an emergent and generous fasciotomy. The key to successful treatment of compartment syndrome after diagnosis is adequate release of the constricting muscle fascia. In most cases, this involves a long incision over the affected compartment and a release of the fascia. Once the skin and muscle fascia are incised, immediate release of pressure is noted as the muscle forcefully bulges through the fascia.

The surgical approach for the lower leg involves long incisions on the medial and lateral sides of the leg (**Fig 11.1-1a–c**). Care should be taken in order to avoid injury, on the lateral side to the superficial fibular nerve, and on the medial side to the posterior tibial artery respectively tibial nerve. In every case, all four compartments should be fully released. Two or 3 days later, the medial wound may often be closed (chapter 10.1), but the lateral wound often requires a split-thickness skin graft (chapter 10.2), as swelling will not have subsided fully yet. Do not attempt to close the muscle fascia,

as recurrence of the compartment syndrome may occur. Moreover, long-term bulging of the muscles through the longitudinally incised muscle fascia will usually not affect the function of the patient's muscle compartment.

Forearm compartment syndrome often involves the anterior compartment but not the posterior one. In selected cases, it is permissible to release only the anterior compartment, if the patient can be assessed clinically after surgery. However, in unconscious patients or in patients who will not undergo subsequent surgery, both compartments should be released at once. The approach utilizes an extensile anterior approach, which may be extended across the wrist in

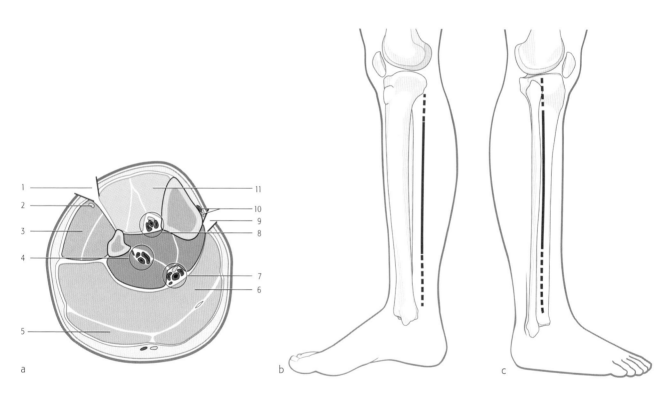

Fig 11.1-1a–c Surgical approach for fasciotomies of the lower leg.
a   Cross section of the mid calf showing surgical planes for decompression.
1   Lateral incision.
2   Superficial fibular nerve.
3   Lateral muscle compartment.
4   Fibular vascular bundle and deep fibular nerve.
5   Superficial posterior muscle compartment.
6   Deep posterior muscle compartment.
7   Posterior tibial vascular bundle and tibial nerve.
8   Anterior tibial vascular bundle and superficial fibular nerve.
9   Medial incision.
10   Saphenous vein and nerve.
11   Anterior muscle compartment.
b   The medial incision begins ~2 cm posterior to the tibia. Possible extensions of the incision are shown by a dotted line.
c   The lateral incision begins at the anterior border of the fibula. Possible extensions of the incision are shown by a dotted line.

order to decompress the carpal tunnel (**Fig 11.1-2a–b**). Dorsally, a mid-line approach may be chosen.

Foot fasciotomies (**Fig 11.1-3a–d**) [2] are performed less commonly than those of the leg or forearm, possibly because this condition may not have been recognized, but also in part, because the sequelae of an untreated foot compartment syndrome are far less debilitating than those of the forearm or leg. There are nine compartments of the foot which are commonly recognized: the medial, lateral and superficial compartments run the length of the mid foot/forefoot. There are four interosseous and one central compartment within the forefoot (**Fig 11.1-3d**) as well as the calcaneal compartment in the hindfoot (**Fig 11.1-3c**). All of these compartments may be accessed by two dorsal and a medial approach.

Unfortunately, fasciotomies are associated with complications. Multiple surgical procedures may be required in order to close the wound (eg, delayed wound closure with elastic vessel loops, split-thickness skin graft, and secondary skin graft) (chapter 10.1, 10.2). Infection rates are high and damage to neurovascular structures may occur if care is not taken in order to avoid them during the fasciotomy. In the presence of a fracture, the bone must be stabilized just as in an open fracture.

11.1.3 Rhabdomyolysis

Rhabdomyolysis is the rapid breakdown (lysis) of skeletal muscle. Most often it is the result of long periods of recumbency while unconscious, but may also occur following blunt or penetrating trauma, or in extreme cases, exercise. Failure to adequately debride all necrotic tissue may also lead to rhabdomyolysis. Recently, rhabdomyolysis has been described as a cause of death in earthquake survivors [3].

Clinical signs include nausea, vomiting, mental status changes from confusion to coma, and dark, tea-colored urine. The latter is caused by the release of the breakdown products of damaged muscle cells such as myoglobin, which are harmful to the kidneys. A dramatic decrease of urine output may follow as a sign of acute kidney failure. Laboratory abnormalities include extremely high concentrations of creatine kinase and transaminases as well as hyperkalemia. A standard urine dipstick may test false positive for blood because the reaction of myoglobin is the same as that for hemoglobin.

If untreated, myoglobin casts accumulate in the nephrons and cause acute tubular necrosis and finally obstructive renal failure.

Treatment involves fluid therapy, combined with diuretics in order to promote high renal flow. Alkalinization of the urine in order to reduce the formation of casts may be beneficial and, in severe cases, hemodialysis may be required. Correction of electrolyte abnormalities and treatment of the underlying cause are important as well. In selected cases, dialysis is mandatory in order for patients to recover from acute renal failure.

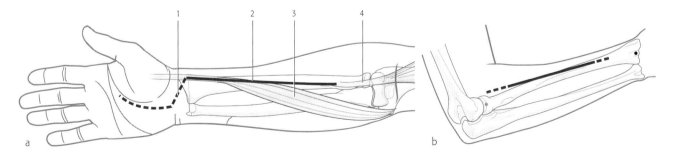

Fig 11.1-2a–b Surgical approach for fasciotomy of the forearm. A possible extension of the incision is shown by a dotted line.
a Anterior skin incision, extensile approach. Landmarks are the flexor carpi radialis muscle and the biceps brachii tendon insertion.
1 Extension for carpal tunnel release (oblique across the wrist flexor crease, ulnar to the thenar crease).
2 Anterior incision.
3 Flexor carpi radialis muscle.
4 Biceps brachii tendon insertion.
b Posterior skin incision. Landmarks are the Lister tubercle (black dot) and the radial head (green dot).

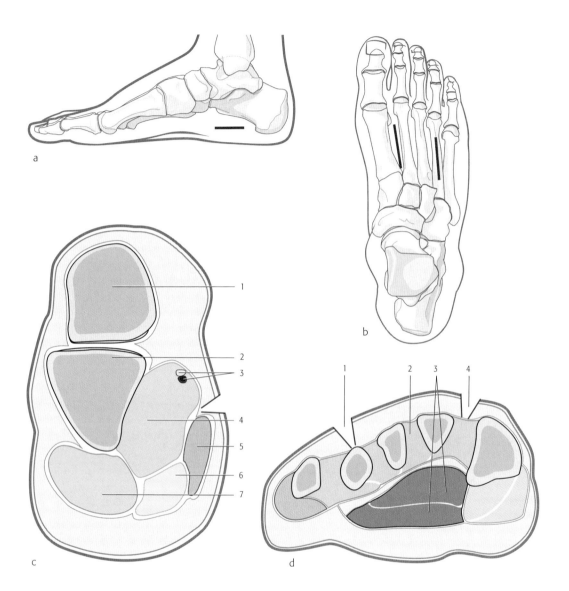

Fig 11.1-3a–d   Surgical approach for fasciotomies of the foot.
a   Note that the medial incision is posterior to the arch of the foot in order to allow decompression of the calcaneal compartment.
b   Dorsal incisions are made between the first and second metatarsal and over the fourth metatarsal bone.
c   Cross section of the hindfoot. The medial approach allows the decompression of all four compartments.
1   Talus.
2   Calcaneus.
3   Posterior tibial vascular bundle and tibial nerve.
4   Calcaneal compartment.
5   Medial compartment.
6   Superficial compartment.
7   Lateral compartment.
d   Cross section of the forefoot. The two dorsal incisions offer access to the four interosseous compartments and the central compartment.
1   Incision over the fourth metatarsal.
2   Four interosseous compartments (green).
3   Central compartment (violet).
4   Incision between the first and second metatarsal bones.

11.1.4 Nerve injury

Nerves may be injured in any kind of soft-tissue trauma. Nerve tissue tolerates stretching far better than bone, but, depending on the extent of damage to the different structures and nerve components, several degrees of injury are observed. A nerve consists of axons surrounded by a myelin sheath. Individual nerve fibers are surrounded by a thin connective tissue called endoneurium. Many individual nerves are grouped into a fascicle (**Fig 11.1-4**). Each fascicle is encapsulated by a connective-tissue layer called perineurium. Blood vessels travel between fascicles and supply the nerve fibers. Several fascicles are grouped together and surrounded by epineurium to form a peripheral nerve.

Sunderland classified nerve injuries according to the individual components that are disrupted (**Table 11.1-1**) [4]:

Grade I injuries, also called neurapraxia, involve injury to the myelin sheath. Neurapraxia presents clinically as a reversible paresthesia. Motor loss may be more severe than sensory damage in these injuries, although incomplete loss of sensation is common. Most neurapraxia injuries occur as a result of local stretching or crushing mechanisms. These injuries are treated expectantly, with a prognosis to full recovery in most cases within 3 months.

Grade II injuries, called axonotmesis, involve disruption of the axon body in addition to that of the myelin sheath. The endoneurium and surrounding structures, however, remain intact. Although the nerve undergoes Wallerian degeneration, nerve recovery is expected to occur in time because the perineurium as a tube is not damaged. Peripheral nerves regenerate at a rate of 1mm per day. In most cases, these injuries are also treated conservatively.

Grade III injuries include disruption of the axon body, the myelin sheath and the endoneurium. These injuries have a poorer prognosis for recovery than less severe injuries of grade I or II. The axon undergoes Wallerain degeneration. Attempts of the nerve to regenerate are hindered by fibrosis and the lack of intact neural tubular structures to guide the regeneration processes.

Grade IV injuries involve injury to all structures except the perineurium. No functional recovery is expected without surgical repair or nerve grafting.

Grade V injuries, called neurotmesis, involve complete transection of the nerve. Nerve repair or grafting is required for the recovery of any function.

Grade of nerve injury	Injured tissue				
	Myelin	Axon body	Endoneurium	Perineurium	Epineurium
I (neurapraxia)	X	–	–	–	–
II (axonotmesis)	X	X	–	–	–
III (axonotmesis)	X	X	X	–	–
IV (axonotmesis)	X	X	X	X	–
V (neurotmesis)	X	X	X	X	X

Table 11.1-1 Sunderland classification of nerve injuries. Table modified according to **Sunderland S** (1951) A classification of peripheral nerve injuries producing loss of function. *Brain*; 74(4):491–516, Oxford University Press.

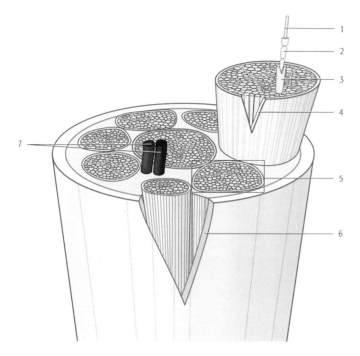

Fig 11.1-4 Peripheral nerve anatomy.
1   Axon.
2   Myelin sheath.
3   Endoneurium.
4   Perineurium.
5   Fascicle.
6   Epineurium.
7   Intraneural blood vessels.

11.2 Complications due to inadequate debridement
Author   David A Volgas

11.2.1   Introduction

"The operative technique is extremely important, for upon the success of the primary operation in removing the causes of infection depends the entire after course of the wound and perhaps the life of the patient."
LTC Joseph A Blake, (US Army Medical Corps) 1919, World War I.

The importance of adequate debridement and its central role in the management of open fractures has been accepted since the early 1900s. However, the consequences of inadequate medical care can be seen even today, whenever prompt medical attention is delayed due to natural disasters, military conflict or lack of medical resources. Therefore, it is important for surgeons to understand the complications that may result from inadequate or delayed debridement.

11.2.2   Superficial infection

Superficial infection (**Fig 11.2-1**) may occur after any surgical procedure, whether emergency or elective. In case of a fracture, there is often an implant beneath the infection and

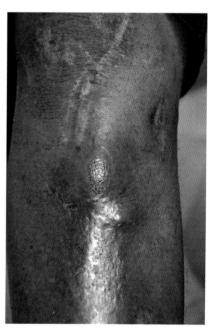

Fig 11.2-1   Clinical photograph of a patient with a superficial abscess, who presented 4 weeks after proximal tibia fracture stabilization with a plate.

the surgeon must be very suspicious of colonization of this hardware. Therefore, the treatment of superficial infection must occur as early as possible, treatment has to be aggressive, usually with a proper surgical debridement (chapter 7.1) and involving irrigation (chapter 7.2) in the operating room.

Aseptic abscesses may mimic superficial infection. Both may present with pain and swelling, but in many cases, the degree of erythema and surrounding induration is less in the case of a sterile abscess. These will usually discharge a fragment of suture and then resolve. Local heat may be beneficial. Oral antibiotics are indicated.

11.2.3 Deep infection

A deep infection may occur following trauma or surgical procedures. It may be the result of hematogenous spread or direct inoculation after inadequate debridement. Direct inoculation, however, is the more common mechanism.

Clinically, postoperative patients typically show slightly elevated temperatures over several days and a high C-reactive protein (CRP) level without any local signs of inflammation. After hospital discharge, they return with pain and often with a draining wound that commenced suddenly and then persisted. Clear drainage is often a result of "subcutaneous" seroma, but is always a reason for concern and the suspicion of a deeper origin. Serous drainage may last longer than

usual in patients on anticoagulation medication, but the surgeon should always be concerned about drainage that continues after 5 days after surgery or drainage, which does not show a clear trend toward decreasing. The discharge may present with purulence or may be a cloudy fluid. Both are most suspicious indicators for a possible deep infection. Alternatively, patients may present weeks or even months after surgical treatment with purulent drainage despite a normal early healing process. In these rare cases, deep infection is believed to have spread hematogenously. Persistent pain in the region of a wound should always raise the suspicion of a deep infection.

Deep infections involve the attachment of bacteria to a surface such as necrotic bone or implants, where the fight against infection is impeded, especially if the bacteria produce a protective biofilm [5]. At present, there are no treatment options for eliminating infection established on an implant except for the removal of the implant. The treatment algorithm for deep infections is shown in **Fig 11.2-2**.

Infected fractures may heal in the presence of an implant, provided the hardware material is not loose and the fracture fixation is stable, but do not always do so. Any loose implant material or dead bone fragment must be removed and, if needed, the stability of fixation should be improved. Leaving the rigidly fixed implant in place and suppressing the infection until the fracture has healed is a valid option until the implant can be removed safely. Therapy with

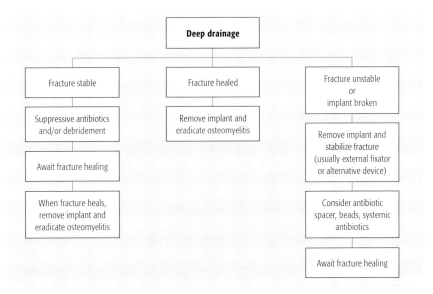

Fig 11.2-2 Treatment algorithm for deep infection involving a fracture.

antibiotics is selected on the basis of cultures taken from tissue samples from the depth, not from superficial skin swabs or cultures from a sinus tract. *Staphylococcus aureus* is often responsive to sulfacycline and/or tetracycline and many infectious disease specialists, who should be consulted in every case, might consider adding rifampicin to the coverage. Intravenous antibiotics over a prolonged period of time are, however, only indicated if the patient has undergone a surgical debridement, but are not expected to cure the infection as long as the implants remain.

Osteomyelitis occurs when bacteria adhere to bone—usually nonviable or necrotic bone—and begin to multiply. Osteomyelitis may develop in a trauma setting either from direct inoculation from the open wound or by spreading from adjacent infected implants. In the case of sequestered necrotic bone, surgical removal must be performed and the dead space managed. When osteomyelitis involves adjacent implants, medical suppression may be carried out as long as the fracture fixation remains stable. However, if fracture fixation is lost, the infected implants must be removed and stabilization must be achieved by other means.

After the fracture has healed and the implants have been removed, the patient's osteomyelitis may still persist. Cierny and Mader described a classification system for osteomyelitis based on four anatomical stages and three host types (**Table 11.2-1a–b**) [6]. This classification is associated with a treatment protocol shown in **Fig 11.2-3a–b**. In general, the surgeon should endeavor to optimize host factors—eg, smoking, control of diabetes, complete or transient cessation of intake of medication interfering with immunosuppression and/or coagulation—prior to undertaking surgical treatment of chronic osteomyelitis (chapter 4.1, 4.3, 4.4). The next step is to adequately debride the bone, including the intramedullary canal and to stabilize the fracture. Finally, after the wound bed is sterile, bone reconstruction may begin. Complete coverage of the treatment of osteomyelitis as well

as delayed union and nonunion, however, is beyond the scope of this book.

While treatment of osteomyelitis may be technically possible in most cases, it may turn out to be very time consuming and require major reconstructive efforts. In some very rare cases, patients may prefer amputation in order to avoid a protracted reconstruction. Moreover, some patients may not be healthy enough to undergo complicated reconstruction while others may not have sufficient vascular supply to support free bone transfers.

11.2.4 Gas gangrene

Debridement is the cornerstone of treatment for severe open or closed soft-tissue injuries (chapter 7.1). When debridement has either been delayed for too long or inadequately performed, significant complications may result, such as infection or even gas gangrene. Gas gangrene is a potentially life-threatening necrotizing soft-tissue infection often occurring as a complication of wound treatment, typically such, with exposure to soil and no or delayed debridement.

In diabetic patients, it may occur without such exposure. It is caused by *Clostridium perfringens*, a gram-positive anaerobic rod bacterium. *Clostridium perfringens* produces a number of exotoxins causing widespread systemic damage including hemolysis or vascular injury as well as destruction of collagen and fascial planes. The time of incubation may be rapid, ie, within hours, or delayed and depends on a low local tissue oxygen tension. *Clostridium perfringens* is sensitive to high-dose penicillin.

The clinical symptoms usually include local crepitation within the soft tissues. Wound exploration may reveal gas, watery discharge, and necrotic muscle. Muscle tissue may be pale, edematous, and may not bleed when cut nor

Anatomical staging	Treatment
I – medullary	Removal of intramedullary nail, intravenous antibiotic (6 weeks)
II – superficial	Decortication, curettage
III – localized	Currettage, delayed bone grafting
IV – diffuse	Excision of necrotic, infected bone, reconstruction

a

Host staging	Definition
A	Healthy host, no major medical problems, nonsmoker
B	Smoker, local tissue compromised, systemic illness
C	Patient with severe systemic illness, ie, not a surgical candidate

b

Table 11.2-1a–b Cierny-Mader classification of osteomyelitis [6]. Patients are described by a combination of anatomical and physiological staging, eg, IIIB. This should not be confused with the Gustilo classification of open fractures.
a Anatomical staging.
b Physiological staging.

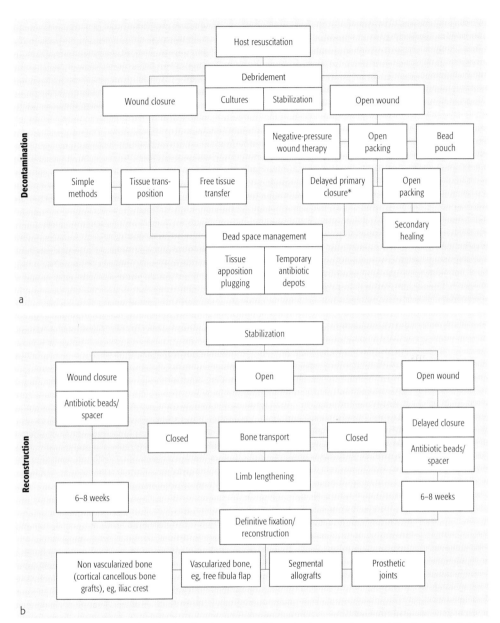

Fig 11.2-3a–b Treatment algorithm for chronic osteomyelitis and subsequent bone stabilization. Controllable host factors such as smoking, diabetes mellitus, and anticoagulative medication should be addressed first.
a The first goal is to decontaminate the wound bed by aggressive debridement and dead space management.
* Delayed primary closure if the wound meets the conditions.
b After the wound is considered clean, reconstruction of the soft-tissue defect and bone defect may be undertaken.

contract when stimulated with electricity. Often, crepitation is associated with free air in the muscles visible on x-rays of the affected extremity. In addition, tachycardia, hypotension, hemodynamic shock, and renal failure may be present. A rapidly progressive course is often seen, and patients may succumb to sepsis within 12 hours [7].

Patients with suspected gas gangrene should be considered critically ill and only immediate and aggressive treatment will save the patient's life. Supportive treatment includes administration of supplemental oxygen and resuscitation with fluids that must be started without delay. Adequate tetanus immunity must be ensured. In spite of the patient's critical situation, surgical debridement must be performed as an emergency. Wide debridement of all involved tissue is required, no dead spaces may remain unexposed and the wounds must remain open. Extensive extremity involvement may even require amputation that may be the life-saving measure in some cases. Since the disease process may continue to involve additional tissue, frequent subsequent debridements are necessary in order to ensure that all necrotic tissues are removed and recesses, which still may harbor *Clostridium perfringens*, are cleansed. Finally, hyperbaric oxygen therapy should be taken into consideration. Clostridia lack superoxide dismutase, making them incapable of surviving in the oxygen-rich environment created within a hyperbaric chamber. This inhibits clostridial growth, exotoxin production as well as the binding of exotoxins to host tissues. Yet, the mortality rate is universal in untreated cases and is 20% even with prompt treatment [8]. In surviving patients, the wound may either be closed at a later date or allowed to heal secondarily by wound contraction and spontaneous reepithelialization.

11.2.5 Functional loss after debridement

Although debridement is vital to a successful salvage treatment, it may include the loss of significant amounts of muscle and/or bone and sometimes tendons. The first concern of the surgeon is to remove all nonviable and necrotic tissue, without regard to "noble" structures (nerves, vessels, etc) and hence to functional outcome. In other words, surgical debridement aims at removing all tissues that have to be removed, and not at preserving function. During the initial assessment and treatment of the wound, the surgeon must take note of muscles and tendons, which have been damaged or debrided. However, after adequate debridement and wound closure, surgeons must turn their attention to the functional restoration of the extremity.

Techniques that may be used to compensate for muscle, tendon and/or nerve damage include supportive measures such as orthotics, limb shortening, or joint arthrodesis, as well as reparative measures including functional transfer of muscle and nerve units and/or tendon transfers. The options available for an individual patient depend on many factors.

Tendon transfers are well described in the upper extremity. In the lower extremity, options are not described as extensively as they are less commonly performed. One useful common transfer technique is the posterior tibialis transfer for acquired foot drop [9]. This transfer, which moves the insertion of the posterior tibial tendon to the dorsum of the foot, may be used in cases of functional loss following anterior compartment syndrome or laceration of the anterior tibial muscle. Sufficient strength to walk without an ankle-foot orthosis may be expected after 6–9 months. Additionally, lengthening of the Achilles tendon may be useful in order to restore a plantigrade foot in cases of pes equinus secondary to tibialis anterior dysfunction.

Arthrodesis may be indicated after irreparable tendon rupture, sciatic nerve injury, or other injuries which leave an imbalance of muscle force across a joint. It is a salvage procedure usually performed after a trial of bracing in the absence of viable muscle transfer options.

Orthotics such as an ankle-foot orthosis may be used in cases of foot drop. A hinged knee brace with a drop-lock hinge may be useful in cases of quadriceps dysfunction. In the upper extremity, wrist extension splints may be useful for radial nerve palsy.

11.3 Complications related to tissue coverage

Authors   Merlin Guggenheim, Claudio Contaldo, Lars Steinsträßer, Sammy Al-Benna, Robert D Teasdall

11.3.1   Complications related to primary closure

The complications associated with primary wound closure include dehiscence, skin necrosis, infection, excessive scarring, and scar contracture. Dehiscence, or wound separation, can either be partial or complete. Dehiscence may be managed with open wound care, primary reclosure, or by reconstruction once the wound is clean. The most common causes for dehiscence are too much tension and suture failure (both a consequence of local ischemia), as well as infection. In case of a localized infection, the removal of one or more sutures may allow the problem to resolve, followed by healing by secondary intention. The same holds true for wound necrosis if the tissue beneath the necrosis or skin slough is healthy and no bare bone or implant material is exposed. Infection may occur whenever there is a break in the skin, and may require debridement and irrigation.

Wounds closed under tension or across areas of tension (joints) may lead to excessive scarring, which occur in two major forms, hypertrophic scarring and keloids. Hypertrophic scars do not extend beyond the edges of the primary scar, as opposed to keloids, which extend predominantly laterally. The cause of these disorders is still unknown, but excessive tension on the wound is felt to be causative in susceptible individuals. A hypertrophic scar may resolve spontaneously. Other methods of treatment include compression of the scar using silicone, intralesional injection of steroids, and ablative therapy (laser, cryotherapy).

11.3.2   Complications related to skin grafts

Graft failure

Causes
The success rate of split-thickness skin grafts should be ~95–100% in an optimal environment with conditioned wounds (chapter 10.2). Unfortunately, this is not always the case, especially in regard to trauma patients and to an aging population with concomitant diseases.

Reasons for graft failure are the following:
- **Poorly vascularized wound beds:** exposed cartilage, tendons, bare bone, and implant material or remaining necrotic tissue resulting from inadequate debridement.
- **Contaminated or infected wound beds:** skin grafts

will not take if local bacterial count exceeds 10,000 organisms per gram tissue. Bacteria, as well as the inflammatory response to bacteria induce the release of enzymes and cytokines at the wound interface that prevent fibrin adherence to the graft. Organisms such as group A β-hemolytic streptococci (eg, *Streptococcus pyogenes*) may result in graft failure even when present in a much lower concentration. Severe wound contamination with *Pseudomonas aeruginosa* also results in poor graft take and, therefore, forms a relative contraindication to skin grafting. In dubious cases, it is recommended to exclude the presence of contamination by bacterial swabs or even by a biopsy of the wound bed after debridement and/or irrigation [10, 11].

Graft take may be compromised by:
- **Inadequate technical handling:** graft desiccation before application, upside-down placement of the graft, excessive stretching of the graft resulting in a "tent-like" deformity without proper contact to the wound bed, too much pressure exerted on the graft after bolstering, or tie-over bandage.
- **Insufficient graft placement and immobilization:** the direct contact of the graft to the wound bed, which is necessary for proper engraftment, may be prevented by hematoma and seroma formation beneath the graft. Movement or shear forces may impede the incorporation of vessels from the graft, and disrupt newly formed vessels should the graft already be revascularized (eg, joints, moving tendon sheaths).
- **Dependent position:** early and undue verticalization of the extremity after skin-graft application will lead to increased orthostatic pressure in newly vascularized, fragile grafts.
- **Concomitant diseases:** peripheral artery occlusive disease, venous insufficiency, lymphatic stasis, diabetes mellitus.
- **Active smoking.**

Of all these causes for graft failure, blood or serous fluid collection beneath the graft as well as shearing and infection of the graft are the most common.

Consequences
Generally, the failure of a skin graft is cumbersome rather than disastrous for both the patient and the surgeon. It usually prolongs the hospital stay and delays final healing time

and, therefore, increases health care costs. Treatment of incomplete graft take usually consists of secondary wound healing. However, in some cases a large portion of the graft sloughs, necessitating reoperation or reevaluation of the wound. Functional loss is rarely associated with graft failure.

Graft contracture

Causes

Contraction of the skin graft occurs in two stages:
- **Primary contraction** is the immediate recoil observed in freshly harvested skin. When the skin is first harvested from its donor site, it contracts immediately after it is released from the surrounding tissue. This reduction in size has been found to range from 9–22%, depending on the thickness of the graft [12]. This primary skin-graft contraction is related to the number of elastin fibers within the graft. It is thought to be the consequence of the passive recoil of elastin fibers within the dermis. Full-thickness skin grafts exhibit the greatest degree of primary contraction due to the inclusion of the elastin-containing dermis in comparison to the thinner split-thickness skin graft, while purely epidermal grafts do not contract.

- **Secondary contraction** occurs during the healing phase, ie, the skin graft contracts, leaving a smaller surface area. The thinner the split-thickness skin graft has been harvested, the greater the degree of secondary contraction will be. This phenomenon is closely related to the percentage of dermis within the graft rather than its actual thickness. Therefore, a graft that includes 75% of the dermis would be predicted to contract less than a graft with 25% of the dermis. Secondary contracture of the skin graft also contributes to hyperpigmentation.

Secondary contraction results from differences in type and number of cellular and matrix components between the dermal layers of the graft and is mediated by myofibroblasts. The dermis suppresses the transformation of fibroblasts into myofibroblasts. The strength of suppression rises with increasing thickness of the dermis. The contraction reduces both the size of the graft at the interface with its recipient bed and the circumference of the graft at its periphery, with each edge of the graft moving towards the center. Split-thickness skin grafts will contract by 20–50% in comparison to the surface initially harvested (**Fig 11.3-1a–b**). The wound bed also exerts an influence on the degree of contraction of the graft. Accordingly, grafting onto rigid tissues (eg, muscle

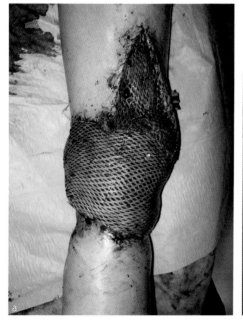
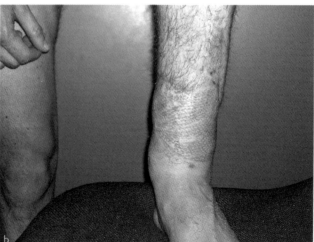

Fig 11.3-1a–b Split-thickness skin graft covering a free gracilis muscle flap.
a   Intraoperative view immediately after skin-graft application.
b   Significant resolution of swelling of the muscle and secondary contracture of the skin graft with good matching to surrounding tissues at the 6-month follow-up.

fascia) results in less contraction in comparison to grafting onto more supple and mobile tissues (eg, deep dermis and subcutaneous fat). Finally, increasing the mesh ratio of split-thickness skin grafts also increases the degree of secondary contraction.

Consequences

A skin graft on top of a flap used as cover for a soft-tissue defect usually remains pliable due to the underlying flap that is padding the graft. Graft contracture very seldom compromises function at the donor site of a flap, because the donor site almost never includes joints. In large abrasion or burn injuries, however, that do not possess the full thickness of the skin, extensive contracture of the skin graft may occur, confining function of joints.

Abnormal sensation in the skin graft

Causes

Initially the graft has no sensation. Reinnervation may set in as early as the first few weeks after grafting. After 1 month, nerves grow into the graft and some sensitivity may return, but has a higher threshold than that of normal skin. Sensitivity first reaches the periphery of the graft originating from the adjacent cutaneous tissue and proceeds centrally. Usually, this process begins during the first months but is not completed for several years following grafting. Split-thickness skin grafts reinnervate more quickly, but full-thickness skin grafts reinnervate more completely. Despite this, reinnervation is almost always incomplete leaving long-term sensory deficits. As a general rule, patients develop protective sensation but no normal perception. Pain is usually the first perceived sensation, followed by touch, heat and cold. Split-thickness skin grafts placed onto intact muscle fascia have better reinnervation than if the muscle fascia has been removed before grafting. The neuroanatomical basis for this difference in the return of sensitivity has yet to be defined.

Consequences

Absent or decreased sensation of a skin graft may be problematic, particularly in weight-bearing areas. The patient will not perceive inadequate pressure or minor injuries, resulting in pressure sores and local infection, respectively. The patient is strictly advised to follow rules in regard to weight bearing. They include not to exceed defined periods of time in a certain position (eg, lying in a supine position, sitting in a wheel chair) as well as wearing customized foot wear and/or prosthesis that discharge the area of interest.

Inhomogeneous pigmentation of donor site and skin graft

Causes

Variations in skin color depend on the following:
- melanin within the epidermis
- oxyhemoglobin within skin vessels
- bile and carotene within the skin.

Permanent hypopigmentation (**Fig 11.3-2**) may occur at donor sites of split-thickness skin grafts. Hyperpigmentation (**Fig 11.3-3**) is a common phenomenon that may occur more frequently in healed skin grafts and less at donor sites. It is due to an overactivity of the melanocytes that may result from melanocyte injury or altered melanocyte control after reinnervation of the skin graft [13]. It has been shown that hyperpigmented skin grafts have an overall increased number of melanosomes within the whole epidermal-melanin unit. Secondary contracture of the skin graft increases the density of melanosomes and contributes further to hyperpigmentation. Accordingly, thinner grafts are more prone to hyperpigmentation than thicker ones. Nevertheless, split-thickness skin grafts may remain pale or white and only

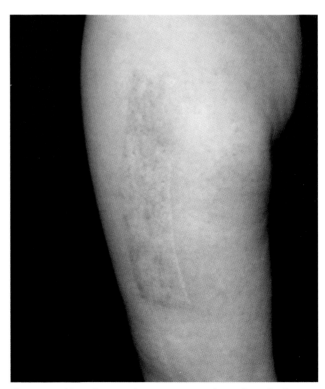

Fig 11.3-2   Hypopigmentation may occur at donor sites of split-thickness skin grafts.

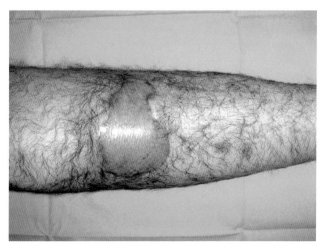

Fig 11.3-3 Hyperpigmentation at the recipient site after split-thickness skin grafting. Clinical photograph at 6 months.

become hyperpigmented with exposure to sunlight. A general recommendation is to keep the graft protected from direct sunlight for at least 12 months after grafting. Hyperpigmentation may be treated with dermabrasion, laser resurfacing, and lotions containing hydroquinone, vitamin A, and dexamethasone as, for example, Pigmanorm®, whereas severe hypopigmentation may be treated using tattoo techniques.

Consequences

Inhomogeneous pigmentation of both the donor site and the split-thickness skin graft itself is an almost exclusively cosmetic complaint. The patient might be limited in having to wear concealing clothing. Therefore, donor sites of split-thickness skin grafts should be in such locations that may be easily concealed whenever possible. Therefore, appropriate donor sites are the upper third of the thigh including the trochanteric region particularly in women, as well as the buttock and the back in men. The scalp may also be a good donor site, particularly in children, where the proportional surface area of the head is larger than in adults.

11.3.3 Complications related to flaps

Partial or total flap loss

Causes

The vast majority of flap loss is caused by macro- and microcirculatory dysfunction that may compromise the pedicle. This is a risk especially in random pattern flaps. Circulatory compromise of a flap may be caused by a variety

of factors, including:
- poor suitability of the flap to this particular patient (noncompliance, comorbidity factors)
- wrong planning of the flap
- improper surgical technique while raising and inserting the flap
- inadequate perfusion conditions (eg, rheology, blood pressure).

Microcirculation will be impaired by:
- inaccurate microsurgical technique (chapter 10.6)
- kinking or compression of the pedicle (eg, hematoma formation, undue tension)
- thrombosis (free flap)
- tension between the flap and the surrounding tissue.

Sequentially, this will result in insufficient venous outflow and inadequate arterial inflow and, ultimately, total loss of the free flap if prompt revision does not achieve salvaging the flap or if kept untreated. In comparison to inadequate arterial inflow, insufficient venous outflow of the flap takes several more days before a well-demarcated necrosis develops [14]. In the latter case, areas of concern are not flaccid, white and avascular, but rather congested, bluish in color with a sluggish circulation. Because the development of necrosis is a slow phenomenon, the elapsing time may allow for some revascularization from healthy surrounding tissues at the wound margin and wound bed. Accordingly, tissue loss predominantly occurs centrally, where revascularization is challenged most.

If pedicled flaps originate from soft tissues adjacent to the traumatized area, they are associated with an increased risk of necrosis (**Fig 11.3-4a–b**) and wound dehiscence because the flap might originate from bruised or crushed skin and muscle. Furthermore, an inflammatory reaction to the trauma, the so-called zone of injury, develops within a few days, which renders the soft tissue's surrounding of the actual defect even more fragile (chapter 10.3.3). Flaps based on several pedicles supplied by retrograde blood flow originating from a major vascular pedicle distally are less reliable than such supplied by a major pedicle proximally with anterograde blood flow to the flap (chapter 10.4, 10.5). This is especially important in posttraumatic defect coverage if the surrounding tissue has directly been traumatized. An alternative to overcome the obstacles of flaps with retrograde blood flow might be the use of fasciocutaneous perforator flaps (eg, pedicled propeller flaps) (chapter 10.4, 10.5) (chapter 12.15) with a well-defined axial pedicle that may better be trimmed to the defect in combination with a superior resurfacing [15].

Postoperative seroma formation that is usually caused by persisting lymphatic outflow may also contribute to flap loss due to the filling of the interspace between recipient site and undersurface of the flap. This will put the flap under tension and possibly compromise its microcirculation.

Inadequate planning of a skin paddle in regard to its underlying muscle may also result in partial necrosis of the cutaneous part of the flap because of scanty perforating vessels to the skin.

Causes for infection that may jeopardize the flap's survival are manifold, including inadequate debridement of a contaminated, dirty, infected or necrotic wound as well as necrosis of the flap that becomes infected [16].

In addition to causes of acute flap loss, delayed tissue loss may occur secondarily, particularly if insensate flap coverage has been performed in weight-bearing areas (**Fig 11.3-5**). Minor injuries that may have remained undetected, will result in pressure sores that most often are superinfected and inevitably develop partial flap loss unless treated (**Fig 11.3-6**).

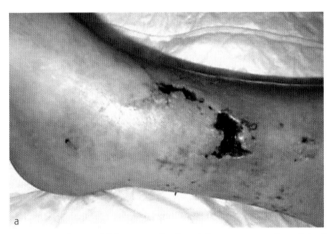
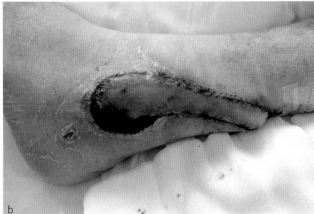

Fig 11.3-4a–b Partial flap necrosis after defect reconstruction of the lower leg.
a Partial necrosis of the randomly perfused distal area of a local skin flap.
b Partial necrosis of the randomly perfused distal area of a regional fasciocutaneous sural flap.

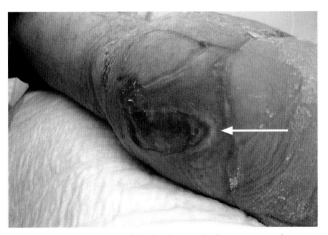
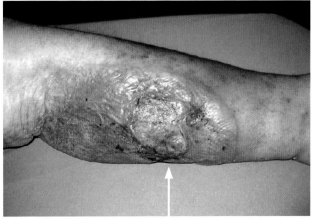

Fig 11.3-5 Pressure sore of the heel (arrow) after coverage of a defect with an insensate, free latissimus dorsi muscle flap and meshed split-thickness skin graft.

Fig 11.3-6 Superinfected ulceration that developed from a minor wound 7 years after coverage of a traumatic soft-tissue defect of the medial calf region (arrow) with an insensate free latissimus dorsi muscle flap and a meshed split-thickness skin graft.

Finally, noncompliance of the patient may be a cause of reconstruction failure, especially during the first postoperative days, when the flap needs to become incorporated within the surrounding tissues by angiogenesis.

Consequences

Total flap loss is disastrous for both patient and surgeon. Partial flap loss is also fatal, particularly if tissue loss occurs over vital structures that require coverage with vascularized tissue. Vital structures include nerves, tendons, or bradytrophic areas such as bare bone, cartilage or nonvascularized implant material. These areas cannot be covered by nonvascularized skin grafts (chapter 10.2). Partial flap loss may cause complete functional failure and require subsequent tissue transfer that is usually more complicated to perform than the previous one, ie, a failed pedicled flap needing to be replaced by a free flap [17].

Wound dehiscence

Causes

This complication may be caused by inadequate perfusion of the flaps' margin and/or of the wound edges as well as infection of the wound. It can result from errors in treatment strategy, ie, wrong timing of surgery, incorrect planning of the flap (eg, tension during flap insertion, inadequate width-to-length ratio) and/or insufficient surgical technique, including inappropriate debridement of the recipient site and flap elevation.

In acute extremity trauma with soft-tissue defect, immediate defect coverage has been associated with a superior outcome, if performed within 48–72 hours in a hospital setting with well-trained orthopaedic and plastic surgeons [18]. Rate of infection and number of operations required in order to obtain the final result are lower, hospital stay and time to bone healing are shorter, and total cost of treatment is less.

However, selected cases will benefit from adequate wound conditioning and deferred coverage, which may even decrease the risk of wound dehiscence, especially if necrosis of the wound margins is not definitively demarcated, debridement has been inadequate, and the surrounding tissues have been heavily traumatized. This change in practice, with a trend to simpler reconstructive techniques may be the result of improved wound-care technology [19].

Pedicled flaps that have an inadequate width-to-length ratio and large, free flaps including several angiosomes and, therefore, randomly perfused areas sometimes might end up with an insufficiently perfused periphery that will even-

tually suffer ischemic necrosis because of the relatively insufficient blood supply by the dominant artery. If flaps are too small for the defect, they will always be under tension and at risk of wound dehiscence (chapter 12.9). Inadequate surgical technique per se may lead to intraoperative injury of the pedicle or elevation of the flap in the wrong plane, which may compromise its survival.

Postoperative wound infection may be another cause for wound dehiscence. Coagulase-negative staphylococci and *Staphylococcus aureus* as normal parts of the resident skin flora are a frequent cause of this type of complication. Of course, heavily contaminated wounds are always at increased risk for infection and wound dehiscence.

Consequences

The consequence of wound dehiscence is cumbersome rather than disastrous. It may lead to salvage procedures, increase the necessary frequency and total time for wound care until healing is completed, prolong hospital stay and eventually increase health care costs.

Overall, wound dehiscence and partial flap loss range from 7–36% for pedicled or perforator flap repair of soft-tissue defects [20–22]. Peripheral vascular disease, smoking, and age have been shown to negatively influence the incidence of these complications. Although age has been demonstrated to be a risk factor for reconstructive failure using free flaps in the lower extremity [17], the overall rate of wound dehiscence and partial flap loss is still considerably lower than in pedicled flaps [16].

Persistent lymph edema of the flap

Causes

Postoperative edema in flaps is a commonly encountered problem, which may develop in large pedicled and free microvascular flaps. It may result regardless of their muscle or fasciocutaneous origin. Flap edema may not only cause cosmetic concerns but also functional disabilities when situated in regions such as the weight-bearing area of the ankle or foot (Fig 11.3-7a–b).

Flap edema in the early postoperative period is a well-known phenomenon, resulting from increased arterial blood flow in association with decreased vascular resistance, reduced lymphatic drainage, and histological changes of the transferred tissue [23]. In particular, edematous flaps are seen on the lower extremities, probably due to persistent, vigorous blood flow into the flap combined with orthostasis, which may considerably uphold flap edema. Denervation of free

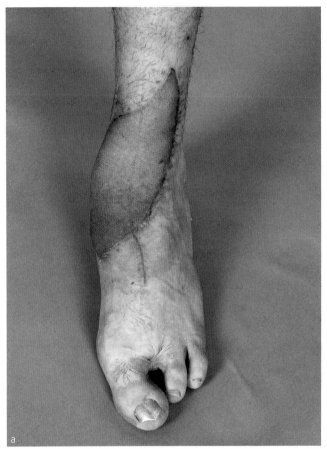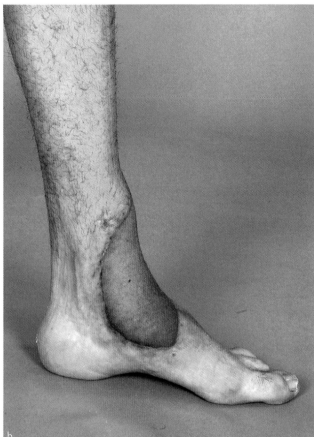

Fig 11.3-7a–b Follow-up 1 year after coverage of an anteromedial lower-leg defect with exposed extensor tendons using a free fasciocutaneous scapula flap. Note the pincushion-like swelling of the flap due to lymphedema.
a   Anterior view.
b   Medial view.

flaps resulting in perivascular sympathectomy will inevitably relieve arteriolar vasoconstriction and reduce muscle tone, facilitating vasodilatation. Interrupted lymph vessels may also contribute to flap edema, since they often may not be able to recanalize adequately within the surrounding tissues and especially across the scar.

Consequences

In order to treat this cosmetic concern and functional disability, compressive garments should be worn at first because the transferred tissue usually recuperates its initial thickness in 6–9 months postoperatively, be it by muscle atrophy, resolution of the edema, or deswelling of skin. Nevertheless, the flap may occasionally remain edematous for a longer period of time [24]. In that case, surgical debulking has been the gold standard in order to reduce the flap's volume and thickness. However, this technique may endanger the flap's vascularization if the patent pedicle is injured. In this regard, muscle flaps are at greater risk because—unlike fasciocutaneous flaps that easily integrate within the surrounding tissues (ie, the wound bed and the wound margin) by angiogenesis—muscle flaps almost always remain dependent on their pedicle. An alternative to surgical fat removal is liposuction and/or skin excision, especially if the fatty tissue is excessive as is sometimes encountered in musculocutaneous or fasciocutaneous flaps. This technique will work better at avoiding injury to the flap's pedicle. Finally, selective embolization of the dominant nutrient artery of the pedicle may be performed, assuming the flap has become well integrated within its recipient bed [25].

Mismatch of the flap with its surrounding tissues

Considerations

While choosing a flap in order to cover a defect, the surgeon must not only take into consideration the purpose of the flap but also whether the transferred tissue will match the new surrounding tissues. Of course, flap selection heavily depends on functional considerations such as restoration of sensation or muscle function, bone reconstruction and pliability. But other aspects must also be taken into consideration when planning a flap, such as matching the flap to its new surroundings in regard to thickness, texture and color. Some surgeons regard these considerations as mere cosmetic aspects but, if neglected, they may cause unpleasant complications.

Bulkiness

Despite muscle atrophy that will develop postoperatively, denervated muscle flaps may still remain bulky (**Fig 11.3-8a–f**) in comparison to well-trimmed, fasciocutaneous flaps (chapter 12.17, 12.18). Although presumably only a cosmetic problem, bulky flaps may prevent the patient from wearing normal footwear and cause a pressure sore to develop on an insensate flap. Strategies to prevent flap bulkiness include:

- selection of thin donor muscles (eg, serratus anterior muscle (**Fig 11.3-9a–b**), where applicable
- insertion of the flap with appropriate tension.

Scarification of the muscle fascia and undermining of margins of the recipient bed as well as the long-term wearing of com-pression garments are other factors that may prevent bulkiness of muscle flaps. Finally, secondary debulking procedures for bulky flaps may be the last option.

Sagging skin

The fasciocutaneous flap tends to lose its elasticity and, consequently, becomes saggy despite being well matched in texture and color (**Fig 11.3-10a–c**) and optimally trimmed during the insertion of the flap. This sagging skin may hinder putting on clothes or prevent the patient from wearing normal foot wear. Furthermore, these flaps tend to heal with a sort of interface between donor site and flap that allows for abundant gliding of the flap. Such a flap that remains completely insensate and is covering weight-bearing areas such as the sole of the foot or stumps will also develop pressure sores. One of the strategies to treat sagging of the flap includes secondary trimming as required. The incorporation of a strong fascia into the flap (fascia lata for anterolateral thigh flaps) or a tendon (palmaris longus tendon for radial forearm flaps) may be used as a suspension.

Mismatch in texture and color

Muscle flaps covered by a split-thickness skin graft may equal fasciocutaneous flap coverage in texture and color (**Fig 11.3-10c**). However, skin grafts covering muscle flaps often remain hyperpigmented (**Fig 11.3-11a–b**). Moreover, the diamond-shaped pattern of the meshed skin graft may permanently remain visible (**Fig 11.3-1b**, **11.3-3**, **11.3-8**, **11.3-9**, **11.3-10**, **11.3-12**).

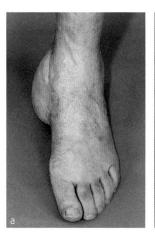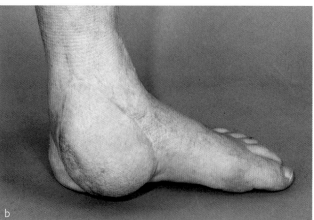

Fig 11.3-8a–f   Note the persisting bulkiness of these denervated free latissimus dorsi flaps even several months after transfer.
a–c   Musculocutaneous flap. Deformity of the medial malleolus that prevents the patient from wearing shoes.
a   Anterior view.
b   Medial view.

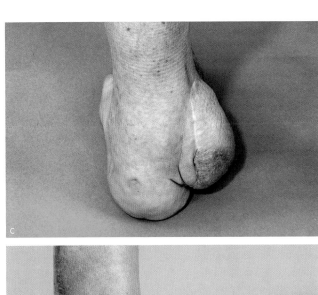
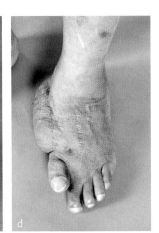
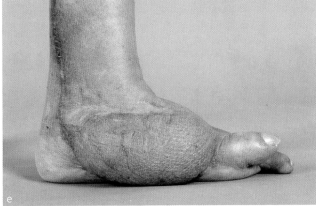
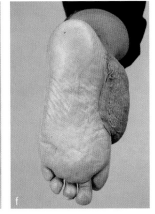

Fig 11.3-8a–f (cont) Note the persisting bulkiness of these denervated free latissimus dorsi flaps even several months after transfer.

c Posterior view.
d–f Muscle flap covered by meshed split-thickness skin graft. Deformity at the medial aspect of the mid foot that prevents the patient from wearing shoes.
d Anterior view.
e Medial view.
f Plantar view.

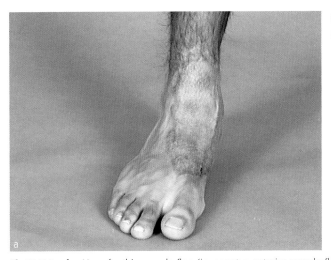
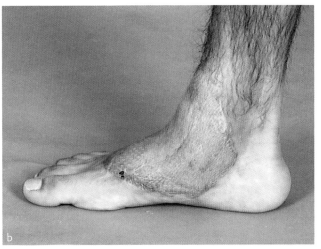

Fig 11.3-9a–b Use of a thin muscle flap (ie, serratus anterior muscle flap) covered with a meshed split-thickness skin graft may provide excellent lining of a defect at the dorsum of the foot. However, the mismatch in texture, pattern, and color of the surface is obvious.
a Anterior view.
b Medial view.

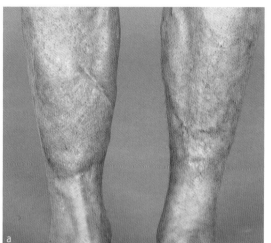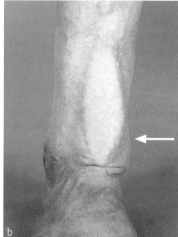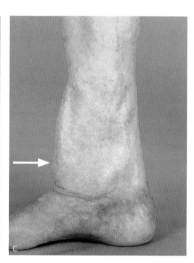

Fig 11.3-10a–c Examples of flaps that match the surrounding tissue nicely in texture and color.
a   Five years after coverage of a lower-leg defect with a free latissimus dorsi muscle flap and a meshed split-thickness skin graft. Anterior view.
b–c Two years after coverage of a lower-leg defect with a free fasciocutaneous scapula flap. The saggy area (arrows) might benefit from surgical thinning and partial resection.
b   Anterior view.
c   Medial view.

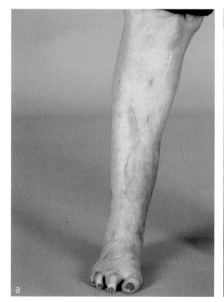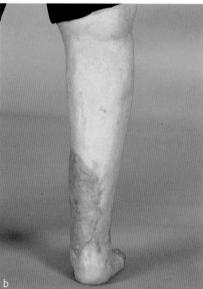

Fig 11.3-11a–b Three years after coverage of a posteromedial lower-leg defect with exposed Achilles tendon using a free latissimus dorsi muscle flap and a meshed split-thickness skin graft. Note the nice contour of the leg and the hyperpigmentation of the graft.
a   Anterior view.
b   Posterior view.

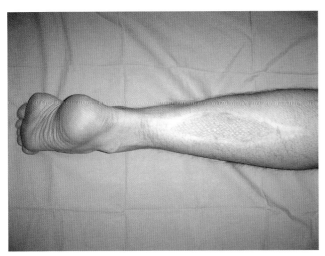

Fig 11.3-12 Clinical photograph 1 year after coverage of a posterior lower leg defect and after bipedicled flap transposition to cover an anteriortibial defect. Permanent diamond-shaped pattern of a skin graft.

11.4 Adherences and scar contracture

Authors   Claudio Contaldo, Merlin Guggenheim

11.4.1   Introduction

Post-traumatic soft-tissue defects may considerably vary in size, composition of traumatized or missing tissues as well as possible exposure of structures. Accordingly, repair of a defect may vary from direct closure to coverage by nonvascularized skin grafts or vascularized flaps in virtually any composition and combination. Depending on the underlying tissues and location as well as on the type of wound closure, respectively wound coverage, adherences or scar contractures may develop. They may not only be cosmetically disturbing but may limit function considerably. The extent and complexity of the defect, the experience of the surgeon as well as factors innate to the patient will determine the appropriate reconstructive approach according to well-defined reconstructive modules (chapter 8.2).

11.4.2   Adherences of skin grafts and flaps

When dealing with a soft-tissue defect, the first question is whether the exposed tissue will tolerate direct closure by approximation of the wound margins or if it may be left to heal by secondary intention. The latter carries a higher risk of scar contracture. Depending on the vascularization of the wound bed, larger defects will need coverage either by skin grafts or flaps. Defects at the level of the deep dermis, subcutaneous tissue, muscle, or fascia may be grafted, since at that level, adherences generally will not impair function, unless the defect extends over a joint. Skin grafts, however, have limitations in regard to cosmetic aspects (eg, mismatch of color, texture, thickness, and suppleness).

Tendons and nerves as well as bare bone or exposed implant material will need to be covered by a flap (**Fig 11.4-1a–f**). Tendons on the dorsum of the hand or the foot, in the Achilles tendon region, as well as in the hollow of the elbow or the knee should be covered with vascularized tissues in order to create some kind of gliding surface. This prevents adherences, which would impair the range of motion considerably or might result in scar contractures or unstable skin coverage due to a decreased take rate of the graft. Unlike exposed tendons and often badly vascularized peritendinous tissue, well-vascularized perineural tissue will allow a skin graft to take. However, adherences of the graft to the nerve may lead to disagreeable neurological symptoms including pain, dysesthesia, or nerve compression syndromes that are less often seen after flap coverage. Therefore, nerves exposed after trauma should always be covered with, respectively buried under, vascularized tissues such as mobilized skin or muscle surrounding the wound or actual flaps.

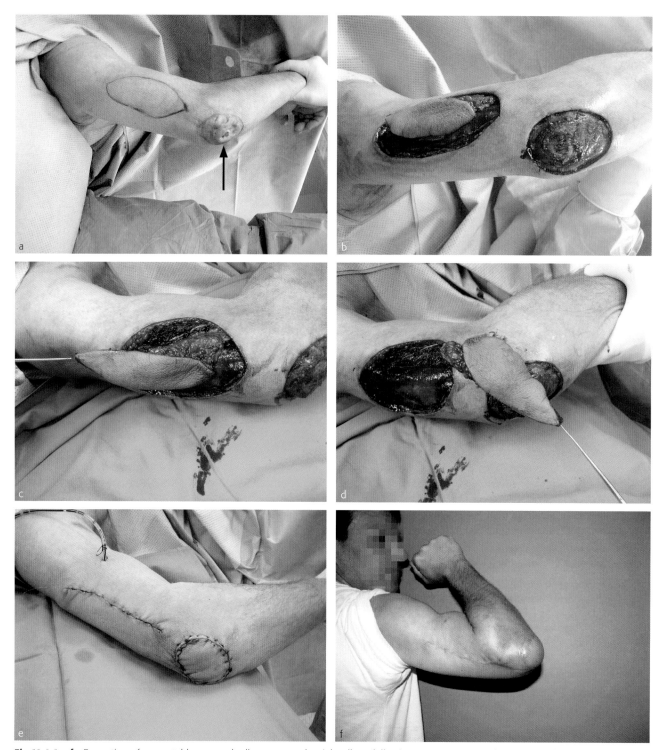

Fig 11.4-1a–f Formation of an unstable scar and adherences at the right elbow following a 3-year course of recurrent inflammation of the bursa olecrani.

a Preoperative state with scar tissue and fistula (arrow) despite multiple surgical procedures.

b–d Radical excision of the scarred tissue and dissection of a distally pedicled fasciocutaneous lateral arm flap tailored to the defect.

e Interposition and insertion of the trimmed island flap into the defect after tunneling beneath the skin bridge.

f At the 6-month follow-up, scarring is adequate and elbow function fully restored.

Tissue defects over bare bone or exposed implant material will rarely or only very slowly develop sufficient granulation tissue, which may be later covered by a skin graft. An increased risk of infection, graft failure, unstable and/or vulnerable scarring and scar contracture will remain. On the other hand, covering exposed bone with a flap will hardly ever impede function and similarly flap coverage of exposed implants will hardly ever result in adherences as the foreign body will rapidly be encapsulated by the vascularized tissue.

A prerequisite to achieving satisfactory results is adequate preparation, ie, conditioning (chapter 9) of the soft-tissue defect prior to coverage. The approach to prevent disturbing adherences aims at reconstructing exposed or sutured tendons and nerves. This particularly holds true for extensive degloving injuries (chapter 3.3) or after burn injuries as well as in non-weight-bearing areas. In order to be successful, thin, pliable and supple tissues that are able to create gliding interfaces are required, which will also help to restore natural anatomical contours [26, 27]. They include super-thin fasciocutaneous flaps [28, 29] or vascularized fascia (eg, fascia temporalis, fascia lata) covered by a split-thickness skin graft with or without dermal substitutes (chapter 10.2) (**Fig 11.4-2a–c**) [26, 27, 30].

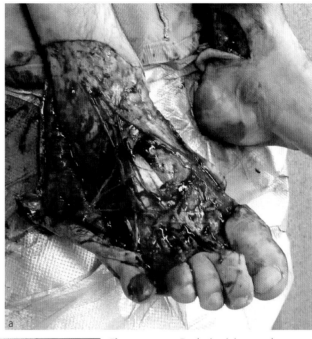

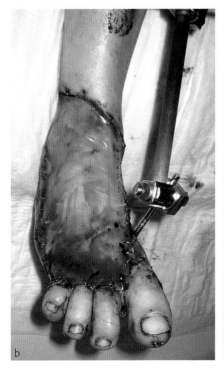

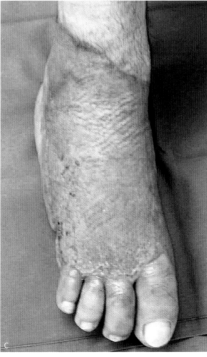

Fig 11.4-2a–c Degloving injury on the dorsum of the right foot that was fixed in a two-staged procedure.
a   Extensive degloving injury of the right foot with full-thickness skin defect exposing the extensor tendons of the foot and toes.
b   After 3 weeks, the vascularized dermal substitute (yellow-reddish spotted pattern) is ready to receive a skin graft. Note that the little toe had to be amputated during debridement.
c   Three months after the application of a meshed, split-thickness skin graft.

11.4.3 Abnormal scar formation and scar contracture

Scar contracture in extremity trauma in general and in hand trauma in particular may result in functional limitations and disability. This problem is, however, more often encountered after burn injuries than after nonburn trauma. Timely management of the burn wound and postburn scars has decisively decreased the incidence of burn scar deformity and contractures of extremities in recent years [28, 31]. The challenging treatment of scar contractures includes physical therapy, temporary splinting as well as surgery (eg, transection of contracture bands, multiple Z-plasties, excision of the contracted tissue and coverage with skin graft and/or dermal substitute or flap, as well as combinations of these treatments). In order to overcome scar contracture, dermal substitutes are increasingly being used to cover both soft-tissue defects originating from trauma or after excision of abnormal scar formation (ie, hypertrophic scar or keloid). However, long-term results in regard to the rate of recontracture are still scarce.

Abnormal scar formation may develop both at the donor site and the recipient site. Associated causative factors include:
- genetics
- race
- gender
- age
- anatomical location.

Locations that appear to have a predisposition for such scar formations are the shoulder region, the intermammary cleft, and the forearm.

Following "overgrafting", ie, if a skin graft overlaps another skin graft, such abnormal scars may also be observed (**Fig 11.4-3**). Although they rarely impair function, such scars may be painful and cosmetically disturbing.

Unlike the abnormal scar resulting from excessive collagen deposition [32], widened scars are much more frequently encountered on the extremities, and are the result of persistent tension and movement at the site of the wound (**Fig 11.4-4**). Although a widened scar is more of a cosmetic problem than a functional one, often it is nevertheless bothersome to the patient, in particular if the reconstruction has functionally been successful. The typical widened scar is flat, wide, often depressed, and usually appears within 6 months after surgery. Treatment consists of scar excision and layered primary closure. Sometimes, larger defects may result from scar excision. These defects will then need some type of

reconstructive surgery, be it a dermal substitute and an unmeshed, split-thickness skin graft or a flap (ie, local, regional, or free flap) that matches best in regard to thickness, texture, and color of the surrounding tissues. Recently, local subdermal injection of autologous fat, ie, lipofilling, has been advocated in order to soften and smooth scars or to correct surface irregularities. Speaking from experience, scars at the donor site of the skin graft or the flap usually are only a minor problem to the patient.

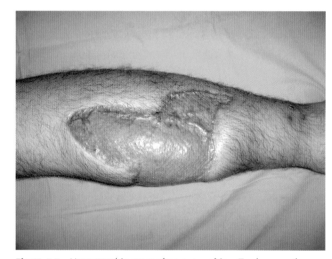

Fig 11.4-3 Hypertrophic scars after overgrafting. Twelve months after reconstruction of a soft-tissue defect of the middle third of the left lower leg caused by trauma. Reconstruction was performed with a free gracilis muscle flap covered with a meshed split-thickness skin graft.

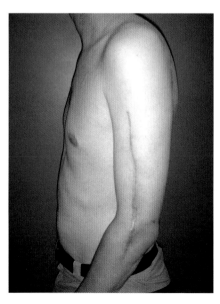

Fig 11.4-4 Widened scar at the donor site of a free lateral arm flap.

References and further reading

[1] **Whitesides TE, Haney TC, Morimoto K, et al** (1975) Tissue pressure measurements as a determinant for the need of fasciotomy. *Clin Orthop Relat Res;* (113):43–51.

[2] **Fulkerson E, Razi A, Tejwani N** (2003) Review: acute compartment syndrome of the foot. *Foot Ankle Int;* 24(2):180–187.

[3] **Vanholder R, Van Biesen W, Lameire N, et al** (2007) The role of the International Society of Nephrology/Renal Disaster Relief Task Force in the rescue of renal disaster victims. *Contrib Nephrol;* 156:325–332.

[4] **Sunderland S** (1951) A classification of peripheral nerve injuries producing loss of function. *Brain;* 74(4):491–516.

[5] **Stewart PS, Costerton JW** (2001) Antibiotic resistance of bacteria in biofilms. *Lancet;* 358(9276):135–138.

[6] **Cierny G 3rd, Mader JT, Penninck JJ** (2003) A clinical staging system for adult osteomyelitis. *Clin Orthop Relat Res;* (414):7–24, Springer.

[7] **Present DA, Meislin R, Shaffer B** (1990) Gas gangrene. A review. *Orthop Rev;* 19(4):333–341.

[8] **Hart GB, Lamb RC, Strauss MB** (1983) Gas gangrene. *J Trauma;* 23(11):991–1000.

[9] **Yeap JS, Birch R, Singh D** (2001) Long-term results of tibialis posterior tendon transfer for drop-foot. *Int Orthop;* 25(2):114–118.

[10] **Krizek TJ, Robson MC** (1975) Evolution of quantitative bacteriology in wound management. *Am J Surg;* 130:579–584.

[11] **Robson MC, Krizek TJ, Heggers JP** (1973) Biology of surgical infection. *Curr Probl Surg;* Mar:1–62.

[12] **Davis JS, Kitlowski EA** (1931) The immediate contraction of cutaneous grafts and its cause. *Arch Surg;* 23:954–965.

[13] **Tyack ZF, Pegg S, Ziviani J** (1997) Postburn dyspigmentation: its assessment, management, and relationship to scarring—A review of the literature. *J Burn Care Rehab;* 18(5):435–440.

[14] **Chen KT, Mardini S, Chuang DC, et al** (2007) Timing of presentation of the first signs of vascular compromise dictates the salvage outcome of free flap transfers. *Plast Reconstr Surg;* 120(1):187–195.

[15] **Pignatti M, Pasqualini M, Governa M, et al** (2008) Propeller flaps for leg reconstruction. *J Plast Reconstr Aesthet Surg;* 61(7):777–783.

[16] **Bui DT, Cordeiro PG, Hu QY, et al** (2007) Free flap reexploration: indications, treatment, and outcomes in 1193 free flaps. *Plast Reconstr Surg;* 119(7):2092–2100.

[17] **Wettstein R, Schürch R, Banic A, et al** (2008) Review of 197 consecutive free flap reconstructions in the lower extremity. *J Plast Reconstr Aesthet Surg;* 61(7):772–776.

[18] **Arnez ZM** (1991) Immediate reconstruction of the lower extremity—an update. *Clin Plast Surg;* 18(3):449–457.

[19] **Parrett BM, Matros E, Pribaz JJ, et al** (2006) Lower extremity trauma: trends in the management of soft-tissue reconstruction of open tibia-fibula fractures. *Plast Reconstr Surg;* 117(4):1315–1324.

[20] **Sananpanich K, Tu YK, Kraisarin J, et al** (2008) Reconstruction of limb soft-tissue defects: using pedicle perforator flaps with preservation of major vessels, a report of 45 cases. *Injury;* 39(Suppl 4):55–66.

[21] **Ma CH, Tu YK, Wu CH, et al** (20 08) Reconstruction of upper extremity large soft-tissue defects using pedicled latissimus dorsi muscle flaps—technique, illustration and clinical outcomes. *Injury;* 39(Suppl 4):67–74.

[22] **Erdmann MW, Court-Brown CM, Quaba AA** (1997) A five year review of islanded distally based fasciocutaneous flaps on the lower limb. *Br J Plast Surg;* 50(6):421–427.

[23] **Lorenzetti F, Salmi A, Ahovuo J** (1999) Postoperative changes in blood flow in free muscle flaps: a prospective study. *Microsurgery;* 19(4):196–199.

[24] **Salmi A, Tukiainen E, Härmä M** (1996) A prospective study of changes in muscle dimensions following free-muscle transfer measured by ultrasound and CT scanning. *Plast Reconstr Surg;* 97(7):1443–1450.

[25] **Heymans O, Verhelle NA, Nélissen X, et al** (2004) Embolization of a free flap nutrient artery to reduce late postoperative edema. *Plast Reconstr Surg;* 113(7):2091–2094.

[26] **Schwabegger AH, Hussl H, Rainer C, et al** (1998) Clinical experience and indications of the free serratus fascia flap: a report of 21 cases. *Plast Reconstr Surg;* 10286):1939–1946.

[27] **Woods JM 4th, Shack RB, Hagan KF** (1995) Free temporoparietal fascia flap in reconstruction of the lower extremity. *Ann Plast Surg;* 34(5):501–506.

[28] **Gousheh J, Arasteh E, Mafi P** (2008) Super-thin abdominal skin pedicle flap for the reconstruction of hypertrophic and contracted dorsal hand burn scars. *Burns;* 34(3):400–405.

[29] **Yilmaz M, Karatas O, Barutcu A** (1998) The distally based superficial sural artery island flap: clinical experiences and modifications. *Plast Reconstr Surg;* 102(7):2358–2367.

[30] **Rose EH, Norris MS** (1990) The versatile temporoparietal fascial flap: adaptability to a variety of composite defects. *Plast Reconstr Surg;* 85(2):224–232.

[31] **Barbour JR, Schweppe M, O SJ** (2008) Lower-extremity burn reconstruction in the child. *J Craniofac Surg;* 19(4):976–988.

[32] **Rudolph R** (1987) Wide spread scars, hypertrophic scars, and keloids. *Clin Plast Surg;* 14(2):253–260.

CASES

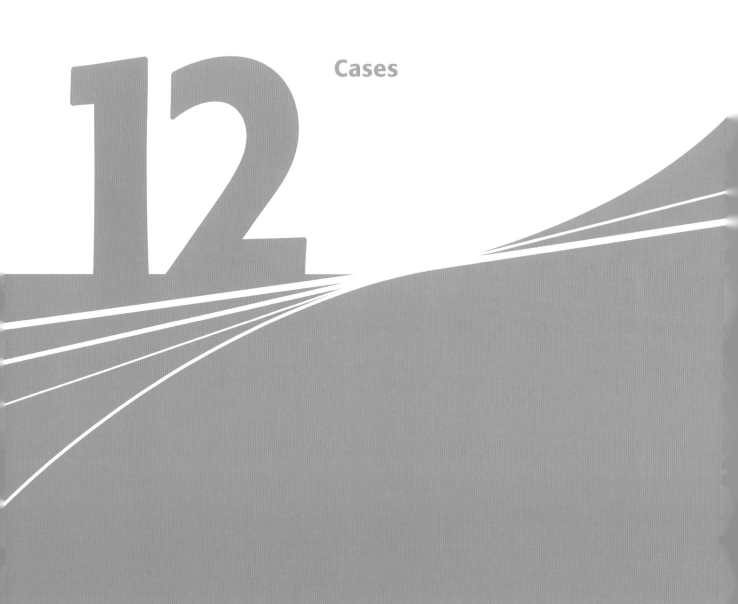

12 Cases

Introduction

Authors   David A Volgas, Yves Harder

In addition to knowing how to perform reconstructive surgery on bone and soft tissues, the surgeon must develop an understanding of when and why to choose a particular option. In most cases, there are many feasible options and only few choices that are absolutely right or wrong. But in any given situation, there may be a solution that is most appropriate.

The following twenty cases depict frequent or exemplary soft-tissue problems of the extremities encountered by the orthopaedic trauma surgeon. However, it should be noted that not all cases require the same level of skills and not all procedures described can be performed by a trauma surgeon. Cases presented in the following section are grouped according to various skill levels. The degree of difficulty in performing the featured surgical procedures increases along with the skill level. Skill level I represents what a general orthopaedic surgeon could perform. Skill level II would be feasible for a trauma surgeon. Skill level III requires a surgeon with some training in soft-tissue coverage, whereas skill level IV requires a surgeon trained in microvascular surgical procedures. The level of required surgical skill is indicated in the table below and in each case.

The focus of these case presentations is on the surgeon's train of thought and decision-making process rather than on surgical techniques. By following the experienced surgeon's thoughts, the reader will learn to understand:
- the process of identifying and selecting feasible options for a certain patient
- the difference between feasible and best options
- when to refer a case to—or ask advice from—a surgeon trained in more advanced reconstructive techniques.

Case number	Skill level	Case type	Location	Indication	Vascular pattern	Type of transfer	Tissue composition	Page
12.1	I	Fracture blisters	Distal tibia	Closed fractue	–	–	–	234
12.2	I	Debridement	Arm	Open fracture	–	–	–	237
12.3	I	Elastic vessel loops	Distal tibia	Open fracture	–	–	–	241
12.4	I	Negative-pressure wound therapy	Distal tibia	Open fracture	–	–	–	243
12.5	I	Split-thickness skin graft	Lower leg	Morel-Lavallée lesion	–	–	–	247
12.6	II	Transposition flap	Distal tibia	Wound dehiscence	Random	Transposition	Fasciocutaneous	250
12.7	II	Bipedicled transposition flap	Distal tibia	Open fracture	Random	Transposition	Fasciocutaneous	256
12.8	II	V-Y advancement flap	Finger	Open fracture	Random	Advancement	Fasciocutaneous	260
12.9	II	Gastrocnemius flap (medial head)	Medial knee	Wound dehiscence	Axial	Transposition	Muscle	264
12.10	II	Gastrocnemius flap (medial head)	Medial knee	Open fracture	Axial	Transposition	Muscle	267
12.11	II	Soleus flap	Anterior leg	Open fracture	Axial	Transposition	Muscle	271
12.12	III	Radial forearm flap	Hand	Open fracture	Axial	Transposition	Fasciocutaneous	275
12.13	III	Distally based sural flap	Medial ankle	Traumatic defect	Axial	Transposition	Fasciocutaneous	279
12.14	III	Medial plantar flap (instep flap)	Plantar heel	Heel ulcer	Axial	Transposition	Fasciocutaneous	283
12.15	III	Free-style perforator flap (propeller flap)	Achilles tendon	Open fracture	Axial	–	Fasciocutaneous	287
12.16	III	Rotation flap	Sacrum	Chronic ulcer	Axial	Rotation	Fasciocutaneous	291
12.17	IV	Lateral arm flap	Lower leg	Open fracture	Axial	Free	Fasciocutaneous	294
12.18	IV	Anterolateral thigh flap	Lower leg	Open fracture	Axial	Free	Fasciocutaneous	299
12.19	IV	Latissimus dorsi/serratus anterior flap (chimeric flap)	Lower leg	Open fracture	Axial	Free	Muscle	302
12.20	IV	Fibula flap	Forearm	Open fracture	Axial	Free	Osteoseptocutaneous	307

12.1 Skill level I: Case 1

Author David A Volgas

Case history

- 54-year-old white male patient
- Independent construction worker without worker's compensation
- Single
- Smoker, 1 pack cigarettes per day
- Consumes 3–4 beer per day
- No other medical problems

The patient was working on a scaffold when it collapsed. He fell ~6 m (20 ft) onto concrete, sustaining an injury to his right leg. Emergency medical personnel started intravenous fluids and administered pain medication in the field. They reduced the fracture by inline traction on site and applied a splint to the leg.

The patient underwent evaluation by the trauma team in the emergency department. No other injuries beside that of the leg were found on primary, secondary or tertiary survey. Findings during the initial clinical examination:

- The right leg showed significant ecchymosis around the ankle, especially medially, indicating considerable intraarticular hematoma in the presence of a closed fracture. Pulses and sensation were normal in the foot except for decreased sensation in the distribution area of the deep fibular nerve, ie, the dorsal area in the first web space.
- There was already marked swelling near the ankle before the initial x-ray studies were complete.
- X-rays revealed a high-energy distal fracture of the leg including a multifragmentary intraarticular pilon fracture (Fig 12.1-1a–b).

Wound conditioning: none.

Present status

The patient was scheduled for surgery the following morning to repair the fibula and place an external fixator across the ankle joint. However, at the time of surgery, when the splint was removed, significant sanguinous fracture blisters were present on the medial side of the ankle (Fig 12.1-2).

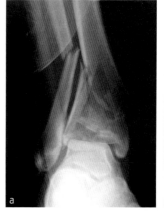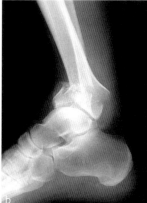

Fig 12.1-1a–b Closed, multifragmentary intraarticular distal tibial fracture (43-C) of the right leg.
a   AP x-ray.
b   Lateral x-ray.

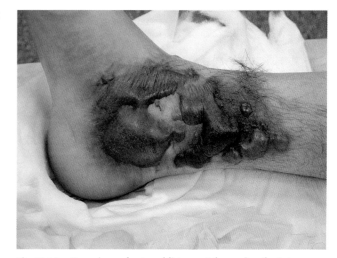

Fig 12.1-2 Sanguinous fracture blisters ~1 hour after the injury on the lateral aspect of the ankle.

Decision making

Open questions

- Should the surgeon proceed with immediate open reduction and internal fixation of the fracture in the presence of fracture blisters? If not, when should definitive management be undertaken?
- How should the fracture blisters be managed?
- If the soft tissue does not recover in time to safely perform definitive fixation, what are the treatment options?

Options and plan

The presence of fracture blisters (chapter 3.3.4) is a sign of significant skin injury. Whenever possible, incisions should not be made through fracture blisters until there is evidence that they are healing. However, the fracture still must be stabilized in order to allow the soft tissues to recover and to prevent further soft-tissue injury. Clearly, in this case, an external fixator is an option.

There is little convincing evidence to support any particular method of management of fracture blisters. The treatment is often based on tradition and personal experience rather than evidence. It is very important that the surgeon realizes that fracture blisters indicate severe injury involving deep soft-tissue compartments. Locally, there is edema, hypoxia and microvascular failure, thus creating a very high risk for further, immediate surgical trauma. Some surgeons prefer to unroof the fracture blister acutely and to cover the wound with a sterile dressing. Yet, one should keep in mind that the liquid of sterile blisters contains a lot of cytokines and growth factors stimulating and accelerating wound healing. Accordingly, the blisters may instead be kept intact until their spontaneous perforation.

There is a window of ~10–14 days during which the fracture can still be manipulated and an anatomical joint reduction achieved. After 2–3 weeks, a callus will already have formed, requiring removal, and hampering reposition and fixation. While the rough bone alignment of the fracture fragments may still be achieved after this period of time, beginning resorption of the fracture ends may preclude accurate positioning of bone fragments. However, to safely undertake an open anatomical reduction, the soft-tissue envelope has to be assessed. If the surgeon is able to flex the ankle dorsally or if pinching the skin around the ankle results in visible wrinkles, this is an indication that the edema has subsided sufficiently in order to safely close the skin after surgery.

In the case of fracture blisters, there should be reepithelialization of the blister within 14 days in most cases. Whenever the color of the skin changes from a deep red to a more normal skin tone and loses the glossy appearance of the acute fracture blister, it is relatively safe to incise through it. Meticulous handling of the soft tissues is required once the definitive procedure is undertaken, including restricted use of retractors, use of sharp rather than blunt dissection, and making the incision longer than normal in order to avoid retracting too hard on the damaged area of the skin (chapter 1). Note that a small incision will require much more traction in order to expose an area of 2 cm from the incision than a longer incision.

Occasionally, the skin does not return to a condition where it would be safe to perform definitive fixation, either because of persistent fracture blisters or edema. Often, these cases are crush injuries or circumferential injuries, which result in extensive internal degloving of the soft tissues and damage to the lymphatic drainage of the limb. In such cases, external fixation may turn out as the definitive treatment. There are some things that may be done during the early phase in order to reduce swelling. Plexipulse® foot pumps are an effective method for rapidly reducing lower extremity swelling, although they are not well tolerated in patients with fractures of the foot and/or ankle. Strict bed rest and elevation of the limb above the level of the heart is usually most effective. Bulky dressings, such as Jones dressing (well-padded bandages to the extremity) may be used as well in order to protect soft tissues whenever a splint is required. Occasionally, the administration of diuretics may accelerate the deswelling process.

Procedure

The patient initially went to the operating room ~16 hours after injury for placement of the external fixator bridging the ankle and for plate fixation of the fibula. Due to the blisters, the external fixator was placed laterally with pins in the tibia, calcaneus and talus (Fig 12.1-3).

Follow-up

Twelve days later, the skin was examined in clinic and found to be suitable for definitive fixation (Fig 12.1-4), which was performed the next day. Intraoperatively, care was taken to minimize any additional soft-tissue trauma by retracting within the fracture.

The fracture healed uneventfully within 4 months (Fig 12.15a–b) and the patient experienced no wound complications. During the first year after injury, he continued to have edema whenever he stayed on his feet for any length of time or experienced pain whenever the weather changed. He did not show any signs of complex regional pain syndrome.

Points to remember

- Soft-tissue injury is normal with fractures.
- Fracture blisters are an outward visible sign of this injury.
- Time should be given in order to allow deep dermal tissues to begin healing.
- Extreme care should be taken not to undermine skin.

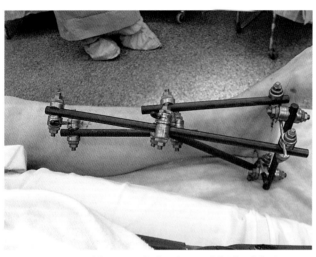

Fig 12.1-3 External fixator applied to the medial side of the leg, spanning the ankle.

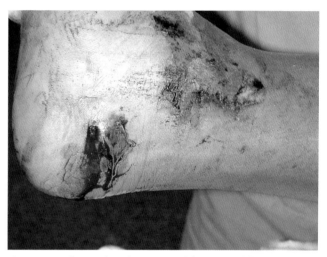

Fig 12.1-4 After 12 days, large parts of the fracture blisters have reepithelialized.

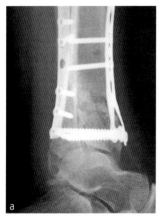
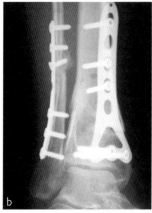

Fig 12.1-5a–b Healed fracture at 4 months.
a   AP x-ray.
b   Lateral x-ray.

12.2 Skill level I: Case 2

Author David A Volgas

Case history

- 24-year-old white male patient
- Coal miner
- Single
- Nonsmoker
- Right-hand dominant
- No other medical problems

The patient was attempting to remove an obstruction from in front of a coal car in a mine. When he removed the obstacle, the coal car rolled forward, pinning both arms under the car. Emergency personnel in the field began intravenous fluids, applied field dressings and splints to both arms, and transported the patient to a level I trauma center, arriving 60 minutes after injury.

The patient was examined on arrival to the trauma center by trauma surgeons and the orthopaedic team. The patient was intubated shortly after arrival for pain control. The initial assessment on presentation to the trauma bay revealed normal chest, abdomen, pelvis, and spine.

Significant findings in the secondary survey included:
- considerable gross contamination in both arms
- extensive crush injury to the right arm extending from elbow to wrist with almost subtotal amputation, absent pulses in the wrist
- crush injury to the left forearm including the first web space and palm of the hand, present radial and ulnar pulses
- subtotal amputation of the left index finger.

Wound conditioning: none.

Present status

In consultation with the trauma and vascular teams the orthopaedic team elected to move immediately to the operating room for a detailed assessment of what was viable, while fluid resuscitation continued. The injuries were rapidly determined to be isolated, since trauma to chest, abdomen or head had already been excluded. No nerve examination could be performed prior to anesthesia because the patient had been intubated in the trauma bay for pain control.

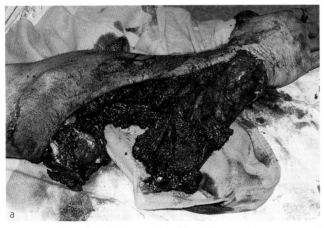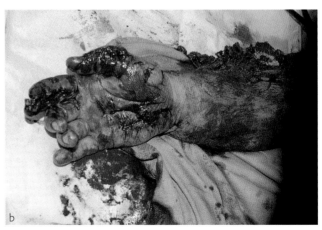

Fig 12.2-1a–b   Clinical photographs of the right arm prior to amputation.
a   Extensive soft-tissue injury and contamination to the right forearm (posterolateral aspect).
b   Extensive soft-tissue injury to the right forearm distally and hand (palmar aspect).

Intraoperative examination of both arms revealed the following:

- pulses not restored after reduction of the right forearm fractures by traction
- very significant muscle damage to the entire flexor and extensor compartments
- abundant muscle tissue crushed and lacerated (Fig 12.2-1a)
- gross contamination of the skin, subcutaneous tissue, muscle, and bone
- numerous lacerations and fractures of the hand (Fig 12.2-1b)
- numerous fractures of both radius and ulna, involving the better part of the diaphyses of both bones, including the distal humerus.

Examination of the left arm revealed:

- large superficial laceration along the posterior forearm (Fig 12.2-2a)
- gross contamination of the wound
- large laceration of the first web space in the hand (Fig 12.2-2b)
- capillary refill in the second digit absent.

Decision making

Open questions

- Which tissue is salvageable?
- What will the likely end result be if there are no major complications?
- Are there any "heroic" measures that might improve the end result?

Options and plan

The initial assessment was that the right forearm was not salvageable. Even if the vessels could have been repaired, the function of the hand and forearm would most likely not have been restored. Making the decision to amputate the dominant arm is always difficult, but in this case, the extensive, contaminated crush injury of the forearm with overwhelming muscle damage, including massive bone trauma and damage to major vessels and tendons in the hand left no other option and led to this decision.

The left arm appeared to be viable, though there was significant damage to the hand. Certainly, the index finger was not viable due to neurovascular damage. There was muscle damage to the forearm, but its extent could not be determined prior to surgical exploration. The arm and hand would require further reconstruction by a hand surgeon in order to optimize functional outcome.

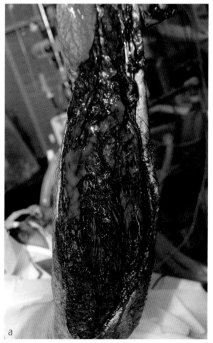
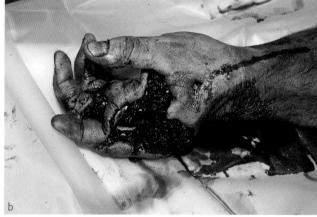

Fig 12.2-2a–b Clinical photographs of the left forearm prior to debridement.
a   Extensive soft-tissue injury and contamination (posterior aspect).
b   Large laceration on the palm of the left hand (lateral aspect).

Having someone knowledgeable about the reconstructive options after emergency debridement facilitates decision making. In this case, the hand surgeon on call was not available for immediate consultation. However, the operating surgeon did discuss the findings with the hand surgeon by phone while still in the operating room immediately after having fully assessed both arms.

Plastic surgeons were not required in this case, because at this stage with grossly contaminated wounds, any type of reconstructive measure was not an option. The vascular surgeons, who were consulted in the emergency department, did not have any hope of salvaging the right arm due to the extensive soft-tissue injury.

Our initial impression was that the patient would need a transhumeral prosthesis for the right arm and be left with a 4-fingered hand on the left, but with reasonably good function of both arm and hand. Yet, this question could not be answered until a full intraoperative assessment of the left arm had been performed.

Certainly the loss of the dominant arm causes the surgeon to think carefully about any drastic measures which might allow salvaging the arm. Nerve grafts, microvascular repair of the arteries, free tissue transfers, and large allografts were all briefly considered in this case. However, even if the finest surgeons working with unlimited resources and sufficient time were to attempt salvage of this arm, the functional result would, nevertheless, be far less than that obtainable with a prosthetic arm. The attempt would, furthermore, involve intensive physical therapy over a long period of time and still would, most likely, only result in a stiff and painful right arm and a hand with negligible function.

Procedure

The orthopaedic team quickly completed a guillotine amputation of the right arm through the distal humeral fracture line. The wound edges were cleaned and vessels ligated. As this was a contaminated wound, the soft tissues to cover the humeral diaphysis were only reapproximated very loosely.

Attention was then directed to the left arm. Crepitus was noted in the proximal forearm, which was later found to be a displaced ulnar fracture (Fig 12.2-3). Meticulous debridement was undertaken, beginning with the skin and methodically working down to the bone (chapter 7.1). Two surgeons working side by side needed ~3 hours to complete the debridement, since the muscle was heavily contaminated with

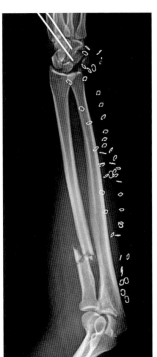

Fig 12.2-3 AP x-ray of the left forearm showing a displaced fracture of the proximal radial bone (after fixation of the carpal fracture).

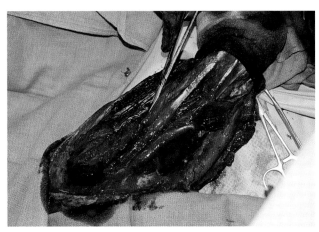

Fig 12.2-4 Systematic, meticulous debridement of the left forearm showing viable musculotendinous tissues.

embedded coal dust (Fig 12.2-4). After the debridement had been completed, the wound was irrigated with 8 l of normal saline (chapter 7.2). Cultures were taken after debridement and irrigation.

Then the left hand was explored and the second metacarpal was found to be fractured segmentally with a dysvascular digit. At the level of the forearm (Fig 12.2-4), the flexor tendons were avulsed from their muscles proximally. Diastasis was noted between the trapezoid and capitate as well as between the trapezoid and trapezium bones. The second ray and the trapezoid bone were resected after discussing the issue with the hand surgeon. The third proximal phalanx was pinned with a K-wire in order to stabilize the mid-shaft phalangeal fracture. The thumb metacarpal was pinned to the carpus also using a K-wire (Fig 12.2-5).

Finally, after debridement, irrigation and fracture fixation, a systematic exploration of the muscles, tendons and nerves was undertaken. Whenever the operating surgeon is not the person who will perform the reconstructive phase of the treatment, he or she must take a thorough inventory of what is intact and functional and what is not, and commu-nicate the findings clearly to the reconstructive surgeon. In this case, the following findings were noted:

- laceration of the extensor tendons to the fourth and fifth digits at the level of the metacarpals
- avulsion of the extensor tendon of the carpi radialis longus muscle from the muscle belly
- all remaining extensor tendons intact
- extensors and flexors to the thumb intact
- avulsion of the second digit flexor tendons from the muscle belly
- exposed radiocarpal and mid-carpal joints dorsally
- nondisplaced proximal ulnar fracture (intraoperative image intensification).

The skin was loosely reapproximated, using elastic vessel loops and staples. A negative-pressure wound-therapy device was applied. The dorsal skin of the hand, which was still bleeding on its edges despite being degloved, was felt to be viable and, thus, was retained in order to cover the wrist joint.

Two days later, the hand surgeon took the patient back to the operating room to search for residual contamination, to make a first-hand assessment of the reconstructive options and to close the wound of the amputated right arm. This was accomplished by shaping the residual muscle to cover the end of the bone, cutting the nerve 2 cm proximal to the bone and burying the nerve stump within the muscle in order to avoid a painful neuroma whenever the patient wears a prosthesis and finally covering the muscle with a split-thickness skin graft. Then the left arm was debrided again and small amounts of residual contamination were found in the muscle. The radial neurovascular bundle to the thumb was found to have been lacerated at the time of the initial injury, but this fact had remained undetected at that time. Despite a lacerated neurovascular bundle to the thumb, the first digit presented with sufficient vascularization and, therefore, it was decided not to repair this vascular axis. Since the skin overlying the wrist was still viable, it was also left. The extensor tendons of the fourth and fifth digits were attached to those of the third digit. After copious irrigation, the skin was reapproximated using elastic vessel loops and staples.

Two days later and after additional wound conditioning with a negative-pressure wound-therapy device, the remaining wounds were closed and covered with a split-thickness skin graft.

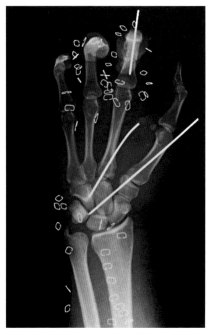

Fig 12.2-5 AP x-ray of the left forearm and hand after fracture fixation.

Follow-up

The patient's wounds have healed uneventfully and, psychologically, he has adjusted well to the consequences of his injury. He was fitted with a conventional prosthesis for his right arm. Today, the left hand is functional for rough motor movements, but the ability for fine motor movements remains limited because of the stiffness of his wrist and fingers. The patient continues to experience considerable phantom pain in the right arm.

Points to remember

- Multidisciplinary interaction (orthopaedic, trauma, vascular, hand, and possibly plastic surgeons) is of major importance.
- The order of priority must be adhered to.
- Infection must be prevented.
- As much function as possible must be preserved.
- The extent of injuries and structures available for reconstruction must be communicated accurately (by initial trauma surgeon to follow-on surgeon).
- This is even more important whenever definitive treatment follows in another hospital (such as in case of military conflict and natural disasters).

12.3 Skill level I: Case 3
Author David A Volgas

Case history

- 26-year-old Hispanic male patient
- Construction worker
- Single
- Nonsmoker
- No other medical problems

The patient was working at a building site when a beam fell and struck him on the distal tibia. The patient was treated at the scene by emergency medical personnel with a clean bandage, splint, intravenous fluids and pain medication.

In the trauma bay, an 8 cm laceration across the anterior tibia, which appeared to reach down to the periosteum, was identified. No fractures were visible on x-rays. The wound was contaminated by fragments of clothing. Initially, the patient underwent debridement of the wound in the trauma bay in order to remove gross contamination. He received tetanus toxoid and broad-spectrum antibiotics.

Wound conditioning: none.

Present status

The patient was taken to the operating room, where his wound was debrided. No gross debris was found in the wound. There was some necrotic subcutaneous tissue, which was debrided. There was a defect measuring 3 cm at its widest. There was soft-tissue swelling and the surgeon assessed that, once the swelling has subsided, the skin would allow primary closure.

Decision making

Open questions
- What are the realistic goals of treatment?
- Which definitive treatment options are there?

Options and plan
The wound did not involve a fracture, so decision making was less complex. The laceration was deep and involved skin, subcutaneous tissue, and to some extent muscle. In addition, there were effects caused by an internal degloving mechanism with shear force across the anterior tibia. Therefore, consideration was given to the possibility that the skin may become necrotic within the next few days. At that point, possibilities for wound closure included:
- primary closure (chapter 10.1)
- wound closure by elastic vessel loops (chapter 10.1)
- application of antibiotic pellets (chapter 9.2).

As this wound is relatively uncomplicated, full recovery is expected. Since the periosteum is intact and there is no fracture, the laceration should heal uneventfully.

Whenever a wound cannot be closed primarily, there are several options a surgeon may take into consideration in order to condition the wound for later closure. First, in heavily contaminated or infected wounds, an antibiotic bead pouch may be used. In this case, this was not necessary. Secondly, a negative-pressure wound-therapy device (chapter 9.3) may be used either alone or in combination with closure by elastic vessel loops and staples (chapter 10.1). Finally, a retention suture technique may be used. Skin grafting or delayed primary closure may be used subsequently in order to close the wound definitively.

Procedure

In this case, wound closure by elastic vessel loops was used in order to help prevent skin edges from retracting (Fig 12.3-1). A negative-pressure wound-therapy device was placed over the elastic vessel loop closure. The patient was taken back to the operating room within 72 hours in order to attempt closure of the wound. By this time, much of the initial swelling had subsided and the wound was approximately half of its original width (Fig 12.3-2). It was now possible to close the wound with sutures (Fig 12.3-3).

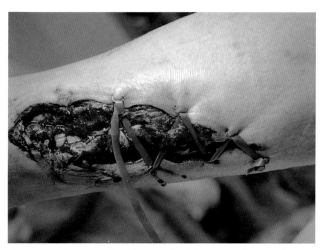

Fig 12.3-1   Intraoperative photograph of the traumatic wound after debridement. Note the method of applying the elastic vessel loops in a "shoestring lacing" technique.

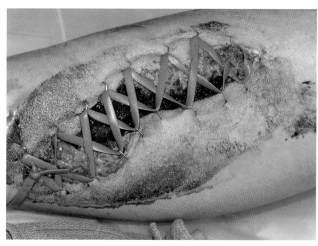

Fig 12.3-2   Intraoperative photograph of the wound after 72 hours of negative-pressure wound therapy and approximation of the wound margins by elastic vessel loops.

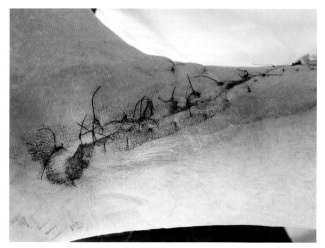

Fig 12.3-3   Intraoperative photograph of the wound demonstrating that delayed primary closure had become possible.

Follow-up

The patient was started on an early range-of-motion mobilization of the ankle in order to prevent scarring and adherence of the tendons to the healing wound. The wound healed uneventfully, without any signs of skin necrosis or infection.

Points to remember

- Elastic vessel loops may be used to assist with closure of fasciotomy wounds or any other type of skin wound that would undergo undue tension if closed primarily.
- The use of elastic vessel loops may help prevent wound retraction, allowing delayed primary closure.
- One of the prerequisites for using this technique is no substantial tissue loss (chapter 10.1), as is the case in the wounds described above (laceration, fasciotomy wound, surgical incision, etc).

12.4 Skill level I: Case 4

Author David A Volgas

Case history

- 43-year-old white female patient
- Unemployed
- Single
- Smoker (1 pack per day)
- Occasional alcohol use
- History of major depression
- Atrophic left kidney (congenital)

The patient was involved in a single-vehicle car accident. She was treated in the field by emergency medical personnel with intravenous fluids, splinting, and a clean bandage. Examination by the trauma surgeons in the trauma bay revealed:
- closed, comminuted fracture of the right distal tibia (Fig 12.4-1a–b)
- marked swelling of the right ankle
- intact neurovascular structures
- scalp laceration.

The patient was taken to the operating room on the night of admission. An external fixator was placed (Fig 12.4-2a–b). The patient was discharged 4 days later to allow swelling to subside prior to definitive fixation. The patient returned to the hospital 10 days from the injury, but initially refused surgery.

She then returned 3 weeks later desiring surgery. Despite the length of time since injury (4 weeks), the surgeon decided to proceed with the surgery as planned because there was still significant intraarticular displacement. The external fixator was removed and an open reduction and internal

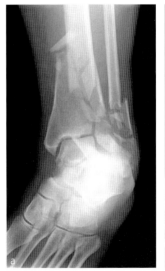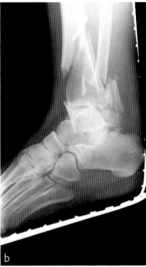

Fig 12.4-1a–b Comminuted distal tibial fracture of the right leg.
a   AP x-ray.
b   Lateral x-ray.

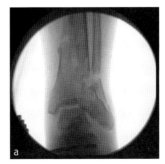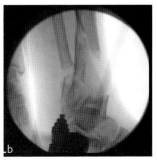

Fig 12.4-2a–b Reduction after placement of an external fixator.
a   AP x-ray.
b   Lateral x-ray.

I
II
III
IV

fixation of the fracture was performed through an antero-lateral approach.

The patient returned to clinic 2 weeks later for suture removal. Onset of necrosis was noted in the skin over the anterolateral wound accompanied by purulent drainage. The wound also showed significant dehiscence (Fig 12.4-3). The patient was readmitted to the hospital for debridement and closure of the wound. After initial debridement, an antibiotic bead pouch was placed (Fig 12.4-4). Four days later, a sural flap (chapter 10.5) was used to cover the defect and a split-thickness skin graft (chapter 10.2) was used to cover the donor site. The patient was discharged on postoperative day 4 on a scheme of home intravenous antibiotics.

The patient returned to the clinic for staple removal after 2 weeks (Fig 12.4-5). She then missed her next appointment and the home intravenous nurse reported that she had disappeared from home. She reappeared 6 weeks later with a partially necrotic flap and recurrent purulent drainage. She was readmitted for debridement of the wound and the necrotic areas of the flap.

Wound conditioning: none.

Present status

During debridement of the epidermis, removing more than 50% of the flap, purulence was found along the plate. The patient was left with an open wound at the edge of the flap, which was ~4 cm wide and could be closed. She also had a skin defect with exposed subcutaneous fat affecting more than 50% of the flap.

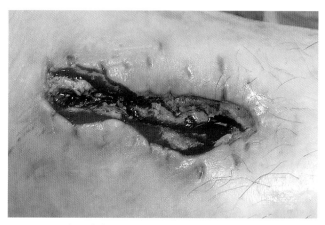

Fig 12.4-3　Clinical photograph showing anterior surgical wound dehiscence.

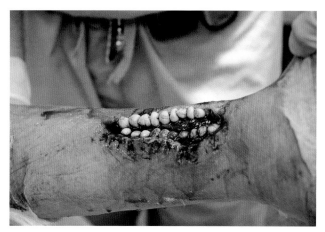

Fig 12.4-4　Intraoperative photograph of the antibiotic bead pouch placed after initial debridement.

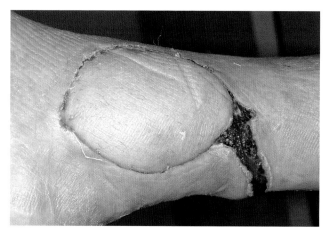

Fig 12.4-5　Clinical photograph showing the sural flap at the first postoperative visit.

Decision making

Open questions
- What are realistic goals of treatment?
- How to overcome noncompliance?
- Which are the initial treatment options?
- Which are the definitive treatment options?

Options and plan

The patient has demonstrated very poor compliance, which has at least partially contributed to an infected wound. Much of her noncompliance was due to fear of surgery and depression, so treatment of this condition is indicated. Repeated attempts to close the wound would be futile without patient compliance. The question of compliance was also relevant for the decision to treat the patient with a negative-pressure wound-therapy device rather than a flap.

There were two goals for treatment of this wound. First, achieving the eradication of the underlying infection as the critical factor for successful treatment of the injury; and secondly, the necessary restoration of intact skin over the wound. Both goals are interdependent. Intact skin is necessary for long-term eradication of the infection and conversely, persistent infection will continue to drain.

Initial treatment options include the removal of the flap that is doomed to failure, an antibiotic bead pouch, negative-pressure wound therapy, split-thickness skin graft, and finally, coverage with a free flap. Given the presence of infection, it is unlikely that a split-thickness skin graft or free flap could prove successful before the infection has been contained.

Options for definitive treatment of the wound remaining after initial treatment of the infection and debridement again include negative-pressure wound therapy, split-thickness skin graft and free flap. Following the principles of the reconstructive modules (chapter 8.2), and after the formation of granulation tissue the most basic procedure with any reasonable likelihood of success was chosen. If the patient should develop recurrent purulent drainage, the plan could easily revert back to antibiotic beads, radical resection of bone or removal of the hardware and placement of an external fixator in order to stabilize the fracture.

Procedure

A psychiatric consult was obtained and a selective serotonin reuptake inhibitor (SSRI) was prescribed. The surgeon spent a great deal of time discussing the problem of noncompliance with the patient. After satisfactory debridement of purulent material and subsequent conditioning of the wound with an antibiotic bead pouch, the patient returned to the operating room for an assessment of the infection and placement of a negative-pressure wound-therapy device (chapter 9.3). The wound appeared clean and no further purulence was detected under the flap. The flap edge along the prior dehiscence was slightly friable and, thus, was debrided, leaving a bleeding skin edge. After irrigation of the wound, a negative-pressure wound-therapy device was placed over the flap (Fig 12.4-6).

The patient remained in the hospital for 7 days with a negative-pressure wound-therapy device in place. After that time abundant granulation tissue was noted (Fig 12.4-7). Consideration was given to apply a split-thickness skin graft, but the patient refused.

Follow-up

After discharge, the patient returned for the first two appointments and then was again lost to follow-up. However, 1 year later, she returned, complaining of contralateral knee pain. Her flap had healed without any further problems (Fig 12.4-8). Her fracture had also healed uneventfully (Fig 12.4-9a–b), her infection had not returned.

Points to remember

- Soft-tissue infections may be very troublesome, especially when patients are noncompliant. Adjustments must be made to treatment options for patient factors including noncompliance.
- Negative-pressure wound therapy is often used to condition wounds for later skin grafting, but it may also be used to stimulate growth of granulation tissue, which will then epithelialize, although this is a much longer process than a skin graft or even a flap.

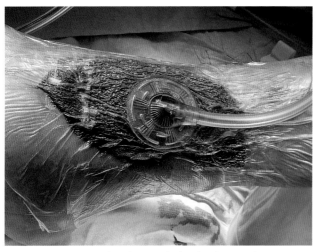

Fig 12.4-6 Intraoperative photograph showing the negative-pressure wound-therapy device in place.

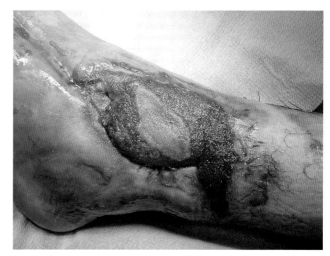

Fig 12.4-7 Intraoperative photograph showing significant granulation tissue over the wound. Local wound care was carried out until the wound had healed.

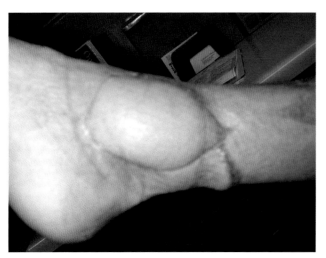

Fig 12.4-8 Clinical follow-up photograph showing the healed sural flap.

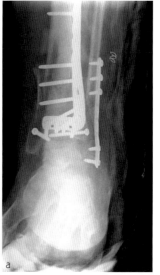
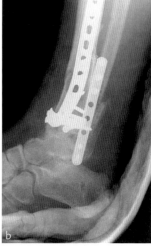

Fig 12.4-9a–b Healing of the distal tibial fracture of the left leg at 1 year. Note that the plates remain and there are no clinical signs of infection.
a   AP x-ray.
b   Lateral x-ray.

12.5 Skill level I: Case 5

Author David A Volgas

Case history

- 38-year-old white female patient
- Housewife
- Single
- Obese
- Nonsmoker
- No other medical problems

The patient was involved in a motor-vehicle collision. She was wearing a seat belt and was the front-seat passenger. Emergency medical personnel at the scene applied a clean bandage and began administering intravenous fluids. Emergency management included fluid resuscitation and an initial debridement of large foreign material from the wound in the trauma bay. The initial clinical examination revealed that both lower extremities were neurovascularly intact.

Findings on the left leg:
- large degloving injury of the left lower extremity (Fig 12.5-1) (chapter 3.3)
- comminuted fractures of the distal femur and distal tibia (Fig 12.5-2a–b, 12.5-3a–b)
- multiligamentous knee injury, which was checked with intraarticular saline, but was found to be closed.

The patient was taken to the operating room on the night of admission for debridement of necrotic tissue, including nonviable skin, subcutaneous fat and muscle. The knee joint was checked a second time and was again found to be closed, although capsule rupture had been suspected as a result of the fracture. On surgical examination of the wound, a true degloving injury was confirmed, with subcutaneous tissue separated from both the underlying fascia as well as the overlying skin (Fig 12.5-4).

Wound conditioning: An external fixator was placed across the knee and ankle in order to rest the soft tissues and stabilize the fractures (Fig 12.5-5). As the patient developed coagulopathy during the period of treatment, negative-pressure wound therapy was not an option. Therefore, the wound was covered with petroleum dressings.

Present status

The wound comprised ~50% of the circumference of the lower leg and 40% of the medial leg just proximal to the knee. The skin bridge, which separated the two defects, had turned necrotic.

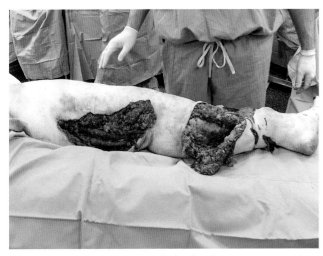

Fig 12.5-1 Initial appearance of the left leg demonstrating massive degloving.

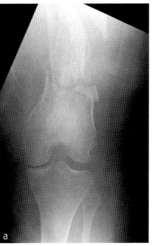
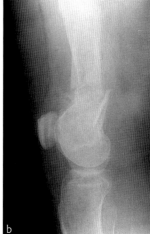

Fig 12.5-2a–b X-rays showing a comminuted supracondylar femoral fracture.
a AP view.
b Lateral view.

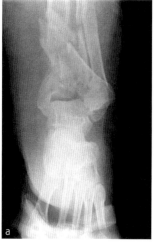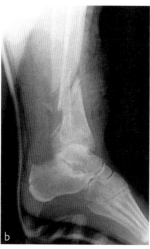

Fig 12.5-3a–b Tibia showing comminution of the metaphysis and significant intraarticular extension.
a AP x-ray.
b Lateral x-ray.

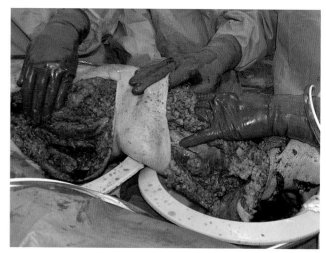

Fig 12.5-4 Intraoperative photograph showing separation of the subcutaneous tissue from the underlying fascia as well as from the skin.

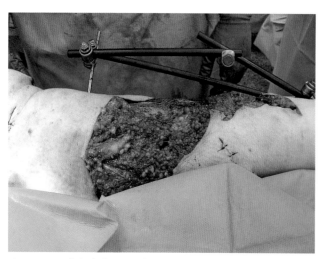

Fig 12.5-5 Clinical photograph showing placement of an external fixator across the ankle.

Decision making

Open questions

- What are the early priorities of treatment?
- Which goals of treatment are realistic?
- What is the appropriate type of skin graft?

Options and plan

The large amount of degloved skin presents several problems at once. First, the skin must be replaced in such a manner as to eventually allow for motion in the knee and ankle joints. Second, the skin loss may interfere with timing or surgical approaches for fracture fixation. Finally, the large volume of skin loss, ~10% of the total body surface, may unsettle surgeons inexperienced in this field. Moreover, "recycling" of the degloved skin needs to be evaluated. If it can be reused, it should ideally be clean and without bruises. It may either be used as a flap or as a graft. In the time that it takes to ensure that the wound bed is not infected, such a skin graft may be refrigerated for up to 10 days.

The goals of treatment are the same as for any periarticular fracture: stable fixation which allows for early range-of-motion mobilization. To accomplish this, the fracture must be repaired as anatomically correct as possible and with a sufficiently stable fixation that will allow early motion. Furthermore, the skin must be replaced by a material that will allow motion. In this case, the fractures were highly comminuted and implied tremendous energy having been absorbed by the bone and adjacent tissues. An assessment of the muscle envelope surrounding the fracture site may be made at the initial debridement and irrigation in order to assist with planning the definitive procedure.

Although an external fixator may be used to temporarily immobilize the fractures, early definitive fixation is desirable in order to allow for early motion of the knee and ankle joints. Should internal fixation be undertaken at an early stage, early skin closure would also be favored in order to protect the implants from infection. However, if the skin is grafted at the initial surgery, additional skin necrosis may declare itself during the next 72 hours, necessitating additional skin grafting. Furthermore, any primary grafts would potentially be compromised by the reduction necessary for fracture fixation a few days later. Therefore, the decision was made in favor of fracture fixation at a second surgical procedure, with skin grafting being carried out during the same procedure.

Procedure

The patient was taken back to the operating room 48 hours later for definitive treatment. Both lower extremities had been draped out. The external fixator was removed, further debridement of necrotic skin was performed, a retrograde intramedullary nail was inserted into the femur, and the distal tibia underwent open reduction and internal fixation with a medial periarticular plate.

Skin was then harvested from the contralateral thigh. The patient being obese, this donor site provided an ample graft. The split-thickness skin graft (chapter 10.2) was meshed at 3:1 for the portions of the skin graft that did not cross the joint, and 1:1.5 for skin that crossed the joint (Fig 12.5-6). This was done in order to allow only little contraction of the graft across the joints, and to make maximum use of the skin graft in the less mobile areas. Posterior graft sections were placed with the joint in maximum extension, while anterior graft sections were placed with the joint in maximum flexion. At the points where graft sections met, the skin graft was tacked down with 3-0 resorbable sutures. The edges of the graft were stapled to intact skin and a negative-pressure wound-therapy device was placed over the entire wound after placing petroleum gauze on the graft. The patient was then returned to the ward.

Follow-up

The patient was discharged 4 days after skin grafting and fracture fixation. Range-of-motion exercises were begun after 5 days. Both fractures healed within 14 weeks (Fig 12.5-7a–b, 12.5-8a–b). A complex knee reconstruction was then performed, repairing the posterolateral corner, the anterior cruciate ligament and a meniscal tear. Rehabilitation for the injury also included aggressive range-of-motion exercises in a brace. The patient was unable to attend physical therapy because of her social situation and developed an

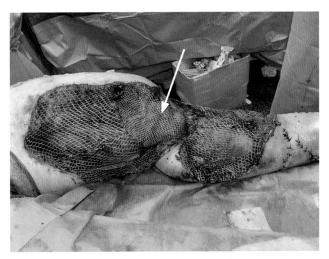

Fig 12.5-6 Intraoperative photograph showing placement of the split-thickness skin graft. Note the smaller mesh ratio for the graft sections crossing the knee joint (arrow).

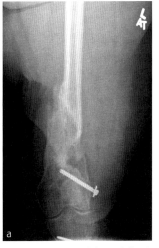
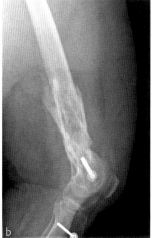

Fig 12.5-7a–b Left knee following removal of the intramedullary nail and multiligamentous knee reconstruction.
a   AP x-ray.
b   Lateral x-ray.

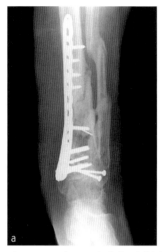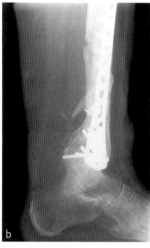

Fig 12.5-8a–b   Healed distal tibial fracture of the left leg 14 weeks after surgery.
a   AP x-ray.
b   Lateral x-ray.

arthrofibrosis. Four years later, she returned to the clinic and had a range of motion of the knee of 20–100°. The skin graft had healed completely. When trying maximum extension, a hard block to extension was felt, but the skin remained loose, indicating that a capsular release would be necessary in order to gain full extension.

Points to remember

- Massive degloving injuries may be treated with split-thickness skin grafts.
- Care must be taken not to contribute to joint contracture by improper technique. Smaller mesh ratios are associated with less coverage, but also less contracture and, therefore, are indicated for grafts which cross the joint.
- Skin that has lost its connection to the underlying fascia is at risk for slough.

12.6   Skill level **II**: Case 1

Author   David A Volgas

Case history

- 35-year-old white male patient
- Unemployed construction worker
- Single
- Smoker, occasional alcohol use, history of cocaine abuse
- No other medical problems

While riding a motorcycle, the patient was involved in a single-vehicle crash. He was unresponsive at the scene and intubated in the field. He was not wearing a helmet. A spine board and air splint were applied in the field and intravenous fluids were administered. The patient was classified as 3T on the Glasgow coma scale and transported to a level I trauma center.

In the trauma bay, the patient underwent the advanced trauma life support (ATLS) protocol, which identified:
- intraparenchymal left frontal lobe hemorrhage
- right pulmonary contusion
- closed fracture of the right navicular bone
- Gustilo type IIIB fracture of the left tibia (**Fig 12.6-1a–b**).

The patient underwent initial resuscitation by the trauma team and emergency ventriculostomy. The wound was debrided and irrigated in the emergency department, but the

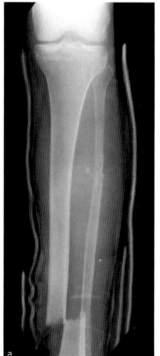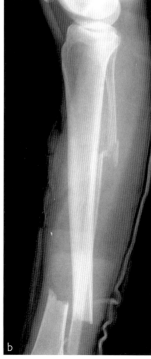

Fig 12.6-1a–b   Left leg showing the displaced Gustilo type IIIB transverse fracture of the distal tibia.
a   AP x-ray.
b   Lateral x-ray.

patient was not deemed stable enough for a full debridement and irrigation in the operating room on the day of admission.

The next morning, the patient was taken to the operating room for formal debridement, irrigation, and fracture fixation by intramedullary nailing (Fig 12.6-2a–b). On the patient's fourth day in hospital, debridement and irrigation were repeated and a negative-pressure wound-therapy device was applied. On the eighth day in hospital, a meshed, split-thickness skin graft was placed over the wound and again immobilized with a negative-pressure wound-therapy device.

After being discharged from the hospital, the patient had a follow-up in the orthopaedic clinic and was found to have a slough of the skin graft and a deep wound infection at the site of the tibial wound. After initially attempting to manage the wound and infection as an outpatient, he was rehospitalized because he continued to have purulent discharge from both the traumatic wound and the proximal surgical incision at the nail insertion site.

Wound conditioning: In this situation, he was taken to the operating room for removal of the intramedullary nail as well as debridement and irrigation of the wound (Fig 12.6-3). Consideration was given to the placement of an external fixator, but the surgeon decided against this since he feared continued infection in the medullary canal and did not wish to cross the knee and ankle joints with a fixator. Intraoperative cultures demonstrated the presence of methicillin-sensitive *Staphylococcus aureus*. The wound was closed over antibiotic beads and intramedullary antibiotics, but the situation of the skin was tenuous. A negative-pressure wound-therapy device was again employed. The patient was discharged with home intravenous antibiotics and a splint in order to allow for dressing changes.

Present status

On a follow-up 2 weeks later, there was an 8 × 3 cm wound with exposed bone. The previous nail insertion site was dry, but there was serous discharge from the traumatic wound.

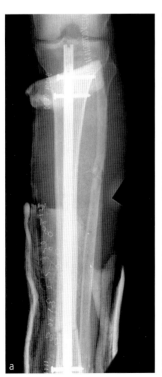 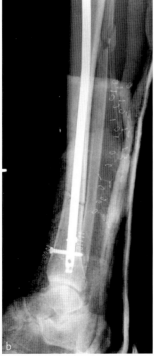

Fig 12.6-2a–b Left leg after reduction and internal fixation using an interlocking intramedullary nail.
a   AP x-ray.
b   Lateral x-ray.

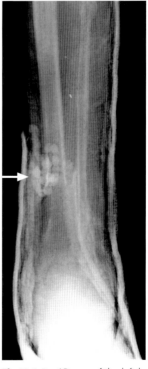

Fig 12.6-3 AP x-ray of the left leg in a plaster cast after removal of the intramedullary nail and placement of antibiotic beads (arrow).

In the past, compliance with wound care by nurses at home as well as cessation of smoking have been issues with this patient. This patient then presented with an unstable fracture, a deep infection, and a wound on the anterior aspect of the mid-distal tibia.

Decision making

Open questions
- What are the priorities for management of this injury: stabilization of the fracture, control of infection and skin coverage?
- What type of coverage should be used for this wound?
- What type of implant should be used in order to provide bone stability?

Options and plan
The three problems—fracture instability, infection, and skin defect—which this case presents, are neither discrete, nor are they separate. Wounds heal much better when the bone is stable. However, implants placed into an infected wound, are likely to become an ongoing source of infection, as bacteria adhere to the implant. This may result in chronic osteomyelitis or, worse, an infected nonunion. Wound closure is much more successful if the wound is not infected or can be converted to a noninfected wound. However, the challenge is to convert an open wound bed or a previously infected wound into a noninfected one.

Therefore, all three problems must ideally be addressed simultaneously. Some surgeons prefer to leave implants in place even in the face of infection as long as they are providing stability to the bone. In this case, however, the nail was removed because there was copious discharge from the nail insertion site.

All in all, the initial plan consisted of a planned staged open reduction and internal fixation of the fracture with primary wound closure after an attempt to decrease bacterial load and achieve near-sterile wound conditions by removing hardware and necrotic material, placing antibiotics beads and administering systemic antibiotics. This plan had to be changed when the primarily closed wound showed dehiscence. At this time, there was not gross purulence at the wound, so the plate was left in place.

In order to provide fracture stability, a variety of options are available. These options include another reamed intramedullary nail, external fixator or plate and screw fixation. An intramedullary nail would have been an acceptable op-

tion, but the patient had had a prior intramedullary infection. The surgeon felt that the risk of an intraarticular infection developing in this patient, who was not diligent about follow-up, was fairly high unless the intramedullary infection was completely cleared.

An external fixator would be an option, but with the history of intramedullary infection, pin-track site problems jeopardizing the stability of the fixation would probably be more likely than if there had been no previous intramedullary infection. One should also keep in mind that wound care would be considerably more difficult with an external fixator in place, and this again would require patient compliance. Nevertheless, an external fixator bridging both knee and ankle to avoid pin placement into the infected medullary canal would have been a reasonable alternative.

Although there is a lack of evidence in the literature concerning rigid versus nonrigid fixation in the face of infection, the surgeon decided to use a rigid internal fixation consisting of a plate and screws. Careful placement of the plate without further periosteal stripping will minimize additional damage to the vascularity of the bone. Also, if the bone should not heal or an ongoing infection makes amputation an option, choosing an implant which does not extend proximal to the level of the prospective amputation will reduce the risk of chronic osteomyelitis.

The choice of fixation used in this case is debatable and there are valid reasons to use another intramedullary nail or an external fixator. Also, the timing of placement of metal implants is debatable. An unstable fracture usually will not heal, especially in the presence of infection. Moreover, infection control is difficult with hardware in place. In this case, the surgeon felt that a short period of instability might allow the infection to be controlled sufficiently in order to reduce the likelihood of infection of the plate. This is certainly a judgment call and needs to be determined on a case-by-case basis.

In order to provide coverage, several options were considered. The soleus muscle may sometimes be used to cover wounds at the junction of the middle to the distal tibial third, but is often too tendinous to provide good cover. Anyway, in this case, during the initial debridement, the soleus muscle was noted to be severely contused.

A local tissue transfer was considered using a randomly perfused fasciocutaneous flap (chapter 10.4). A reverse-flow sural flap was also considered (chapter 10.5.2), but the surgeon felt that it would require more postoperative care than a local fasciocutaneous flap in the context of limited compliance. Furthermore, during the placement of the plate, an attempt was made to identify the sural artery in case the primary closure failed. However, it could not be located by Doppler ultrasound.

A plastic surgery consult was obtained. An angiogram was taken, which showed single-vessel runoff in the leg. The plastic surgery consultant was unwilling to place a free flap because of the history of vascular injury, smoking, infection, and noncompliance. Moreover, in such a situation, an end-to-side anastomosis may even induce a so-called steal phenomenon (chapter 10.6) from the distal end of the anastomosis into the flap, which could finally jeopardize the vascularity of the foot. Finally, amputation was considered, primarily because of the patient's poor compliance.

After considering all these options, a local transposition skin flap was determined to have the greatest chance of success with the least risk.

Procedure

The patient returned to the operating room for definitive management of the unstable fracture and soft-tissue defect. The bone was stabilized with a locking plate (Fig 12.6-4a–b). A silver-impregnated dressing was applied, with a negative-pressure wound-therapy device. A week later, the silver dressing was removed and the wound examined (Fig 12.6-5). A randomly perfused fasciocutaneous flap was transposed to the defect (Fig 12.6-6a–b). The donor site was covered with a split-thickness skin graft (Fig 12.6-7a–b). Cultures were obtained during surgery and following debridement. Although the cultures were negative, the patient remained on intravenous antibiotics throughout the course of treatment. He was discharged on home intravenous antibiotics for 6 weeks.

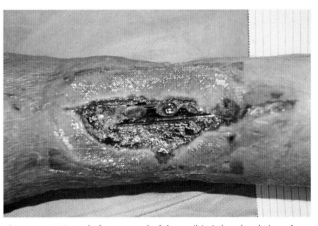

Fig 12.6-5   Wound after removal of the antibiotic beads, plating of the fracture, and subsequent wound dehiscence. The shiny apposition within the soft tissues originated from silver-containing dressings.

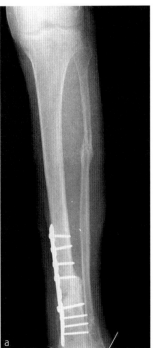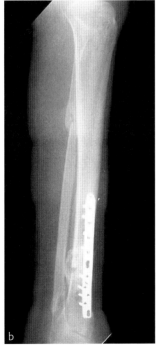

Fig 12.6-4a–b   Left leg after reduction and internal fixation using plate and screws. Note the callus formation indicating relative fracture stability. The fibular fracture has healed in the meantime.
a   AP x-ray.
b   Lateral x-ray.

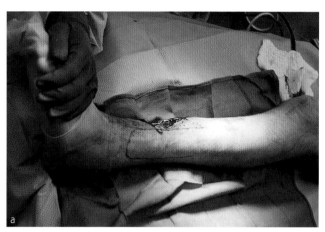
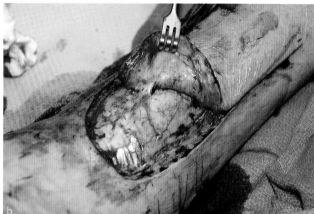

Fig 12.6-6a–b   Outline and elevation of the local skin flap (ie, transposition flap).
a   Outline of the pedicled skin flap with a width-to-length ratio of 1:3.
b   Flap elevation in an epifascial plane with regard to muscles and tendons.

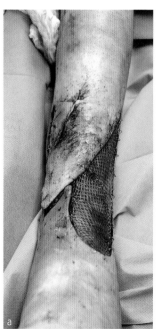
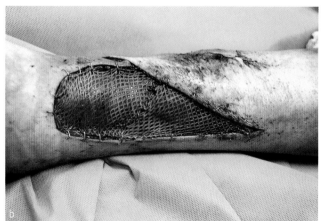

Fig 12.6-7a–b   After transposition and insertion of the flap and grafting of the donor site with a meshed split-thickness skin graft.
a   AP view.
b   Lateral view.

Follow-up

The fasciocutaneous flap healed completely within 2 weeks (Fig 12.6-8a–b). After 10 months, the fracture had healed, there was no more discharge, and the patient was back to work (Fig 12.6-9a–b). He was able to walk without pain.

Points to remember

- Complex problems may often be reduced to relatively simple choices by clearly defining the goals of reconstruction and the methods available to accomplish each goal.
- It may not always be possible to carry out initial plans after all the facts are discovered or complications develop.
- Be prepared to use a variety of reconstructive techniques when approaching any problem. The safest procedure must be offered in order to have the highest chance of healing. Unfortunately, these procedures are not always the simplest ones.
- Give as much consideration to the personality of the patient as to that of the fracture when choosing a plan.

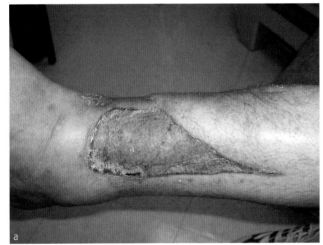

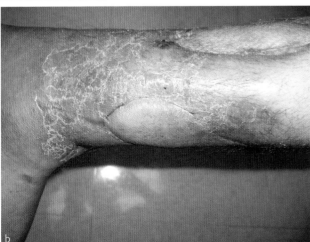

Fig 12.6-8a–b Healed flap and donor site.
a   AP view.
b   Lateral view.

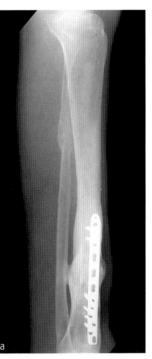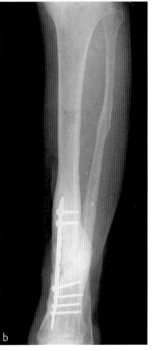

Fig 12.6-9a–b Healed left tibial fracture with abundant callus formation at the 10-month follow-up. Note that two screws have been removed because they began to back out.
a   AP x-ray.
b   Lateral x-ray.

12.7 Skill level II: Case 2
Author Yves Harder

Case history

- 34-year-old white male patient
- Laborer
- Married
- Smoker
- No other medical problems

The patient was involved in a motorcycle crash with a car at high speed. There was no loss of consciousness. The patient sustained a Gustilo type II fracture of the junction mid-distal third of the tibia.

Following transport to a level I trauma center, the patient was surveyed by the trauma surgeon on call. Clinical and para-clinical examination revealed the above mentioned isolated trauma of the right leg (Fig 12.7-1a–b). Accordingly, debridement and irrigation of the wound was performed, followed by fracture stabilization using an intramedullary nail. Subsequently, the patient had to undergo an exchange of the intramedullary nail (Fig 12.7-2a–b) as the fracture had failed to heal. One year later, the fracture still had not healed (Fig 12.7-3a–b). The nail was removed and a plate fixation with screws was used to stabilize the bone after treatment of the nonunion. Thereafter, the postoperative course was complicated by wound dehiscence located over the fracture site with exposure of bone and plate. The wound measured ~4 × 3 cm.

Wound conditioning: The wound was treated with petroleum gauze based dressings changed every 3 days for 2 weeks as an outpatient. Negative-pressure wound therapy was used for another 2 weeks.

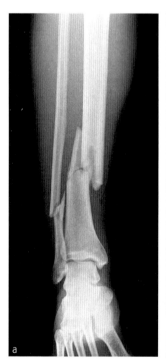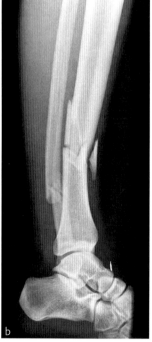

Fig 12.7-1a–b Open, multifragmentary fracture at the junction between middle and distal third of the right lower leg (42-C).
a AP x-ray.
b Lateral x-ray.

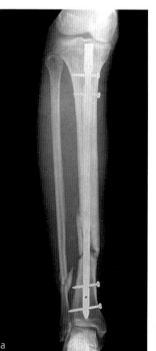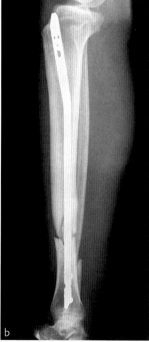

Fig 12.7-2a–b Three months after stabilization of the right tibia with an intramedullary nail. Note the absence of bone healing.
a AP x-ray.
b Lateral x-ray.

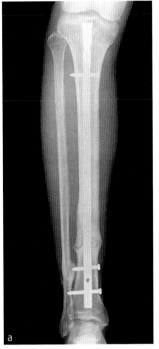
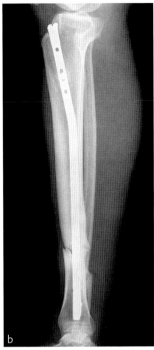

Fig 12.7-3a–b Fracture of the right lower leg immediately before extraction of the nail and plate fixation showing a hypertrophic nonunion.
a   AP x-ray.
b   Lateral x-ray.

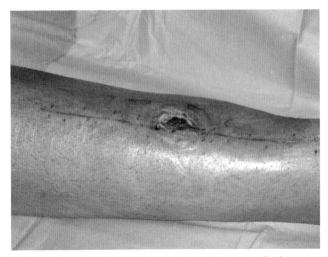

Fig 12.7-4 Clinical photograph of the leg with a longitudinal scar along the tibial crest. At the transition of the middle to the distal third of the leg, supposedly well-vascularized wound of ~4 cm in diameter with macroscopically clean granulation tissue.

Present status

- Soft-tissue defect at the anterior aspect of the right lower leg between the middle third and the distal third of ~4 cm in diameter.
- Macroscopically the granulation tissue seems clean with visible plate and palpable bone (Fig 12.7-4).

Following debridement and irrigation, the surgeon found healthy tissue but bone devoid of periosteum as well as an exposed plate with screws. The swabs taken superficially and deep within the wound after debridement and irrigation revealed no bacterial contamination. The surrounding tissues were soft and appeared to be healthy.

Decision making

Open questions
- What are realistic treatment goals in a young, healthy, active smoker without comorbidities?
- What coverage option offers the greatest chance of success?

Options and plan
The primary goal in this case is the functional restoration of the limb, which requires bone union. However, in order to achieve bone union, complete soft-tissue coverage must be obtained.

Because of the exposed plate and the presence of a nonunion, it is necessary to provide well-vascularized tissue to close this skin defect. Dressing changes alone are not likely to result in rapid closure of the wound and would ultimately result in an infection of the implant material and underlying fracture site. Negative-pressure wound therapy did not produce adequate granulation tissue to support a split-thickness skin graft (chapter 10.2) and, in the face of an exposed plate, its continued use is unlikely to be successful. In the long run, the resulting scar would remain unstable or the patient would possibly develop a fistula, indicating chronic infection such as osteitis.

Both the small size of the defect as well as the elasticity and quality of the adjacent skin allow for a local flap with tissues adjacent to the defect (chapter 10.4). Reliable muscle flaps from the calf, ie, gastrocnemius and soleus muscle have their dominant pedicles within the proximal area of the leg. Accordingly, they would not reach a defect at the transition zone of the middle and distal third of the lower leg. The distally based soleus/hemisoleus flap is not very reliable in

I
II
III
IV

a smoker. Furthermore, its donor site has been heavily traumatized and must therefore be associated with fibrotic changes. Although always an option, coverage by a free flap is not always required, especially if infrastructure is limited or surgical experience for microsurgical techniques unavailable. A fasciocutaneous flap such as the distally based sural flap would be possible from the point of view of the defect localization (chapter 10.5), yet this flap is rather unreliable, particularly in smokers. The free-style perforator flap (chapter 10.4) based on a perforating vessel adjacent to the defect is usually more reliable and, therefore, an option for such defects, as is the local transposition flap (chapter 10.4), in this case a bipedicled or bridge flap (Fig 12.7-5a–b).

Procedure

Four weeks after decortication and plate fixation of the nonunion, a debridement of the soft-tissue defect at the anterior tibial crest was performed, including the radical excision of granulation and scar tissue within the wound. Then, the surgical scar at the anterior tibial crest was incised. A parallel counter-incision was performed at the lateral aspect of the right lower leg to elevate a randomly perfused, bipedicled fasciocutaneous flap with a length of 15 cm and a width of 6 cm (width-to-length ratio of almost 1:1 due to both pedicles) (chapter 10.3). The flap was elevated in a subfascial plane. In order to increase its width, stab incisions were performed to "mesh" the flap's fascia. Thereafter, the flap was easily transposed to the skin border at the anterior tibial crest in order to cover the soft-tissue defect. Tension-free skin closure was performed using intradermal and transcutaneous stitches (Fig 12.7-6a). At the lateral aspect of the leg, the resulting donor-site defect was covered with a meshed split-thickness skin graft harvested on the ipsilateral thigh (Fig 12.7-6b).

Follow-up

The postoperative course was uneventful and both flap and bone healed without further surgery (Fig 12.7-7a–b). The

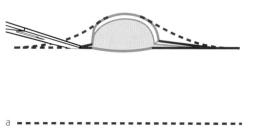 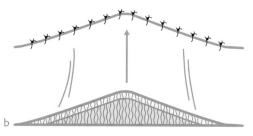

Fig 12.7-5a–b Schematic drawing of a bipedicled (proximal and distal inflow) skin flap transposed medially into the defect.

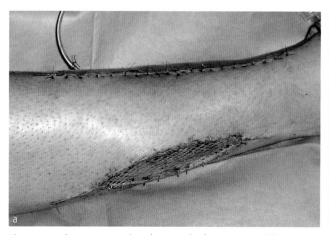 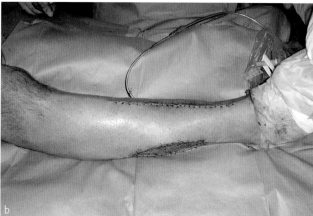

Fig 12.7-6a–b Intraoperative photograph after excision of the granulation tissue and transposition of the bipedicled flap.
a   Tension-free closure using subdermal and transcutaneous stitches.
b   The donor site is covered with a meshed split-thickness skin graft.

skin graft take was 100%. After 10 weeks, the patient was walking without crutches, bearing full weight on the healing tibia. At 6 months, the fracture had completely healed (Fig 12.7-8a–b).

Points to remember

- Soft-tissue problems may develop much later than the initial trauma, after repeated surgery. Revision surgery in the area of prior trauma carries a high risk for complications. This may sometimes be ameliorated by adjusting the surgical approach. In this case, if the surgical incision for the plate had been placed over the anterior tibialis muscle, a split-thickness skin graft might have solved the issue of wound dehiscence.
- In some selected cases, soft-tissue coverage may easily be accomplished using healthy local tissues if available.

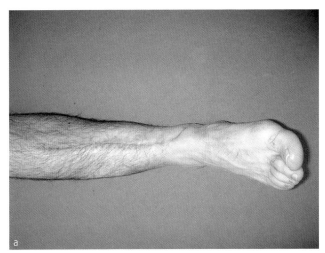

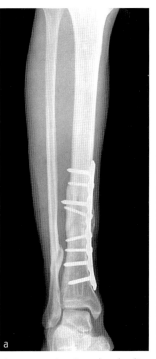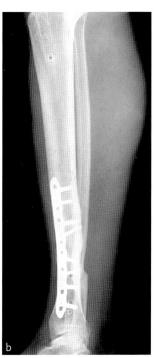

Fig 12.7-8a–b Complete healing of the fracture at 6 months.
a   AP x-ray.
b   Lateral x-ray.

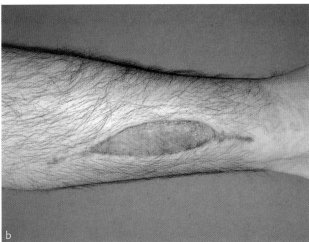

Fig 12.7-7a–b Follow-up at 6 months.
a   Well-healed anterior tibial scar.
b   Perfectly integrated split-thickness skin graft.

12.8 Skill level II: Case 3

Author Angelo M Biraima

Case history

- 32-year-old white male patient
- Construction worker
- Right-hand dominant
- Single
- Nonsmoker
- No other medical problems

When working with a wood saw the unprotected left hand got caught in the saw. The patient sustained an amputation of the distal phalanges of the index and thumb.

Paramedics provided a clean bandage and placed the two amputated fingertips in a plastic bag surrounded by ice-cooled water.

In the trauma bay, the conscious patient was examined by the trauma surgeon. There were no other injuries except for those of the left hand, namely:

- transverse cut of the thumb 2 mm distal to the eponychial fold (Fig 12.8-1)
- transverse amputation of the index finger at the level of the proximal interphalangeal joint
- abrasion of the palmar skin (Fig 12.8-2)
- avulsed nerves (Fig 12.8-3) at the amputated part of the index finger.

An x-ray confirmed the clinical assessment with amputation of the distal part of the thumb's tuft and amputation through the proximal interphalangeal joint of the index finger (Fig 12.8-4).

Wound conditioning: none.

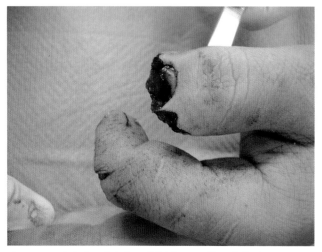

Fig 12.8-1 Left thumb before debridement (dorsal view).

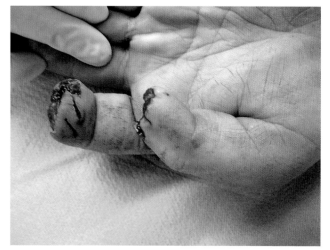

Fig 12.8-2 Left index finger before debridement (palmar view). Note the abrased skin.

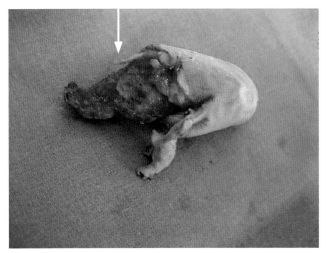

Fig 12.8-3 Avulsed part of the end phalanx of the left index finger. Note the stripped digital nerve (arrow).

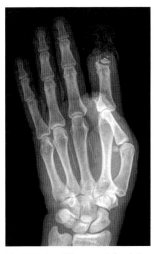

Fig 12.8-4 AP x-ray of the left hand showing the amputation through the tuft (phalanx) of the thumb and through the proximal interphalangeal joint of the index finger.

Present status

After adequate debridement, the visible nail bed of the thumb was 2 mm long and well supported by the remaining bone. The index finger showed avulsed digital nerves over at least 4 mm length. The palmar soft tissues were stripped off the bone to the level of the distal interphalangeal joint, but sufficient in length in order to allow primary closure of the wound. The cartilage of the proximal interphalangeal joint of the index finger was exposed.

Decision making

Open questions

- Which fingers can be salvaged?
- If a finger cannot be salvaged, at what level to amputate?
- How to cover the soft tissues?

Options and plan

The patient should be able to use his hand for heavy work and continue his profession as a construction worker. Protective sensation at the fingertip is important. Maximum length of the amputated fingers should be preserved without compromising wound closure or defect coverage.

In trauma hand surgery, one of the primary goals is to treat the injuries in such a way that will avoid immobilization of the fingers, especially if there is no fracture or crush injury.

Definitive wound closure should be aimed for by any means, allowing the patient to start passive and active movements of his hand and fingers. In clean cut injuries, very distal replantations up to the level of the distal interphalangeal joint are possible. Initial assessment after debridement showed considerable avulsion injury of the end phalanx of the index finger with torn nerves and vessels, making a successful replantation very unlikely.

Exposed bone and cartilage need coverage with vascularized tissue. Secondary healing would considerably increase the risk of infection that could threaten the preservation of the entire finger. Many flaps have been described for small fingertip injuries, allowing immediate coverage with local tissue.

Procedure

Index finger: Debridement of the index finger included shortening of the stump to the level of the proximal interphalangeal joint as the avulsed tip could not be saved. This allowed the remaining palmar skin to be used as a turn-up flap cover for the head of the proximal phalanx, creating no tension.

Thumb: All crushed tissue from the palmar side of the thumb was excised and the bone thoroughly washed out. To length-en the visible nail bed, a quadrangular area proximal to the eponychial fold was deepithelialized, thereby allowing the free skin edge to be pushed back by about 2 mm (Fig 12.8-5, 12.8-6). Then a palmar based advancement flap with the apex at the proximal interphalangeal joint crease was mobilized and moved distally to cover the bone (Fig 12.8-7 to 12.8-9) (chapter 10.4.2). The flap was fixed with a needle to the bone and the skin closed with simple, interrupted sutures. The thumb was covered with a paraffin-gauze dressing. A splint was applied in order to protect the flap and the needle fixation for 10 days.

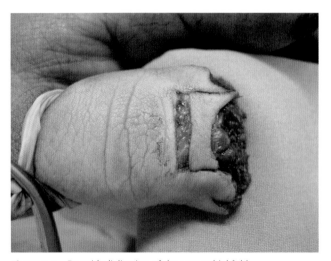

Fig 12.8-5   Deepithelialization of the eponychial fold.

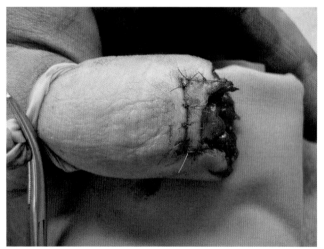

Fig 12.8-6   Lengthening of the visible nail bed after mobilization of the eponychial fold.

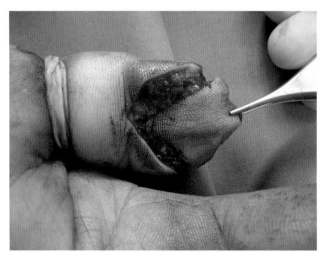

Fig 12.8-7   After making incisions for the V-Y advancement flap, some septa in the apex have to be cut to gain additional length.

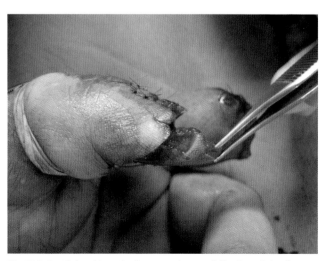

Fig 12.8-8   Gain of length after complete mobilization of the flap.

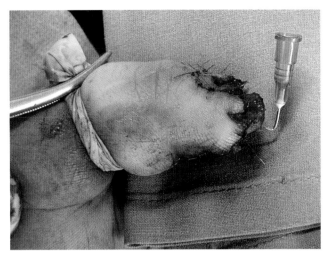

Fig 12.8-9 Temporary fixation of the flap with a needle to the underlying bone.

Follow-up

Six months after the operation, the patient had good protective sensation and experienced no pain when working. He was pleased with the cosmetic result of the remaining nail of the thumb (Fig 12.8-10a–b).

Points to remember

- Most fingertip injuries, as long as they are not accompanied by large avulsion injuries, allow the surgeon to close the wound directly by advancing local tissue, thus providing early functional aftertreatment.

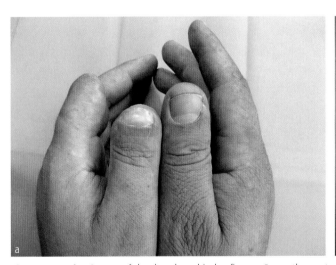
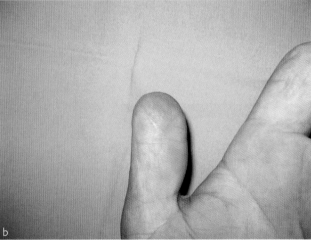

Fig 12.8-10a–b Aspect of the thumb and index fingers 6 months postoperatively.
a   Note the slightly dystrophic growth of the nail that has insufficient bone support.
b   Nearly invisible scars of the V-Y advancement flap (palmar view).

12.9   Skill level II: Case 4
Author   David A Volgas

Case history

- 38-year-old white male patient
- Registered nurse
- Married
- Nonsmoker
- Occasional alcohol use
- No other medical problems

The patient was riding a motorcycle at ~60 mph (96 km/h) when another motorcycle collided with his from behind. The patient lost control of his vehicle and crashed. There was no loss of consciousness. Prehospital treatment included the application of splints for both legs.

The initial assessment on the day of injury included:
- Gustilo type II fracture of the left fibular head with dislocation of the posterior knee (Fig 12.9-1)
- Gustilo type II right bimalleolar ankle fracture
- fractures of the right ribs 2–4.

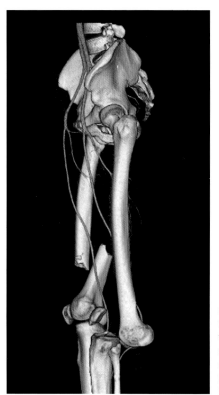

Fig 12.9-1   3-D reconstruction of the initial CT scan showing the knee dislocation exerting pressure on the popliteal artery.

The patient underwent closed reduction of the knee dislocation. CT angiography was performed and excluded vascular injury. Yet, pressure on the popliteal artery was noted (Fig 12.9-1). After closed reduction of the knee dislocation, pulses at the level of the foot were again palpable. During the initial hospitalization, an open reduction and internal fixation of the right ankle as well as debridement and irrigation of both legs were performed.

Three weeks after the initial injury, the patient underwent a multiligamentous knee reconstruction and placement of a splint including a hinge (Compass®) to protect the reconstruction by medial and lateral stabilization of the knee joint.

Two weeks later, the patient presented to the treating physician with an obvious infection of the medial surgical incision and breakdown of the 8 cm long wound. The patient had knee pain, erythema and swelling around the wound and purulent discharge. Clinical examination at this time demonstrated failure of the posteromedial ligamentous reconstruction and an open knee joint.

Wound conditioning: The patient underwent three surgical debridements to remove necrotic tissue and sterilize the joint. An antibiotic bead pouch was left in the wound at the time of the last debridement. Cultures grew pan-sensitive *Staphylococcus aureus*.

Present status

After surgical debridement of the wound, there was an 8 × 6 cm skin defect over the medial joint line with exposed joint (Fig 12.9-2). The defect in the knee joint capsule measured 4 × 5 cm. The medial meniscus, medial tibial plateau, and medial femoral condyle were visible through the defect. The defect was located just anterior to the site of the tibial collateral ligament repair and its inferior border was the medial meniscus. The tibial collateral ligament repair was intact, but the capsule had been excised.

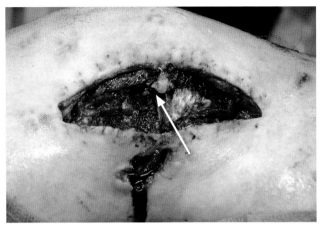

Fig 12.9-2   Medial incision over the knee showing subtotal loss of the joint capsule (arrow).

Decision making

Open questions

- What are realistic goals of treatment?
- Is the end result likely to be an arthrodesis or mobile knee joint?
- Is it realistic to expect a cure of the infection in the presence of a graft?
- What are the definitive treatment options?
- If the knee is salvageable, what coverage procedure will have maximum rehabilitation potential and offer maximum chances of eradicating the infection, if bacteria remain on the graft? Which will have the best cosmetic result (clothing wear, bulk, etc)?
- If the knee is not salvageable, is coverage needed when the limb is shortened?

Options and plan

While after debridement the wound appeared to be clean, there was no guarantee that there were no residual bacteria attached to the autograft, which had been used for reconstruction of the tibial collateral ligament, or the resorbable screw used in that repair. Furthermore, the patient presented with a septic knee. At the final debridement, the cartilage appeared normal, but the outcome of the articular cartilage was questionable. However, the patient was a young healthy patient, who adamantly refused an arthrodesis except as a salvage procedure. Therefore, given the lack of clinical evidence against an attempt to retain the native joint and the patient's strong preference for it, the decision was made to proceed with reconstructive efforts.

The question now was how to address two problems, a large skin defect and an open joint without medial capsule or attachment for the medial meniscus. The surgeon felt that simply placing a muscle flap over this defect would not allow the open joint capsule to seal and, moreover, would likely lead to a fistula. Also, the loss of the capsule makes retention of joint fluid, and thus nutrition of the articular cartilage, difficult, if not impossible. Furthermore, without an intact capsule, the medial meniscus would remain unstable with a tendency to displace into the joint. Therefore, a replacement of the capsule was deemed to be the method of choice.

There is no literature to guide the selection of which material to use for the replacement of the joint capsule, but there are several options, including autologous fascia, lyophilized grafts or collagen grafts, whether human or bovine. Because a pedicled muscle flap, ie, gastrocnemius flap was planned, an autologous fascial graft from the ipsilateral leg was chosen.

Survival, integration, and finally function of any nonvascularized implant, whether autograft, allograft or xenograft, depends on a clean environment and host versus graft reaction. In this case, several cycles of debridement and irrigation had been performed in order to reduce germs in the wound bed to a maximum before applying the fascial graft.

The issue of how to cover the skin defect was easier to resolve. This area of the leg is very amenable to coverage with a medial gastrocnemius flap (chapter 10.5.3). The initial injury is more than 6 weeks old. Surrounding tissues have not only experienced direct trauma, but also infection and repeated surgical manipulation resulting in some contraction and loss of suppleness. The soft-tissue defect exposing the fascial graft ended up being about 8 × 6 cm large, requiring a very proximal mobilization of the gastrocnemius muscle. Other surgical options would include distally based fasciocutaneous flaps or a muscle flap such as from the vastus lateralis muscle, or a free flap. Whether the use of free muscle flaps is beneficial in view of the established infection and in comparison to fasciocutaneous free flaps is still a matter of debate. Negative-pressure wound therapy is not an option in the face of exposed cartilage and knee capsule repair using a nonvascularized fascial graft. Further prolonged negative-pressure wound therapy would run the risk of desiccating the joint.

Arthrofibrosis is common after knee dislocation with or without ligamentous repair. Motion is critical in order to prevent this. In this case, the selected treatments were planned with early range-of-motion mobilization in mind. The fascial repair of the capsule would be tensioned with the knee in flexion in order to repair the anterior portion of the defect and then brought to extension for the posterior portion of the repair, thus ensuring that it would not be stretched to the point of failure in flexion or extension. Likewise, attention would be given to the insertion of the gastrocnemius flap to make sure that it could accommodate flexion and extension of the knee.

Procedure

The patient was taken to the operating room 3 days after the last debridement. Antibiotic beads, which had been left in the wound during the previous debridement, were removed. The joint was inspected. The articular cartilage was more or less normal. The decision was made to use an autologous fascial graft to close the capsular defect and thereby attempt to salvage joint mobility. A medial approach to the gastrocnemius muscle was made. The deep fascia was incised longitudinally in order to expose the musculature within the deep posterior muscle compartment. A section of the deep fascia measuring 6 × 5 cm was excised posterior to the longitudinal incision (Fig 12.9-3). This fascia was used to reconstruct the joint capsule in order to guarantee tightness and stability (Fig 12.9-4).

Nonresorbable suture was used to attach the medial meniscus to the fascial graft and then the fascial graft to the intact capsule distally. The graft was secured proximally to bone and periosteum also using nonresorbable suture (Fig 12.9-5). Thereafter, the medial head of the gastrocnemius was elevated and rotated in order to cover the fascia, which now formed the capsule (Fig 12.9-6). A split-thickness skin graft was placed over the flap and immobilized with a negative-pressure wound-therapy device for 3 days (Fig 12.9-7).

Follow-up

The patient began range-of-motion exercises 3 days after surgery. The flap healed uneventfully. The surgeon was very concerned about failure of the fascial graft sealing the joint. However, no subcutaneous fluid was noted postoperatively and the fact that the patient eventually developed a joint effusion proved that the joint capsule had sealed. Initially, the patient returned to full weight bearing with a relatively good range of motion. Nevertheless, he did not return to work because of chronic pain.

No signs of infection were noted during the follow-up period, but the patient developed posttraumatic arthritis and pain, which eventually required a knee arthrodesis ~18 months later. The arthritis may either have been the result of the initial injury or of the septic knee.

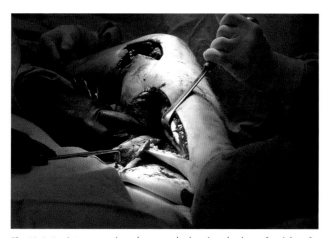

Fig 12.9-3   Intraoperative photograph showing the large fascial graft obtained prior to elevation of the medial gastrocnemius muscle.

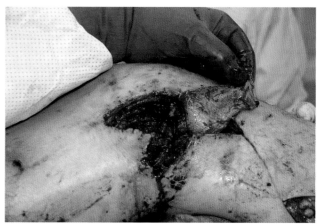

Fig 12.9-4   Fascial graft used to repair the defect of the joint capsule.

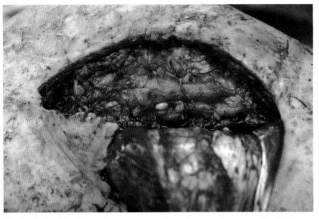

Fig 12.9-5   Fascial graft sutured in place in order to cover the joint, with the medial head of the gastrocnemius muscle ready for insertion into the defect.

Points to remember

- Soft-tissue trauma not only involves skin but other structures such as a joint capsule. No two cases are alike and surgeons should carefully assess the injury and the prerequisites for successful outcome. In this case, the surgeon recognized that if the joint capsule did not seal, nutrition to the articular cartilage would be compromised.
- Whenever a nonvascular graft such as an autologous fascial graft or allograft is used, the graft bed must be sterile. The concept of early coverage sometimes needs to be modified if avascular material is being used in the coverage.

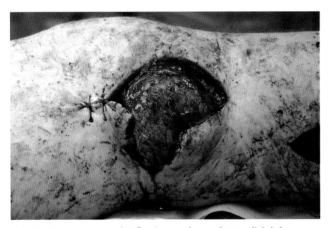

Fig 12.9-6   Gastrocnemius flap inserted over the medial defect.

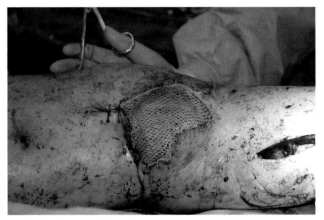

Fig 12.9-7   Split-thickness skin graft covering the gastrocnemius muscle flap.

12.10   Skill level II: Case 5
Author   David A Volgas

Case history

- 46-year-old white male patient
- Tire maintenance worker
- Married
- Smoker
- No other medical problems

This patient repairs and services large tires for heavy equipment. He was attempting to inflate a tire he had just repaired, but did not realize that the safety equipment designed to protect him was not installed properly. The tire exploded when it slipped off the rim. In the field, emergency personnel started intravenous fluids, applied a clean bandage and splint to the leg and placed an oral airway. The patient was transported to a level I trauma center.

The patient was examined by trauma surgeons in the trauma bay. Facial fractures, airway compromise, and lung contusion were identified. Emergency management included endotracheal intubation and ventilation.

The secondary survey and x-rays revealed:

- laceration across the left hip (joint not open)
- moderate edema and ecchymosis around the left knee, laceration across the lateral tibia extending anteriorly to below the tibial tubercle on the left (Gustilo type IIIB fracture)
- closed mid-shaft femoral fracture on the right
- open comminuted distal femoral fracture and comminuted proximal tibial fracture on the left (Fig 12.10-1a–b)
- both lower extremities with intact neurovascular status
- large hematoma in the right calf.

A bedside debridement and irrigation was performed in the trauma bay by an orthopaedic resident. Aggressive fluid substitution was performed, beginning in the trauma bay. Over the next 24 hours, the lactic acidosis and base deficit had corrected. The extent of lung contusion was not felt to be significant.

The patient was taken to the operating room on the morning after admission for formal debridement and irrigation, followed by retrograde intramedullary nail fixation of both femurs and fixation of the left proximal tibia with a less invasive stabilization system (LISS) (Fig 12.10-2a–b). The soft-tissue laceration was incorporated into the surgical approach to the lateral tibial plateau. Care was taken not to undermine the skin around this traumatic wound, nor to handle it with forceps or retractors except as necessary.

Wound conditioning: The wound was loosely closed at the end of the initial procedure with sutures and a negative-pressure wound-therapy device was installed.

Present status

Skin that had looked questionably viable during the first debridement was now clearly necrotic and, hence, was debrided after 72 hours. The surgeon then applied an antibiotic bead pouch and asked for help with coverage (Fig 12.10-3). Antibiotic beads were placed during the second debridement.

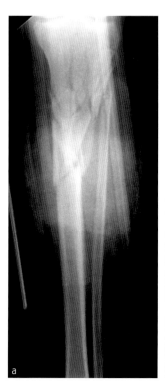 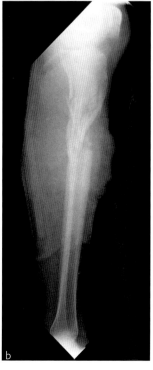

Fig 12.10-1a–b Comminuted fracture of the left proximal tibia.
a AP x-ray.
b Lateral x-ray.

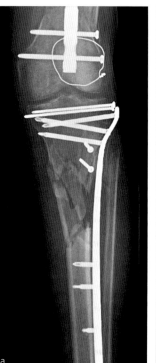 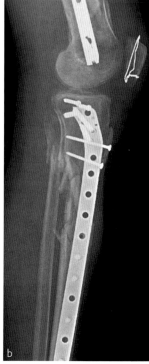

Fig 12.10-2a–b Left tibia after plate fixation with the less invasive stabilization system (LISS). Cerclage of the transverse fracture of the knee cap and retrograde intramedullary nail fixation of the femur.
a AP x-ray.
b Lateral x-ray.

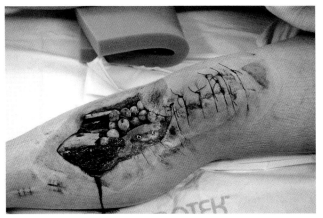

Fig 12.10-3 Anterior view of the proximal tibia with soft-tissue defect of 6×10 cm showing the placement of antibiotic beads after the second debridement of soft tissues and bone.

Decision making

Open questions

- With the presence of significant local injury, would a free muscle transfer be better than a local muscle flap?
- If bone grafting becomes necessary, should this be staged or performed at the time of coverage?

Options and plan

The lower extremity assessment project (LEAP) study concluded that local flap coverage had a much higher complication rate than free muscle transfer in cases with severe osseous injury. However, there are new data from military cases, which suggest that local flaps may be equal to free muscle transfer. During the previous procedure, the surgeon had carefully examined the gastrocnemius muscle in order to assess its viability. However, an arteriogram had not been performed previously, as the surgeon preferred a visual inspection of the muscle (four "C"s) (chapter 2.4, 5.1). If the muscle had shown substantial bruising, lacerations, or had failed to meet the criteria of the four "C"s, the surgeon would have decided to defer to the plastic surgeons for a free flap transfer (eg, muscular, fasciocutaneous), despite the delay. However, the judgment of the surgeon was that there was less risk involved using a regional muscle flap than by delaying definitive coverage for 5–7 days.

The medial gastrocnemius flap (chapter 10.5.3) was chosen in this case because it is based on an artery proximal to the defect and its arc of rotation included the area of the defect.

In regard to the management of the segmental bone defect in the proximal tibia, muscle is known to provide a good source for osteoprogenitor cells as many trauma surgeons have observed by substantial bone growth in a bone defect covered by healthy muscle. In this case, there was great concern for the possibility of residual bacterial contamination, despite aggressive debridement and placement of the antibiotic bead pouch. Therefore, primary bone grafting was felt to pose an increased risk. The muscle flap was expected to heal within 2–4 weeks and could afterwards be carefully raised from its recipient bed in order to allow placement of a bone graft if spontaneous bone healing had not occurred. Therefore, the surgeon decided to delay bone grafting until it was evident that the wound was not infected and that no spontaneous bone healing had occurred.

Procedure

Six days after the injury, the patient was again taken to the operating room, this time for definitive coverage of the 6 × 10 cm defect, which also involved considerable bone loss (Fig 12.10-4). A gastrocnemius muscle flap elevated from the medial side of the calf was inserted into the defect. At the time, some sequestered and necrotic bone was identified and excised, leaving 50% of the diaphyseal circumference of the bone (Fig 12.10-5a–b). After debridement and irrigation, deep swabs were taken, but cultures showed no growth of bacteria. The muscle flap was laid directly onto the bone bed (Fig 12.10-6a–b) and covered with a split-thickness skin graft (Fig 12.10-7) (chapter 10.2).

Follow-up

The patient was followed in clinic for 28 months. The open fracture with considerable bone defect healed without the need for a subsequent bone graft. The patient had returned to his job without any functional restrictions. At that time, there was no discharge from the wound (Fig 12.10-8a–b).

Points to remember

- It is often difficult to accurately assess the full extent of soft-tissue viability at the time of the first debridement. In such cases, a second look after 48–72 hours is indicated.
- Early fracture fixation may be performed at the first operation if adequate soft tissue exists to cover the implants, even if the skin cannot be closed. Otherwise, definitive fixation should be delayed until soft-tissue coverage may be obtained.

- In such an extensive defect of composite tissue including skin, muscle, and bone, muscle flaps are probably better suited than fasciocutaneous flaps because the muscle can both fill the dead space and prevent infection. Furthermore, the muscle may even be a very good source of osteoprogenitor cells, possibly precluding the need for a subsequent bone graft, provided that ~50% of the cortical bone is still there.
- In case plastic surgeons are available, the use of a tailored free flap consisting of muscle or muscle and skin may be considered. As in all surgical flap procedures, a flap must be selected with an adequate pedicle. When planning the flap, also keep possible subsequent surgery in mind, such as revision surgery, bone grafting, joint replacement, etc.

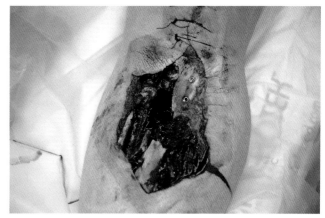

Fig 12.10-4 Tibial wound after removal of antibiotic beads. Note the large bone defect with ~50% of the posterior cortical circumference remaining.

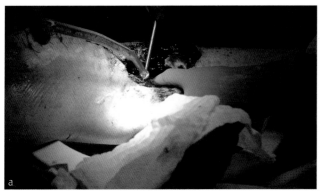
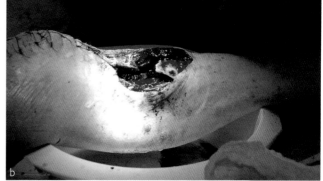

Fig 12.10-5a–b Clinical photograph of the wound after final debridement.
a   Debridement of necrotic bone.
b   Tibial defect showing the large bone defect. Note that there is ~50% of the cortical circumference missing anteriorly.

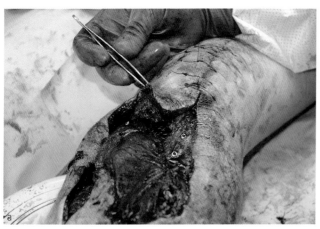
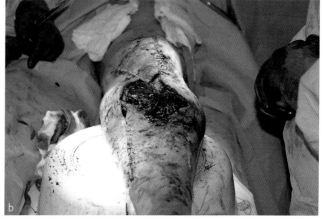

Fig 12.10-6a–b Clinical photograph of the wound after placement of the flap.
a   Forceps lifting skin, which demonstrates that soft-tissue attachments have remained and may be preserved.
b   Flap inserted over the bone defect.

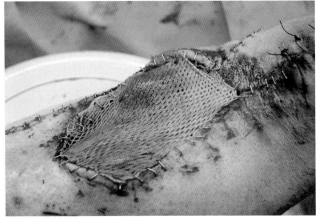

Fig 12.10-7 Intraoperative view after placement of the meshed split-thickness skin graft covering the gastrocnemius muscle.

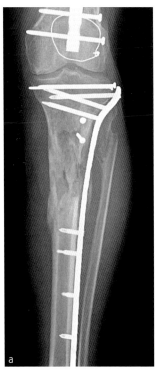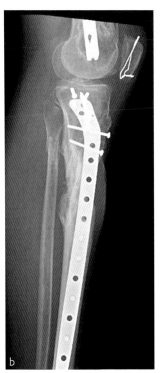

Fig 12.10-8a–b Follow-up of the left leg at 28 months. Healed fracture.
a AP x-ray.
b Lateral x-ray.

12.11 Skill level II: Case 6

Author David A Volgas

Case history

- 26-year-old Hispanic male patient
- Construction worker
- Married
- Smoker
- No other medical problems

The patient was injured at work when he was struck by a moving pipe. He was treated with a clean bandage and splint in the field by emergency medical personnel. On presentation to the emergency department, the diagnosis was:
- isolated injury to the left leg
- intact neurovascular bundles.

Initial debridement of the open wound over the tibia was accomplished in the trauma bay while the secondary assessment was under way.

The patient was examined in the trauma bay by a junior resident, but photographs were taken to discuss with more senior staff. A 6 cm oblique wound across the fracture medially was noted. The mid-shaft fracture of the left lower leg was classified as a Gustilo type IIIB fracture. The wound was not reexamined until the patient was taken to the operating room (Fig 12.11-1).

On the night of admission, the patient was taken to the operating room as soon as the tertiary survey was complete and any further injuries had been excluded. The wound underwent debridement of small amounts of nonviable subcutaneous tissue. The wound was irrigated with 8 l of normal saline. An intramedullary nail was inserted into the tibia in order to stabilize the bone. The surgeon reevaluated the options for coverage of the bone. The skin around the wound appeared viable and the defect could be closed to within 1 cm (Fig 12.11-2).

Wound conditioning: The surgeon decided that an attempt should be made to perform delayed primary closure after conditioning the wound by negative-pressure wound therapy (chapter 9.3) and closure by elastic vessel loops and staples (Fig 12.11-3) (chapter 10.1). Wet gauze was placed within the depth of the wound, pressing against the bone in order to help prevent desiccation.

Present status

The patient had a wound which potentially could be closed on a delayed basis if the acute swelling resolved promptly. The patient was returned to the operating room 48 hours later for reexamination of the wound (Fig 12.11-4) and definitive closure. However, the skin remained edematous and rigid. Delayed primary closure could not be achieved. The fracture was exposed for ~5 cm. Edema had not resolved.

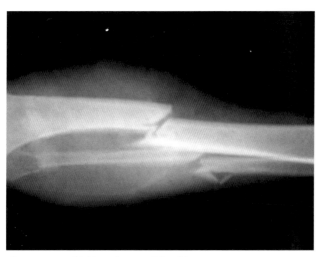

Fig 12.11-1   Initial lateral x-ray of the tibia.

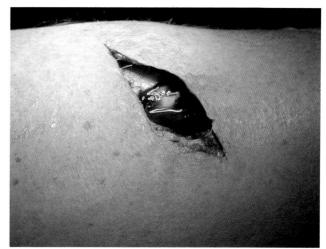

Fig 12.11-2   Traumatic wound after the initial debridement and intramedullary nailing of the tibia.

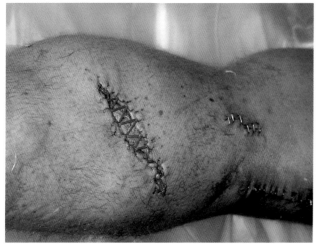

Fig 12.11-3   Wound margins initially approximated with elastic vessel loops and staples.

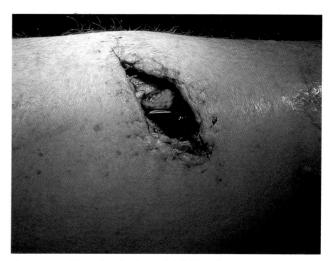

Fig 12.11-4   Wound at the time of definitive closure.

Decision making

Open questions

- What is the ideal time in which to achieve definitive coverage?
- What type of coverage should be used?

Options and plan

Ideally, the wound should be covered definitively at the time of the initial surgery. In this case, the surgeon felt that, although there was local swelling, the use of elastic vessel loops and staples, combined with negative-pressure wound therapy would offer a good possibility that the wound would be closed within 72 hours without any procedures higher up on the reconstructive ladder (chapter 8.2).

Published results strongly suggest that early wound closure involves fewer complications. Although primary closure is to be preferred, in many centers this is not always possible because, on the one hand, they cannot keep surgeons trained in flap surgery available at all times and, on the other hand, the wound sometimes does not declare itself immediately. Definitive closure within 72 hours is considered ideal whenever primary closure is not possible.

In cases where the wound is located over the middle third of the tibia, a soleus flap may offer satisfactory coverage. However, if there is marked comminution or obvious damage to the soleus muscle, a free flap should be selected.

A soleus flap may easily be rotated to cover the defect present in this case (chapter 10.5.3). At the time of the initial debridement, the soleus did not appear to be badly damaged, and, therefore, was taken into consideration. In this case, the surgeon chose a soleus flap (Fig 12.11-5 to 12.11-10), having considered the alternatives discussed above.

Procedure

A soleus flap was performed using the proximally based hemisoleus muscle. A split-thickness skin graft was then applied with a negative-pressure wound-therapy device to secure the skin graft. A posterior splint was applied to immobilize the skin graft.

Follow-up

This patient's fracture healed within 14 weeks and did not require additional bone grafting. The flap healed without sequelae.

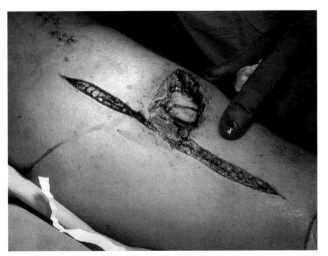

Fig 12.11-5 Wound after debridement of wound edges and incision for soleus flap.

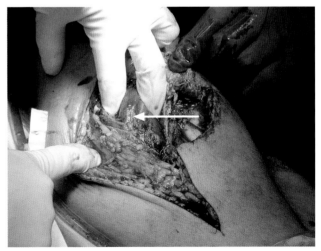

Fig 12.11-6 Soleus muscle (arrow) isolated between the surgeon's fingers.

Points to remember

- Many coverage options are available for a given wound. Rather than simply choosing the most basic option, the surgeon should attempt to select the option which best provides a high likelihood of success, the most durable coverage and the best environment for bone healing. In cases where the skin is without a healthy subcutaneous layer, especially over bone or hardware, the more advanced option is preferable. In this case, the skin, which initially had been closed by an elastic vessel loop technique, did not have a healthy subcutaneous tissue.

- Whenever a regional muscle flap might need to be considered, the surgeon should check for any potential damage to the muscle. Such damage should already be assessed at the initial debridement and irrigation.

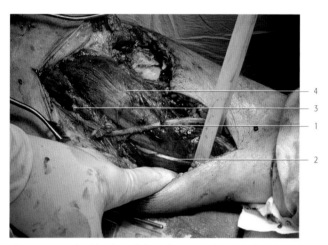

Fig 12.11-7 Identification of the soleus muscle. Note the saphenous nerve (1) crossing the field and the plantaris tendon (2) continuing longitudinally between the gastrocnemius (3) and soleus (4) muscles.

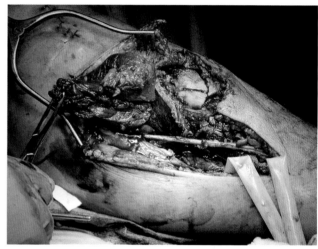

Fig 12.11-8 Soleus muscle transected and reflected to cover the bare tibia.

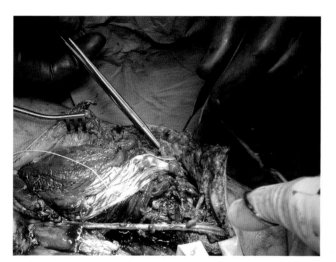

Fig 12.11-9 Soleus muscle flap that is being inserted into the recipient bed.

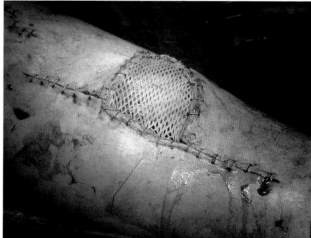

Fig 12.11-10 Soleus muscle flap in place and overlying split-thickness skin graft.

12.12 Skill level III: Case 1

Authors Timo Schmid, Esther Vögelin

Case history

- 16-year-old white male patient
- Student
- Right-hand dominant
- Landau-Kleffner syndrome (infantile acquired condition of unknown origin consisting of aphasia and epilepsy) treated with Valproate® (valproic acid) medication
- Single
- Nonsmoker

While constructing an explosive device of unknown composition with his friend, the blasting charge exploded in the patient's hands. The patient was treated by emergency personnel in the field with a clean bandage and splinting, intravenous fluids and analgesics, as well as intubation for airway management. He was transported to the hospital by helicopter.

Upon admission to the emergency department, the patient was examined by a multidisciplinary team consisting of trauma surgeons, hand surgeons, and ophthalmologists. The following clinical findings were reported:
- both eyes presented with perforations to the ocular globes
- superficial soft-tissue injury of the left knee
- severe hand injuries

- arm injuries
- no life-threatening chest or abdominal injuries.

Wound conditioning: none.

Present status

In the operating room on the night of admission, the patient was found to have the following injuries of the right upper extremity (Fig 12.12-1a–b, 12.12-2):
- several superficial wounds on the upper and lower arm with multiple foreign bodies
- traumatic subtotal amputation of the little finger at the level of the proximal interphalangeal joint
- full-thickness skin defect including the dorsal aspect of the mid hand as well as at the index, middle and ring fingers with concomitant fractures of the proximal interphalangeal joint of the middle and ring fingers
- intact palmar skin
- normal neurovascular structures of the index, middle, and ring fingers
- uninjured thumb.

The left hand also showed severe injuries, the management of which, however, will not be discussed as part of this case.

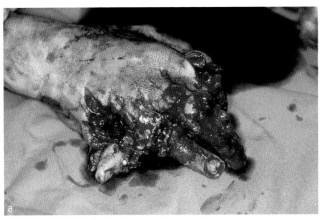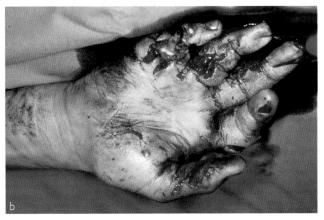

Fig 12.12-1a–b Clinical photograph of the right hand on admission.
a   Dorsal view showing the soft-tissue defect of the index, middle, and ring finger as well as subtotal amputation of the little finger.
b   Palmar view showing adequate perfusion of the thumb, index, middle and ring finger as well as multiple superficial wounds.

Decision making

Open questions

- Is secondary healing an option?
- Does the defect have to be covered?
- What type of tissue shall be used for defect coverage (vascularized or nonvascularized tissue)?
- Is it possible to jeopardize perfusion of the fingers by sacrificing one of the main arteries of the forearm?
- Is decreased tendon gliding to be expected?

Options and plan

The hand includes many important and susceptible structures within a very small area. Preserving viable bone as well as tendinous and neurovascular structures is important for the restoration of function. However, destroyed, nonviable tissue has to be removed aggressively in order to prevent nonunion, excessive scar tissue or late infection, regardless of its later potential function. It is a delicate balancing act between the preservation of important structures (such as intact but devascularized digital nerves or tendons) and the debridement of contaminated or dead tissues (such as bone fragments or cortical fractions, joints, soft tissues). The borders of healthy, vascularized tissue are sometimes very difficult to define, particularly very early after the trauma, ie, before demarcation of necrotic tissue. Therefore, it may be necessary to postpone final soft-tissue coverage until after a second or third look.

With the possible functional outcome in mind, debridement and a plan for reconstructive surgery have to be addressed for the subtotal amputation of the little finger and the injuries to the hand and arm. The aim is to maximize function of the hand in the long term.

In some situations involving, for example, the critical general state of the patient or gross contamination of the hand, reconstruction (tendon, bone, nerves) and final soft-tissue coverage must be postponed until after repeated debridement, thus becoming a two- or multi-step procedure. Technical and infrastructural difficulties should only cause a delay of reconstruction in exceptional cases. However, in this case, provisional closure by means of a synthetic skin (eg, Epigard®) or negative-pressure wound therapy over a paraffin gauze has proven effective in keeping the wound environment clean or even conditioning the wound if tendons, nerves and/or vessels are exposed. In some situations, the use of skin grafts or skin substitutes can offer provisional wound closure.

In some rare cases of complex hand injuries, skin grafts may be a definitive option for covering exposed muscles, dermis, or tendons with maintained paratenon in an area where only very little mobility is required and/or minimum mechanical stress is applied.

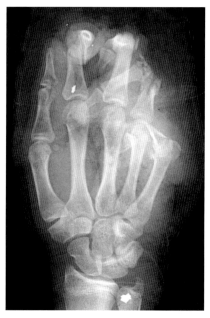

Fig 12.12-2 AP x-ray of the right hand. Note the destruction of proximal interphalangeal joints of the index and ring finger, the intraarticular proximal interphalangeal joint fracture of the middle finger as well as the extensive bone defect of the little finger.

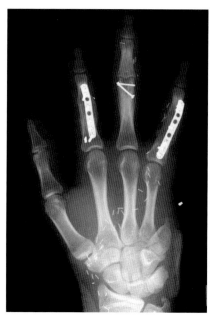

Fig 12.12-3 AP x-ray of the right hand. Arthrodesis of the index and ring finger and fixation with 2.0 mm plates. Middle finger: Osteosynthesis of the intraarticular proximal interphalangeal joint fracture of the proximal phalanx with screws.

The right hand presents with an intact thumb. The intraarticular fractures of the index finger and of the ring finger include a bone defect and the destruction of the proximal interphalangeal joint, though the fractures may heal after bone grafting and arthrodesis. Stable fixation of the intraarticular fracture of the proximal interphalangeal joint of the middle finger by means of conventional open reduction and internal fixation is important, because the ring and little fingers have been severely injured, respectively amputated. The goal must therefore be to reconstruct a functional 4-fingered hand of good quality in order to restore opposition of the thumb to the remaining fingers (Fig 12.12-3).

The full-thickness soft-tissue defect of the right hand measures ~8 × 3 cm and exposes the extensor tendons and the metacarpal bone over the middle and ring finger, including the implant material for fracture fixation. Secondary healing, therefore, is not an option. Skin grafts would not adhere or revascularize on exposed tendons devoid of paratenon. Furthermore, a well-functioning hand needs tendons surrounded by a gliding layer.

In addition, complex injuries as described here often require secondary interventions or salvage procedures, such as bone grafting to treat delayed or nonunion of the bone, tenolysis or hardware removal due to limited range of motion. Hence, well-vascularized tissue such as a flap is needed in order to cover the tendons, the reconstructed bones and their hardware as well as the dorsum of the mid hand and fingers. Taking the right forearm into consideration, only a pedicled flap from the same extremity would be able to replace like with like. Nevertheless, the donor-site defect and the need for bilateral reconstruction must be taken into consideration. A free-style perforator flap may be an option, if the skin of the forearm has remained uninjured (chapter 10.4). Otherwise, free flaps are always an option, as long as the arterial supply to the hand is not reduced to one artery or considerably diminished. This could induce a so-called steal phenomenon, ie, perfusion of the flap at the expense of the hand or some fingers, particularly if a muscle flap with a high perfusion demand (high-flow flap) is applied (chapter 10.6).

Thin flaps such as fasciocutaneous flaps and low perfusion demand flaps (low-flow flaps) (chapter 10.6) (eg, lateral forearm flap, anterolateral thigh flap, thoracodorsal perforator flap), fascial flaps (eg, temporal fascia) plus split-thickness skin grafts, or muscle flaps (eg, serratus anterior flap, gracilis flap) are preferable options. They not only resurface well the affected limb, but also may provide a better tendon sheath with high gliding capacities.

Procedure

The patient was taken to the operating room for initial debridement and irrigation. Both hands underwent debridement and reconstructive surgery to address the amputations and bone injuries (Fig 12.12-3).

The large dorsal soft-tissue defect (size 8 × 3 cm) of the middle and ring finger of the right hand was covered with a pedicled fasciocutaneous radial forearm flap with retrograde perfusion (chapter 10.5). This was carried out once sufficient inflow to the hand via the ulnar artery had been confirmed by an Allen test (chapter 10.5.2).

The flap was elevated including the cephalic vein (superficial venous system), passed dorsally above the tendons of the first extensor compartment and, subcutaneously, pulled to the dorsum of the hand. The flap was trimmed to fit the dorsal defect, ie, the middle and ring finger, resulting in a cutaneous syndactyly. The donor site was covered with a meshed split-thickness skin graft (Fig 12.12-4a–b) (chaper 10.2).

All possible effort has been put into reconstruction and restoration of function of the left hand, in order to provide two "functional instruments" for daily professional life.

Follow-up

On the right hand, active and passive mobilization was initiated rather early after surgery by hand therapy, taking into consideration primarily the rate of soft-tissue healing and solidity of bone fixation. Complete healing of the flap was uneventful, allowing for the division of the cutaneous syndactyly 3 weeks after initial surgery. Another 3 weeks later at the follow-up (Fig 12.12-5), it was decided to reduce the bulky flap volume by fat removal procedures and scar revisions. This was repeated at the 9-month follow-up (Fig 12.12-6).

At the 1-year follow-up, the remaining joints of the right-hand fingers presented with nearly full range of motion except for the arthrodesed proximal interphalangeal joint of the index and ring finger. Perfusion and sensation were normal. There was good grip strength of 40 kp using the Jamar dynamometer on his right dominant hand. The patient was last seen at a 6-year follow-up and showed good function of both hands that allowed full activity (Fig 12.12-7).

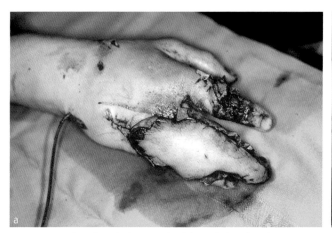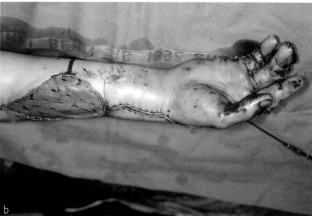

Fig 12.12-4a–b Clinical photograph of the right hand and forearm after soft-tissue coverage.
a   Distally based radial forearm flap including cutaneous syndactyly of the middle and ring finger.
b   Flap donor site covered with an unmeshed split-thickness skin graft.

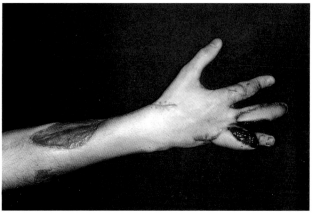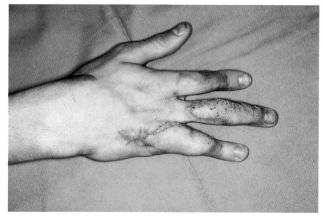

Fig 12.12-5 Right hand 3 weeks after separation of the syndactylized middle and ring fingers.

Fig 12.12-6 Right hand at the 9-month follow-up. State after scar revisions.

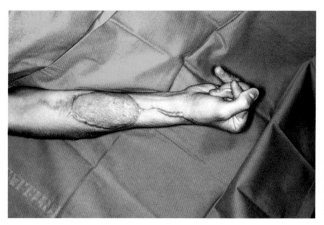

Fig 12.12-7 Clinical photograph of the right hand at the 6-year follow-up. Active flexion of the fingers including the arthrodesed index and ring fingers. Good flexion of the middle finger after intraarticular proximal interphalangeal joint fracture repair. Donor site of the radial forearm flap with hypertrophic scar of the unmeshed skin graft.

Points to remember

- Early, thorough debridement in concert with reconstructive procedures may lead to good functional results.
- The radial forearm flap is a useful flap for coverage of extensive soft-tissue defects of the distal forearm and of the hand with exposed tendons, vessels, and/or nerves. One of its major disadvantages is the sacrifice of the radial artery. In other words, perfusion of the hand depends entirely on an intact distal ulnar-radial arterial communication as well as the anterior and posterior interosseous arteries.
- The radial perforator flap is a good alternative to the classic radial forearm flap, although its perfusion depends on one or more perforators that render the flap less predictable. Furthermore, the flap has a limited arc of rotation, at most reaching the metacarpophalangeal joints but not the fingers in comparison to the posterior interosseous flap.
- Maximum effort to reconstruct mutilating hand injuries as best as possible is of utmost importance, particularly in patients who suffer from diseases (such as in this case epilepsy) or lose vision/go blind from the trauma. Yet, such information is often not known by the surgeon during damage-control or initial reconstruction. Reconstruction must focus on the long term. A mobile and sensitive 3- or 4-fingered hand may be better than to save all severed, injured parts of a mutilated hand.

12.13 Skill level III: Case 2
Author   David A Volgas

Case history

- 24-year-old white female patient
- Computer graphics designer
- Married, two small children
- Nonsmoker
- No other medical problems

The patient was attempting to strap a child into the child seat in the back of the car, when the car started to roll backwards, knocking the patient to the ground. The medial side of the lower leg was dragged along the ground. Prehospital treatment included clean bandage, short leg air splint, and intravenous fluids, given by paramedics.

The patient was examined by trauma surgeons on presentation to the trauma bay. Chest, abdomen, pelvis, and spine were normal.

Findings at the right lower extremity:
- superficial abrasion along the medial side of the lower leg with punctate bleeding (Fig 12.13-1)
- full-thickness skin defect measuring 8 × 6 cm
- deep abrasion of the medial ankle with loss of the medial malleolus and exposure of the mid-tarsal joints (Fig 12.13-1)
- wound contamination with gravel and dirt
- ruptured tibialis posterior tendon (Fig 12.13-2)
- intact tibial nerve and posterior tibial artery
- loss of the medial malleolus confirmed by an AP x-ray (Fig 12.13-3).

The patient was taken for emergency debridement and irrigation on the day of admission. The assessment after adequate debridement revealed:
- skin defect with exposed bone and joint measuring 8 × 10 cm
- exposed peritenon of the extensor tendons
- repairable rupture of the tibialis posterior tendon
- intact medial neurovascular structures.

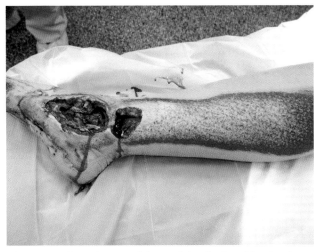

Fig 12.13-1   Open fracture of the medial malleolus with extensive skin defect and abrasion of the medial distal two thirds of the lower leg.

Wound conditioning: An antibiotic bead pouch (Fig 12.13-4) was placed on the wound in order to keep the exposed bone and tendon moist as well as the wound sterile.

Present status

On the third day postinjury, the patient returned to the operating room for a second debridement. In the operating room, the wound was found to be stable with the defect essentially the same as after the last debridement.

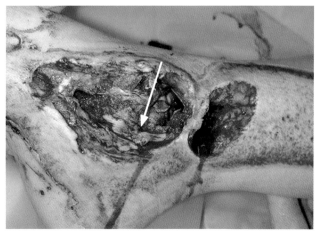

Fig 12.13-2 Close-up of the injury at the time of admission: rupture of the tibialis posterior tendon (arrow).

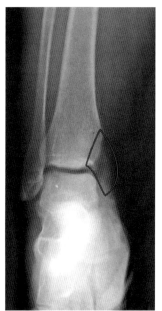

Fig 12.13-3 AP x-ray showing the loss of the medial malleolus. Note the template outlining the missing bone (red line).

Decision making

Open questions
- What is the functional goal for this patient and her injury?
- Is the malleolus salvageable?
- Do the muscles work?
- What are definitive treatment options?
- Does this defect have to be covered?
- Is secondary healing an option?
- How shall this defect be covered?
- What to use: nonvascularized or vascularized tissue?
- If vascularized tissue, pedicled versus free flap and fasciocutaneous versus muscle flap?
- What type of bone stabilization should be chosen?

Options and plan
The functional goal should be to restore near-normal ankle function with a closed soft-tissue envelope that allows wearing a shoe.

In this case, the soft-tissue injury may be managed with a tissue transfer of some type and should result in a durable, flexible skin cover. Shoe wear may be affected until the flap matures, but the end result should be excellent. The rupture of the tibialis posterior tendon is repairable and will not result in substantial functional impairment. The bone defect may probably be managed with a bone graft or by immobilization.

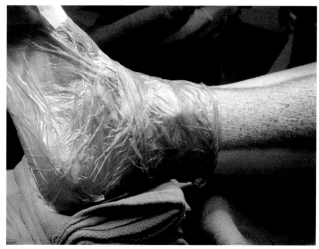

Fig 12.13-4 Wound dressing after aggressive debridement and application of an antibiotic bead pouch.

The soft-tissue defect is large, and healing by secondary intention would be a very time-consuming option. Furthermore, there would be an increased risk of infection if granulation was allowed. In order to cover the bone, joint, and hardware, vascularized tissue is required. Skin grafts will not take in a nonvascularized recipient bed such as metal or exposed joint. Due to adherences, a skin graft will lose mobility when placed on tendons without peritenon. Last but not least, as the graft will show a significant tendency to contract, this may further reduce the range of motion if placed across a joint.

In this case, all traumata are localized on the medial side of the leg. Therefore, the pedicle for a sural flap is not compromised as the donor site of the flap is located posteriorly. There are abrasions along the entire medial side of the leg, which would likely interfere with the pedicle of the posterior tibial artery in case of a free tissue transfer. Perhaps this might even compromise the healing of the incision needed to expose the recipient vessel for a free flap or requiring the dissection of the anterior tibial artery. The defect size is certainly within the limits of a regional fasciocutaneous flap. Since the fasciocutaneous sural flap was felt to have a low risk of morbidity and a reasonably good probability of healing, this option was chosen (chapter 10.5.2). As always, the option with the greatest chance of success was chosen, preferably replacing like with like, ie, skin and subcutaneous tissue together.

Bone stabilization is also an issue in this case. Certainly, if no suitable allograft had been available, this might have precluded the reconstruction of the medial malleolus. However, an allograft was available and selected in order to achieve a good long-term result. Otherwise, with the lateral ligaments being intact as in this case, the ankle might have been quite stable without medial bone support. As this young woman is quite active, stability might have become questionable in the long run. Of course, if the ankle would have developed arthritis, an ankle arthrodesis would have been an option.

Procedure

The decision was made to proceed with a repair of the posterior tibialis tendon, using unbraided suture, which decreases the surface area to which any residual bacteria could adhere (Fig 12.13-5). Cultures were again taken, which proved negative.

A 1:1 x-ray of the contralateral ankle was used to create a template of the medial malleolus using a sterile piece of plastic. This template was fashioned with a notch on the metaphysis in order to provide better axial stability and prevent shear (Fig 12.13-6). The cadaver bone was marked using the template (Fig 12.13-7) and the resulting allograft was secured using a plate (Fig 12.13-8).

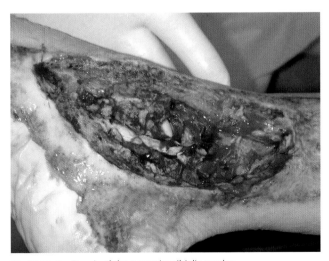

Fig 12.13-5   Repair of the posterior tibialis tendon.

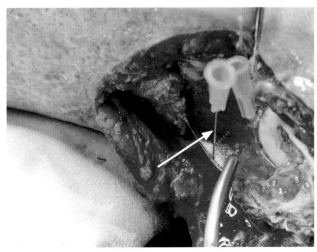

Fig 12.13-6   A template was fashioned from sterile plastic based on a 1:1 x-ray of the contralateral ankle. The template (arrow) was then temporarily placed in the defect to confirm size and shape.

After localizing the intended flap's pedicle with a handheld Doppler device, the fasciocutaneous sural flap—using a 9 × 6 cm skin paddle—was elevated and placed over the wound. Local tissue was not available with which to close the joint capsule, so the deep fascia of the fasciocutaneous flap was tightly sutured over the capsular defect. No attempt was made to reconstruct the deltoid ligament. An external fixator with a kickstand (Fig 12.13-9) was applied in order to help protect the flap yet still allow access to change the dressings over the more proximal abrasions. The donor site of the flap was closed using a meshed split-thickness skin graft (chapter 10.2). Since this flap was pedicled, no special assessment beside clinical observation was necessary. The leg was kept immobilized for 5 days. The external fixator was removed after 4 weeks.

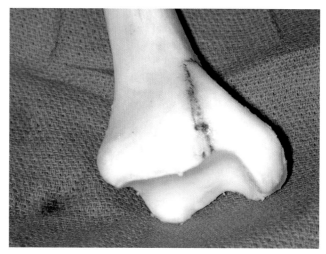

Fig 12.13-7 Cadaver bone marked according to the template. In a next step, it was cut with a saw.

Follow-up

The patient developed a pes equinus contracture over the next few months (Fig 12.13-10) and this necessitated a tendo-Achilles lengthening. At the latest follow-up (6 years postinjury), the patient walked with only a minimal limp, had mild, aching pain in the ankle after being active on it all day. The range of motion was 15° of dorsal flexion, 30° of plantar flexion, and x-rays showed solid union of the bone graft without any signs of osteitis or presence of any sequestra. This mild discomfort allowed the patient to remain employed and to run a half marathon race.

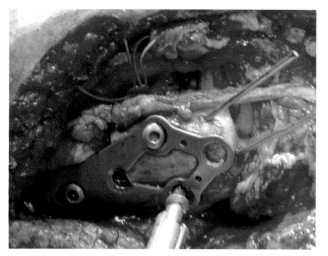

Fig 12.13-8 Stabilization of the cadaver bone graft after provisional K-wire fixation and definite plate and screw fixation.

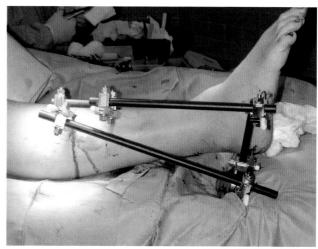

Fig 12.13-9 External fixator fitted with a kickstand in order to help protect the flap and still allow access to the injured tissues.

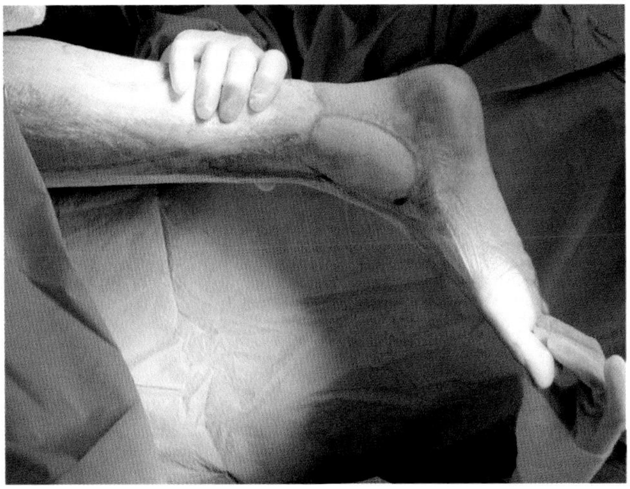

Fig 12.13-10   Pes equinus contracture at the 6-month follow-up.

Points to remember

- Defining the expected functional outcome is an important early step. In this case, the decision that the patient should be able to return to near-normal function guided the subsequent decision to use a sural flap in reconstructing this soft-tissue defect.
- This patient developed a complication, an Achilles-tendon contracture, which was recognized in time and treated appropriately. Complications are inevitable in reconstructive surgery, but if anticipated, recognized, and treated appropriately, a satisfactory result may still be achieved.

12.14 Skill level III: Case 3

Authors   Angelo M Biraima, Pietro Giovanoli

Case history

- 56-year-old white male patient
- Computer scientist
- Married
- Heavy smoker, exertional dyspnea
- Various medical problems, including microprolactinoma
- Obese (BMI 52.3)

The patient underwent repeated abdominal surgery complicated by a leakage of a bowel anastomosis and subsequent septic shock, which required a transfer to an intensive care unit in another hospital. During the prolonged hospitalization, the patient developed a pressure sore on his left heel.

The soft-tissue defect on the heel was initially managed by trauma surgeons with negative-pressure wound therapy, with dressing changes every 3–4 days (Fig 12.14-1). Weeks later, the general condition of the patient had improved. However, the skin defect was still considerable (Fig 12.14-2) and showed no tendency to heal, so that revision by a plastic surgeon was required.

This revealed the following:
- full-thickness skin defect measuring 3 × 5 cm
- thick layer of fibrinous tissue partially covering the defect
- induration of the surrounding subcutaneous tissue
- no signs of granulation tissue in the wound bed
- no signs of epithelialization in the periphery
- absence of palpable pulses in the ankle region
- x-ray without signs of osteomyelitis, but calcaneal spur visible on the lateral x-ray (Fig 12.14-3).

Laboratory findings showed anemia and malnutrition with hypoalbuminemia and hypoproteinemia.

Wound conditioning: Surgical debridement of all necrotic and poorly vascularized tissue almost down to the bone was performed (Fig 12.14-4). The soft-tissue defect was temporarily covered with a negative-pressure wound-therapy device in order to prepare the wound ground as best as possible. Three weeks later, the wound appeared clean with healthy granulation tissue indicating that the wound healing capacity of the patient was slowly recovering.

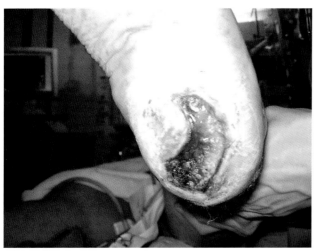

Fig 12.14-1 Plantar aspect of the left heel on admission showing a 3–4 cm large soft-tissue defect covered with fibrin.

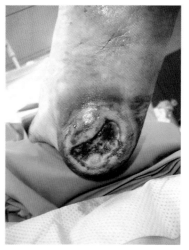

Fig 12.14-2 Clinical photograph several weeks after repeated local bedside debridement and wound conditioning by negative-pressure wound therapy.

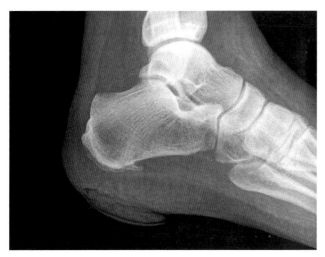

Fig 12.14-3 Lateral x-ray of the calcaneus showing a spur but no signs of osteomyelitis.

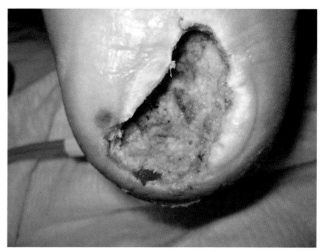

Fig 12.14-4 Clean wound after surgical debridement and first dressing change after negative-pressure wound therapy. Scarce bleeding and some granulation tissue visible.

Present status

After excision of all necrotic tissue, the following resulted:
- soft-tissue defect of 4 × 5 cm (Fig 12.14-5)
- underlying calcaneal bone still covered with sparse but hypoperfused fat tissue
- cultures positive for *Staphylococcus aureus* and *Staphylococcus epidermidis*.

Decision making

Open questions
- What are realistic goals of treatment?
- What are the definitive treatment options?
- What type of coverage is needed, nonvascularized or vascularized tissue?
- What about timing? Is it a one-step or staged procedure?
- Is antibiotic therapy necessary?

Options and plan

In the long run, the patient should be able to walk again wearing normal footwear. Therefore, the type of coverage should provide durable, healthy skin that will withstand mechanical stress in the weight-bearing area of the heel.

The patient is recovering from a large open wound related to complicated abdominal surgery with sepsis and subsequently has developed severe malnutrition and anemia. Treatment of the severe malnutrition and anemia is critical to the management of the soft-tissue defect.

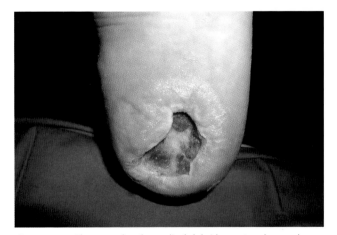

Fig 12.14-5 Three weeks after radical debridement and wound conditioning by negative-pressure wound therapy, the wound has developed some granulation tissue, which covers about half of the wound surface.

Primary antibiotic therapy is not necessary, as a low-grade wound contamination is not a contraindication to defect coverage with a well-vascularized flap. The general and nutritional state of the patient, however, will be decisive for the timing of flap coverage and the start of a therapeutic antibiotic regimen based on intraoperative cultures.

Considering the size of the defect, healing by secondary intention would be very time consuming and most uncertain in its result. Wounds with exposed avascular tissue (ie, stripped tendons, bare bone, or implant material) cannot be covered with nonvascularized skin grafts, while the size of the defect per se is not a decisive argument in favor of skin graft or flap.

Relative indications for a vascularized flap:
- previously ambulatory patient
- need for healthy, sensitive and mechanically resistant tissue cover within the weight-bearing area of the heel
- healthy tissue adjacent to the heel defect.

Options for a vascularized flap:
- Fasciocutaneous flap: This is based on the medial plantar artery feeding the instep area of the foot (chapter 10.5.2). This skin is mechanically resistant and sensitivity can be maintained after transposition into the defect. The donor site of the flap is not within the weight-bearing area of the foot (arch of the foot) and may be covered by a split-thickness skin graft, though scarring may be considerable.
- Free flap: This is especially suitable if a large bone defect needs filling. In this specific case, however, this flap would be rather complicated but could serve as back-up option.
- Muscle flaps: Without overlying skin paddle, these would be entirely unsuitable in this case, as they would need to be raised and rarely have sufficient mechanical resistance or the necessary sensitivity unless the cutaneous nerves of the free flap are connected to local cutaneous nerves. These flaps also tend to be very bulky and may prevent the patient from wearing footwear.

Procedure

With a handheld Doppler device, the left posterior tibial artery as well as the medial plantar artery were identified within the arch of the foot. After reexcision of the wound margins, a skin paddle originating from the instep area of the foot was outlined to match the defect. The dissection of a fasciocutaneous flap including the plantar fascia was started at the distal end of the outlined skin paddle and continued in a retrograde manner, identifying the perforator between the abductor hallucis and the flexor digitorum brevis muscles (Fig 12.14-6). After elevation of the flap, the medial plantar nerve was identified and, after isolation of its cutaneous portion to the skin paddle, intraneural dissection was performed. Next, the incision was extended in direction of the medial malleolus and dissection of the tibial vascular bundle was started (Fig 12.14-7). To extend the reach of the flap, the origin of the abductor hallucis muscle was transected. The remaining skin between the donor site (instep area) and the recipient site was undermined in order to form a subcutaneous tunnel and the flap was moved into the defect (Fig 12.14-8). The donor-site defect was covered with a meshed split-thickness skin graft.

Follow-up

One year after the operation the patient had good protective sensation in his left heel and was walking without pain. The flap matched well with the surrounding skin and the split-thickness skin graft was stable (Fig 12.14-9).

Points to remember

- Before such a tissue defect can be covered, a careful assessment of the whole patient and local conditions is mandatory. This applies to nutritional and vascular status

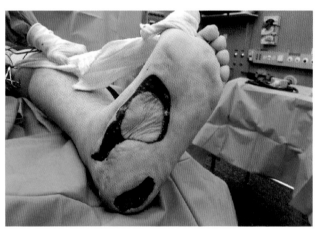

Fig 12.14-6 Intraoperative view of the medial plantar flap (instep flap) after circumferential incision.

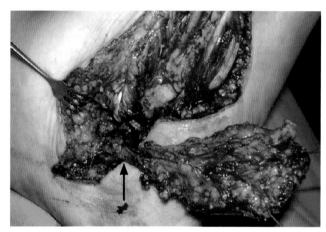

Fig 12.14-7 Isolated flap with its neurovascular pedicle proximally (arrow).

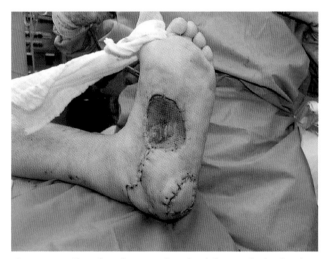

Fig 12.14-8 Flap after placement into the defect on the heel and coverage of the donor site with a meshed split-thickness skin graft. No signs of venous congestion.

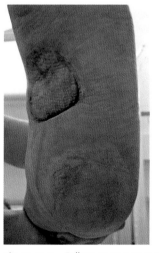

Fig 12.14-9 Follow-up at 1 year. Very nice and smooth integration of the flap into the neighboring skin of the heel, while the donor site is still prominently visible.

in particular. Furthermore, the timing of surgery and type of tissue transfer must be adapted individually to the local situation and the expectations of the patient (eg, with regard to outcomes for return to sensation and weight bearing).

- Choose the option providing the best chances of achieving the desired result and not necessarily the simplest one (chapter 8.2).

- Whenever possible, replace like with like (chapter 8.1).
- Formation of hypertrophic tissue may be seen at the borders of the skin graft—a problem resulting from bad skin match and considerable contraction of the split-thickness skin graft. As long as this occurs in the non-weight-bearing area, it rarely causes problems. The use of a split-thickness skin graft from the opposite side (glabrous, mechanically stable skin) may overcome this problem.

12.15 Skill level III: Case 4

Authors   Jörg Grünert, Rafael Jakubietz

Case history

- 54-year-old white female patient
- Facility manager
- Single
- Smoker
- Obese (BMI 31)
- No other medical problems

The patient sustained a closed injury of the ankle joint without fracture and was immobilized in a splint for ~2 weeks. She developed a pressure sore with full-thickness necrosis and exposure of the Achilles tendon, which was treated with wet-to-dry dressings twice a day and a short leg splint. On presentation to the plastic surgeon, the examination revealed:

- full-thickness soft-tissue defect measuring 3 × 4 cm over the Achilles tendon
- exposed and partially desiccated Achilles tendon
- hardenend wound edges
- no signs of infection
- normal sensation and perfusion of the foot with palpable pulses, in particular of the dorsalis pedis artery.

Wound conditioning: Aggressive and radical debridement was performed under general anesthesia with resection of ~20% of the Achilles tendon's circumference at the posterolateral aspect and irrigation with copious amounts of fluid. Subsequent bacteriological cultures were negative. Wet-to-dry dressings were applied.

Present status

There was a full-thickness soft-tissue defect measuring 4 × 5 cm (**Fig 12.15-1**). The remaining Achilles tendon was completely exposed.

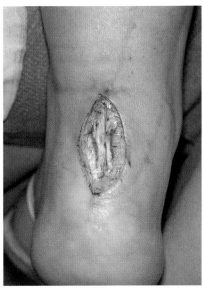

Fig 12.15-1   Soft-tissue defect with exposed Achilles tendon after debridement.

Decision making

Open questions
- Which are the goals of reconstruction?
- Is the tendon salvageable?
- How should the soft-tissue defect be managed before definitive coverage?
- How and when should definitive closure be performed?

Options and plan
The goal of treatment is 3-fold:
1. Part of the tendon should be salvaged and the remaining ~50% of the tendon's cross section should still allow for normal daily activities and weight bearing.
2. Resilient coverage of the soft-tissue defect and recovery of a normal range of motion of the ankle joint. The soft-tissue cover must be supple and provide adequate padding of the remaining tendon, without being too bulky so as not to interfere with normal footwear. The transferred tissue must resist the constant friction caused by footwear, while preserving the gliding properties of the tendon.
3. Any local or regional tissue transfer or flap should not impair perfusion nor sensation of the foot.

Chronic wounds are often colonized by numerous strains of bacteria. Coverage attempted in the face of an active infection is doomed to failure. Reducing bacterial load mainly depends on adequate and aggressive debridement. In order to further condition the wound, negative-pressure wound therapy has been shown to decrease bacterial count (chapter 9.3). Alternatively, wet-to-dry dressings performed twice a day serve the same purpose (chapter 9.1). However, this procedure is painful, labor intensive, and time consuming.

Prior to definitive closure, cultures should preferably be negative and adequate debridement and copious irrigation must be repeated as the first step of the reconstructive procedure.

Possibilities of soft-tissue reconstruction in case of an exposed tendon include:
- pedicled or free flaps
- pedicled perforator flaps (chapter 10.4)
- fasciocutaneous or muscle tissue.

The soft-tissue defect with an exposed, nonvascularized tendon mandates reconstruction with well-vascularized tissue that preferably fits into the defect and does not interfere with the gliding of the tendon under motion.

Skin grafts, therefore, are not an option as they will not take well on poorly vascularized tissue but would adhere and tether the tendon.

Local or regional pedicled flaps are technically easy and mostly appropriate. Muscle flaps are rather bulky, tend to adhere to the underlying tendon and, in addition, would require skin-graft coverage that would be insensate and nonresistant in regard to mechanical stress.

The fasciocutaneous flap seems to fulfill all requirements. Moreover, the fasciocutaneous flap replaces like with like, ie, skin which resembles the missing tissue. It is resistant to mechanical stress and the fascial component of the flap provides a gliding surface which allows normal motion of the Achilles tendon. Fasciocutaneous flaps elevated as perforator flaps are preferred. They should be supplied by one vascular bundle only in close vicinity to the defect (chapter 10.4). This should be the case, particularly when considerable rotation of the flap is required. Depending on the size and orientation of the defect, either a rotation flap or a propeller flap can be used (chapter 10.4.3). Adjacent structures such as muscle and nerves can be spared. If no adequate perforating vessels can be identified preoperatively and confirmed intraoperatively, the sural flap may serve as a backup option (chapter 10.5.2, 12.13). However, the sural nerve has to be sacrificed resulting in an insensate area of the lateral border of the foot (ie, dermatome of the sural nerve).

Basically, microvascular tissue transfer is always an option, but technically demanding, often time consuming and associated with some degree of donor site morbidity, depending on the flap that is elevated. Therefore, it should only serve as back-up option.

Procedure

About 4 weeks after initial debridement and having excluded any contamination, the reconstructive procedure was undertaken. With a handheld Doppler device, a dominant perforating vessel originating from the fibular artery was identified lateral to the Achilles tendon and selected as the flap's pedicle, ie, pivot point for the propeller flap (Fig 12.15-2). The total length of the flap proximal to the pedicle included the distance between pedicle and distal wound margin (Fig 12.15-2) (chapter 10.4.3). In prone position, the debridement and irrigation was repeated without tourniquet, in order to excise all tissue with dubious perfusion. Flap elevation was initiated with a medial incision opposite to the preoperatively identified perforating vessel. Having found the vessel in a subfascial plane (ie, below the muscle fascia) it was dissected (Fig 12.15-3), and good flow in the artery was identified by Doppler ultrasound. As the perforating vessel serves as the pivot point, any misjudgment could render the flap too short, although the length of the flap may still be adapted at this point of the procedure.

After elevation of the entire flap (Fig 12.15-4), both concomitant veins and the feeding artery require further careful dissection in order to allow even blood flow during the subsequent twisting of the pedicle. Now the flap can easily be rotated 180° into the defect and tailored to the size needed (Fig 12.15-5, 12.15-6). Potential tethering of the pedicle has to be prevented by further dissection of the vessels. The

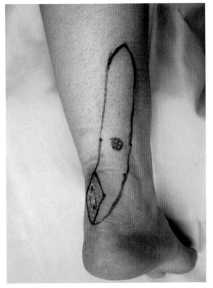

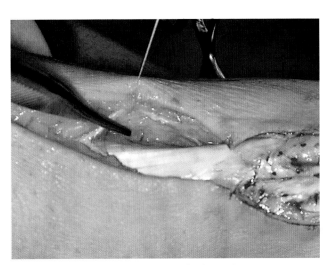

Fig 12.15-3   Perforating vessel (tip of the forceps).

Fig 12.15-2   Preoperative planning of the flap based on the dominant perforating vessel identified with a handheld Doppler device.

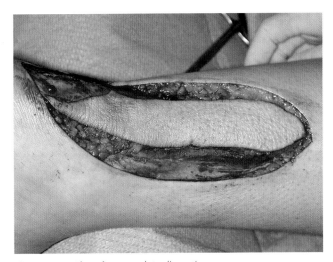

Fig 12.15-4   Flap after complete dissection.

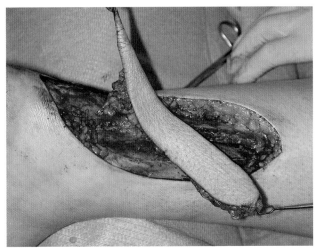

Fig 12.15-5   Clockwise propeller-like rotation of the flap.

resulting defect at the donor site required the application of a meshed split-thickness skin graft (Fig 12.15-7) (chapter 10.2). Circular dressings have to be avoided and easy visual access to the flap should be possible. A splint prevents direct pressure on the flap and immobilizes the ankle. Ambulation is allowed after ~2 weeks when the wound has safely healed.

Follow-up

The out-hospital course was uneventful. At the 4-month follow-up, the patient presented with a functional ankle and a cosmetically acceptable result (Fig 12.15-8).

Points to remember

- Fasciocutaneous perforator flaps need to be part of the armamentarium of the surgeon dealing with soft-tissue defects, especially on the extremities.
- There are many styles of perforator flaps. Which of them is chosen for a given case is a matter of wound location and geometry.

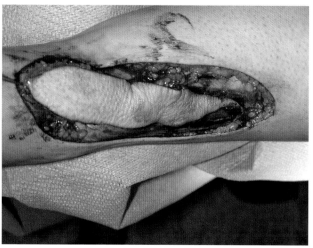

Fig 12.15-6   Insertion of the flap after 180° rotation. Tension on the twisted vessel must be avoided.

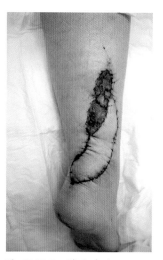

Fig 12.15-7   Clinical picture 5 days postoperatively. The skin graft covering the remaining defect, which was placed to help avoid undue tension, has taken well.

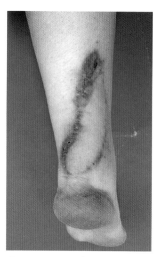

Fig 12.15-8   At the 4-month follow-up, the flap is well integrated without any bulkiness but with widened scars.

12.16 Skill level III: Case 5

Author   Mirjam Zweifel-Schlatter

Case history

- 32-year-old white female patient
- Working full-time as a bank accountant
- Single
- T10-paraplegia
- Underweight (1.68 m, 50 kg, BMI 17.7)
- No other medical problems
- Very conscious about her appearance

The patient had sustained a fracture of her thoracic spine 10 years ago, resulting in T10-paraplegia. She spends ~14 hours a day sitting in a wheelchair. About 7 years after the accident, the patient developed a small, superficial pressure sore over the coccyx, which she treated conservatively with hydrocolloid dressings. Surgery to correct the unstable scar and the chronic pressure sore over the coccyx was declined. She did not attend medical follow-up until a year later, when her family doctor finally referred her to a specialist.

The patient initially presented to the plastic surgeon with the following results on examination:
- fever (38,7°C)
- foul-smelling circular wound of 8 cm in diameter over her sacrum extending down to the coccyx with exposed bone and purulent discharge diagnosed as a stage 4 ulcer (Fig. 12.16-1)
- buttocks and wound completely insensate.

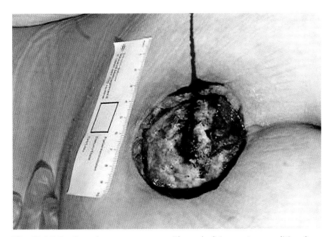

Fig 12.16-1   Sacral pressure sore with underlying osteomyelitis of the sacrum and coccyx in a young paraplegic, malnourished, and anemic patient.

Laboratory findings: Hgb 10.2 g/dl, WBC 15000, CRP 180 mg/l, albumin 22 g/l as sign of chronic infection and malnutrition.

Wound conditioning: The patient was admitted to hospital for wound debridement and cultures. Two debridements were performed. The softened, osteomyelitic coccyx was excised. Biopsies were taken from the remaining debrided sacral bone and sent for histological and microbiological examination to confirm osteomyelitis and guide antibiotic therapy.

Present status

After the repeated debridement, the findings were:
- skin defect over the sacrum with exposed sacral bone of 10 cm in diameter
- excised coccyx
- no rectal fistula (ruled out by endoscopy).

It is important to note that the assessment of the wound does not stop at its margins. The patient generally showed:
- signs of malnutrition, ie, hypoproteinemia and hypoalbuminemia
- chronic anemia induced by the chronic infection.

Decision making

Open questions
- How to achieve stable soft-tissue coverage enabling the patient to sit and to return to work?
- How to achieve the eradication of osteomyelitis of the remaining sacrum?

Options and plan
In this case, the soft-tissue defect may be managed with a tissue transfer of some type and must result in a durable cover in order to support weight bearing while sitting. A stable and long-lasting skin envelope, however, can only be achieved with a successful treatment of the underlying osteomyelitis. Treatment of osteomyelitis and of the soft-tissue defect are inseparable. Osteomyelitis cannot be cured without soft-tissue coverage, but the soft-tissue coverage cannot be expected to survive in the presence of a persistently leaking sinus. Successful reconstruction further depends on good wound-healing capacity. Therefore, it is

paramount to resolve the present state of malnutrition. Accordingly, a staged approach is considered.

Reasons for choosing a staged approach:
• Treatment of malnutrition is imperative prior to any reconstructive surgery of a substantial defect as there is a high risk of wound healing complications, which would compromise both the recipient and the donor site.
• Treatment of the osteomyelitis of the sacrum: Appropriate antibiotics should be given, based on cultures obtained from bone biopsy. An infectious disease consult is indicated.
• Antimicrobial drugs will effectively reach the osteomyelitic zone only after coverage of the exposed bone with vascularized flap tissue.

After radical debridement of a pressure sore, a large wound often remains. The debrided and exposed cancellous sacral bone oozes substantially. In order to condition the wound, simple saline-gauze dressings are initially preferred to negative-pressure wound therapy until the serosanguineous discharge has stopped. Then, a negative-pressure wound-therapy device is applied, which decreases the frequency of dressing changes and enhances granulation tissue formation.

Once the wound is "clean" and the nutritional status has recovered, definitive treatment options can be discussed, which must address a safe defect reconstruction and eradication of the infection of the underlying bone.

Well-vascularized muscle flaps potentially supply more blood and therefore more oxygen to the infected area and possibly more antibiotics to the wound in comparison to fasciocutaneous flaps. As yet, however, no comparative study to prove this assumption has been published. Muscle flaps, in addition, are voluminous, able to obliterate cavities and to plug dead spaces. On the other hand, muscle is not very pressure resistant and the initially bulky reconstruction (sometimes falsely considered as additional padding for the weight-bearing area of the coccyx) is prone to failure. Muscle flaps are excellently suited to fill cavities, but in case of sacral pressure sores, there is no cavity or dead space because the wound surface is flat, or even slightly convex.

Local fasciocutaneous or dermal flaps, however, are good options in order to cover the sacral defect with pressure-resistant and well-vascularized tissue.

The next consideration is how to design the flap. All resulting scars should lie outside of the weight-bearing zones as otherwise they would tend to break down in a wheelchair-

dependent patient. It is advisable to design a flap that will not preclude the subsequent elevation of another flap in case the first one should fail.

In this case, a monolateral rotation flap (chapter 10.4.2) from the buttock was chosen. It offers stable coverage of the sacral wound and the scars will lie outside the weight-bearing areas, which is another advantage of a rotation flap in comparison to a pedicled perforator flap (chapter 10.4.3) based on the superior gluteal artery. While elegant as a procedure, the resulting scars after having raised such a perforator flap would run across the buttock. The rotation flap is elevated without muscle fascia and, therefore, is more elastic and easier to rotate into the defect. In case of recurrence, which is likely in such a young paraplegic patient, the rotation flap may be raised a second time and pulled further medially, ie, remobilization of the flap.

Alternatively, it would still be possible to use an ipsilateral gluteal muscle flap that has not been elevated yet. Last but not least, the contralateral buttock remains completely untouched and is available for future interventions if needed.

Procedure

Two weeks after the initial debridement and wound conditioning with negative-pressure wound therapy (chapter 9.3), the wound bed showed ample granulation tissue, which was a sign of good wound-healing potential and at the same time showed that the high-protein drinks have improved the nutritional status. The cultures of the bone biopsy have grown *Escherichia coli*. The patient was operated in a prone position, starting with the excision of all undermined wound margins and granulation tissue about the sacrum (Fig 12.16-2). According to the size of the resulting defect, a large rotation flap was planned (chapter 10.4.2) and outlined on the skin with a high-riding arch that extends proximally over the posterior iliac border down to the greater trochanter laterally.

Elevating the flap in this manner ensures that the flap can easily be rotated into the defect without any tension, preventing it from being pulled medially, which would endanger the blood supply (Fig 12.16-3). Elasticity of the flap is increased considerably, if it is elevated without the often rigid muscle fascia, which might inhibit the rotation of a large flap into the defect (Fig 12.16-4).

Antibiotic treatment should be started shortly before surgery according to the antibiogram. Postoperatively, the patient was nursed in an air-cushioned bed for 5 weeks and care was taken to avoid pressure on the flap until the patient can get back into the wheelchair. During the first 3 postoperative weeks, hip flexion of more than 30° was not allowed in order to prevent any tension on the flap, which might endanger wound healing.

Occupational therapists and physical therapists performed specific assessments of the patient. Accordingly, the back of the patient's wheelchair was adjusted and she was given a different supporting cushion.

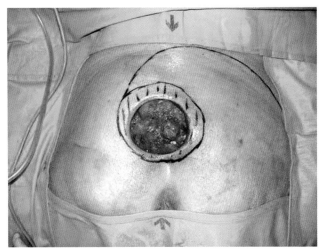

Fig 12.16-2 Two weeks after debridement and negative-pressure wound therapy, and after taking first measures to improve the nutritional status. The wound seems clean and shows ample granulation tissue. The undermined wound edges (shaded area) are excised prior to coverage with a large rotation flap. Note the design and dimension of the flap with a high-riding arch of rotation.

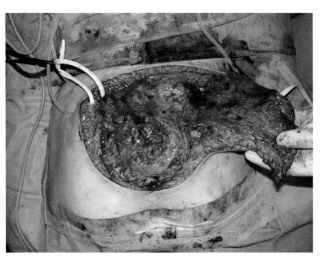

Fig 12.16-3 The rotation flap is elevated without the rigid fascia of the underlying muscle.

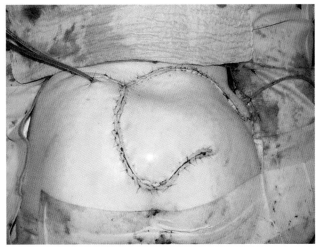

Fig 12.16-4 Final state after rotation and tension-free insertion of the flap into the defect.

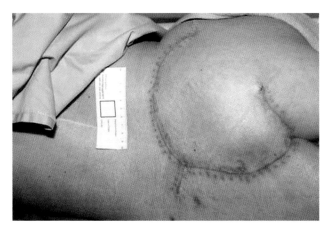

Fig 12.16-5 The patient is fully mobilized and shows a stable reconstruction 3 weeks after flap surgery.

Follow-up

With the described regime, recovery was uneventful and no wound-healing problems were encountered (Fig 12.16-5). At the last follow-up nearly 4 years after reconstruction, the patient showed a stable soft-tissue coverage of the sacrum without recurrence of either pressure sore or osteomyelitis. The former full-time working woman had decided to cut down commitments in order to be able to rest and get out of the wheelchair in between hours. She was a highly-motivated and compliant patient, which may have contributed to the lack of recurrence.

Points to remember

- Successful treatment of a sacral pressure sore with osteomyelitis always starts with radical wound debridement and subsequent wound conditioning prior to definitive coverage.
- Malnutrition must be corrected prior to definitive coverage.
- Fasciocutaneous flaps often suffice to reliably cover such a defect.
- Stable reconstruction of the weight-bearing area with a rotation flap provides durable coverage and function. Well-planned flaps and mobilization without tension are the keys to initial success.
- In order to avoid cumbersome pressure sores and for long-term success, perfect patient compliance and good education are prerequisites, not only in case of debilitated or paralyzed, overweight, or malnourished patients with comorbidities, but also in case of patients with pressure sores resulting from long bed rest after trauma.

12.17   Skill level IV: Case 1

Authors   Maxime Servaes, Yves Harder

Case history

- 25-year-old male patient
- Flight engineer
- Engaged
- Sportsman
- Smoker
- No other medical problems

The patient crashed on his motorcycle into a security barrier at high speed. There was a prolonged extrication, taking nearly 1 hour to evacuate the patient.

Clinical findings in the trauma bay included:
- Glasgow coma scale score 15/15
- no other apparent lesions except for the injuries to both lower legs.

Clinical and radiological findings of the right lower leg:
- considerable swelling with axial displacement of 45°
- bluish discoloration of the calf
- stocking-like dysesthesia of the foot
- cold and pale foot, no palpable distal pulses
- at the middle third of the leg an anteromedial wound

measuring 12 × 6 cm with a large, proximally-based skin flap
- displaced, comminuted tibial and fibular fracture (Gustilo type IIIC fracture) (Fig 12.17-1a–b).

Clinical and radiological findings of the left lower leg:
- two small wounds at the anteromedial aspect of the lower leg
- no neurovascular deficit
- displaced, comminuted tibial and fibular fracture (Gustilo type II fracture) (Fig 12.17-2a–b)
- one wound on the thigh measuring 3 × 4 cm.

The right lower leg was realigned under analgesia and pulses recovered rapidly. The patient was taken to the operating room and both tibial fractures were stabilized using intramedullary nails with static locking. On the right side, anteromedial and anterolateral fasciotomies were performed to release all four muscle compartments (chapter 11.1). At that time, arterial bleeding was detected at the posteromedial aspect of the fracture site, matching a transection of the posterior tibial artery. The vascular surgeon on call performed a segmental repair of the artery using an autologous reversed saphenous vein graft. The skin flap covering the wound at the middle third of the lower leg was assessed intraoperatively to be viable and sutured back into place. All other wounds were left open because of the swelling, including the ones on the other leg. Postoperative angiography of the right leg confirmed patency of the three arteries including the repaired posterior tibial artery.

Wound conditioning: On the second day, the patient was taken back to the operating room for another irrigation and debridement of all the wounds of the right leg. Medially, the fasciotomy wound was partially closed with the help of staples and elastic vessel loops (chapter 10.1). A negative-pressure wound-therapy device was placed over the larger wound and changed every 3 days (chapter 9.3). One week later, another debridement and irrigation was performed including the excision of the now necrotic skin flap (chapter 7). On the twelfth day, the lateral fasciotomy wound could be closed.

Present status

Fifteen days after the injury the patient was first presented to the plastic surgeon for advice. The patient presented with an anteromedial soft-tissue defect of the right leg that was clean and covered with ample granulation tissue in the periphery except for the exposed, necrotic appearing tibia in the center of the defect (Fig 12.17-3). X-rays of the right leg showed adequate stabilization (Fig 12.17-4a–b). Bacterial swabs revealed bacterial contamination of the granulation tissue with a mixed flora including *Pseudomonas aeruginosa*, *Streptococcus mitis*, α-hemolytic streptococci, and coagulase-negative staphylococci, which were sensitive to common antibiotics. According to the infectiologist, systemic treatment with ciprofloxacin and ceftazidime was initiated to protect the bone.

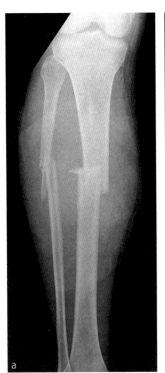
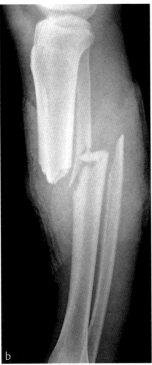

Fig 12.17-1a–b   X-rays of the right lower leg on the day of injury showing a Gustilo type IIIC fracture.
a   AP view.
b   Lateral view.

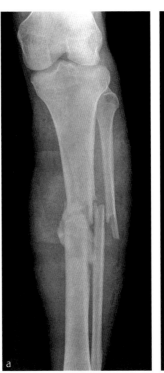
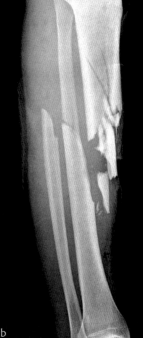

Fig 12.17-2a–b   X-rays of the left lower leg on the day of injury showing a Gustilo type II fracture.
a   AP view.
b   Lateral view.

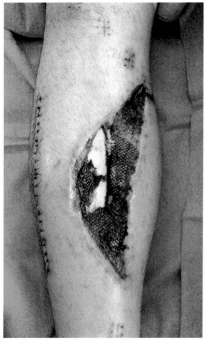

Fig 12.17-3   Right leg with a soft-tissue defect of 15 × 6 cm including a 5 × 2 cm area of exposed tibial bone 2 weeks after injury.

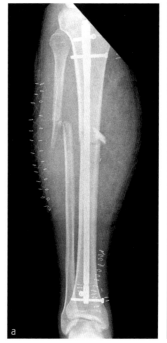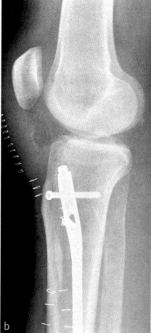

Fig 12.17-4a–b   X-rays of the right lower leg 15 days after injury. Adequate stabilization of the Gustilo type IIIC fracture.
a   AP view.
b   Lateral view.

Decision making

Open questions
- What type of coverage provides the lowest risk of complications (eg, nonunion, infection)?
- How to get the timing of coverage right?

Options and plan
Delayed primary closure in this case is not possible because of the loss of tissue. Healing by secondary intention using various types of dressings including negative-pressure wound therapy is not recommended because it is very unlikely that granulation tissue will form over exposed bone, ie, bone without periosteum, while there is an increased risk of infection resulting in osteomyelitis, which would eventually compromise bone healing.

A considerable soft-tissue defect in a young patient with exposed, bare bone needs to be repaired with a vascularized flap. At this point, three issues must be discussed:
- origin of the flap
- composition of the tissue used for repair
- timing of coverage.

There was considerable energy involved in the initial injury as evidenced by the development of vascular injury and compartment syndrome. It is therefore reasonable to assume that the surrounding tissues such as local muscle and subcutaneous tissue were also exposed to such significant energy. In view of this fact, an appropriate coverage procedure has to be selected.

Local rotation flaps such as a soleus or sural flap are associated with a high rate of complications in the case of severe trauma to the lower extremities. A free muscle flap is not necessary because there is neither a bone defect to be plugged nor gross infection to be treated. Furthermore, the muscle flap would need to be covered by a skin paddle (too bulky a coverage) or a split-thickness skin graft (imperfect match of color and texture) (chapter 10.2). Since the soft-tissue defect is confined to the skin, a fasciocutaneous free flap tailored to the defect, such as a free lateral arm flap, would be ideal (chapter 10.6). The repair to the motto "like with like" results in a good match of color and texture. A free flap would utilize vessels that were not in the zone of injury (chapter 10.3.3), which would be advantageous in this patient.

Flaps in general, but free flaps in particular, are associated with an increased failure rate when applied between 3–5 days and 4–6 weeks following trauma, which equals an increased inflammatory state within the zone of inquiry (chapter 10.3). Accordingly, some surgeons advocate immediate flap coverage or delayed coverage beyond the 4–6 week period.

Procedure

After 5 weeks, the soft-tissue coverage was planned, using a fasciocutaneous free flap from the lateral aspect of the nondominant left arm. A new, preoperative arteriography confirmed the distal patency of the anterior tibial and fibular arteries as well as the successful repair of the posterior tibial artery and served as a roadmap for the anastomosis.

First, the arm flap was planned using a handheld Doppler device. A tailored skin paddle of 15×6 cm to match the defect was outlined. It was centered on perforating vessels of the collateral posterior radial artery (Fig 12.17-5). Second, the lateral arm flap was dissected in a subfascial plane. Simultaneously another team isolated the anterior tibial artery and its concomitant veins. Third, the flap was anastomosed end-to-end to the recipient vessels with standard microsurgical techniques. Finally, the flap was trimmed and sutured

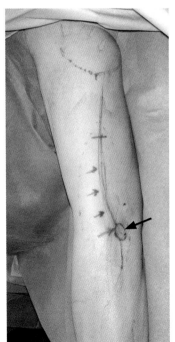

Fig 12.17-5 Anatomical landmarks of the lateral arm flap showing the outlines of the deltoid muscle (white arrows) as well as the intermuscular septum (blue line) and the lateral epicondyle (black arrow). The perforator arteries are indicated with blue arrows after localization with Doppler ultrasound.

into the defect except for a small area close to the pedicle in order to avoid any tension and inevitable congestion of the flap. The donor site was closed primarily. One week later, the remaining wound was closed under local anesthesia.

Follow-up

The postoperative course was uneventful, in particular in regard to the integration of the flap as well as the healing of the donor site. Gradual verticalization was initiated, beginning on the fifth postoperative day. After uneventful wound healing including the secondary closure of the distal surgical wound, the aftercare consisted of an intensive rehabilitation program. The patient was motivated and compliant. A significant edema on the right lower leg in connection with the flap necessitated regular lymphatic drainage and the wearing of surgical stocking.

Four weeks after flap surgery, ie, 10 weeks after trauma, partial consolidation of the tibial fractures was observed on x-rays, allowing for partial weight bearing (10 kg). Complete bone union of the right lower leg was observed 3 months after the accident (Fig-12.17-6a–b) and the patient started with full weight bearing. The flap showed good integration within the adjacent tissues and a perfect match of thickness, texture, and color (Fig-12.17-7a–b). The donor site did not reveal any functional sequelae. Physical therapy was initiated to begin muscle strengthening in order to compensate for atrophy.

Points to remember

- This case demonstrates the importance of early multidisciplinary planning. Although the end result of a healed fracture with no infection was obtained, the course of healing was delayed and undue risks were taken because there was no early multidisciplinary plan.

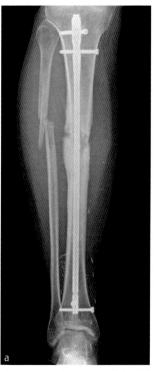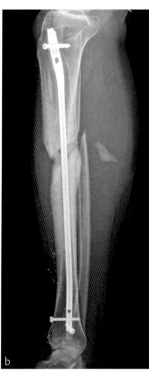

Fig 12.17-6a–b X-rays of the right lower leg 6 months after the accident, showing bone union.
a AP view.
b Lateral view.

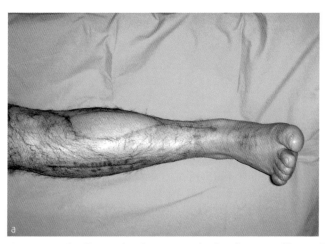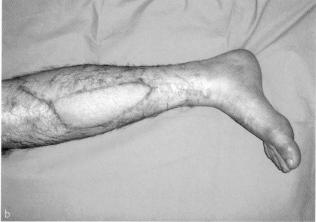

Fig 12.17-7a–b Six months after surgery, the flap shows good integration and a good match of thickness, texture, and color.
a Anterior view.
b Medial view.

12.18 Skill level IV: Case 2

Author Stefan Langer

Case history

- 69-year-old white male patient
- Pensioner
- Married
- Nonsmoker
- Arterial hypertension

The patient was riding a bicycle at reduced speed when he was hit by a car. He was transported to the hospital with a splint in place to stabilize the leg.

On presentation to the trauma bay of a tertiary hospital the patient was examined by the surgeon on duty. The patient was conscious and presented with the following isolated injury of his right lower leg:
- axial deformity
- bruised but intact skin envelope on the distal half of the leg
- palpable pulses on the dorsum of the foot and posteriorly to the medial malleolus
- normal sensation distally
- closed distal tibial and fibular fracture (42-B3.3).

After 2 days of bed rest and elevation of the leg, open reduction and internal fixation of the tibial fracture was performed using a plate and screws. The patient was administered a perioperative antibiotic (second-generation cephalosporin) that was continued for 7 days due to the extensive initial swelling. The patient further received subcutaneous heparin as thromboprophylaxis.

The initial postoperative course was uneventful. From approximately day 3 on, the patient developed a circumscribed discoloration of the skin on the right lower leg, which resulted in skin necrosis. Two weeks after initial surgery and complete demarcation of the necrosis, the patient was referred to a level I hospital with a specialized trauma unit.

Initial clinical investigation showed a well-demarcated, full-thickness skin necrosis of 4 × 6 cm that was located on the medial side of the surgical incision (Fig 12.18-1).

Wound conditioning: Radical excision of all necrotic skin was essential. At the same time, exposure of the hardware was inevitable.

Present status

After irrigation and debridement, the soft-tissue defect ended up being much larger in comparison to the circumscribed skin necrosis, ie, ~4 × 8 cm. Implant material was clearly exposed but clean, and there was no evidence of loosening, which was confirmed by an x-ray (Fig 12.18-2a–b). According to the consulting trauma surgeon, replacement was not necessary but additional bone grafts were recommended to increase the likelihood of bone healing.

Decision making

Open questions
- What are realistic goals of treatment?
- What are the definitive treatment options?
- How should the defect be covered?

Options and plan
This fracture should heal within 6 months without significant late sequelae. The ankle may require a long time to recover its entire range of motion.

The persisting soft-tissue defect still revealed exposed bone and implant. Coverage using a negative-pressure wound-therapy device (chapter 9.3) in order to create granulation tissue was unlikely to succeed since bone and implant do not provide adequate vascularity to support this. Therefore, the soft-tissue defect needed to be covered with vascularized tissue.

Vascularized tissue may be obtained from many sources. Local flaps might provide adequate tissue (chapter 10.4). The defect was too distal for a muscle flap (gastrocnemius or soleus flap) to provide coverage (chapter 10.5). A fasciocutaneous flap such as a sural flap could also have been an option. Free flaps could have been used as well, either from the lateral arm, radial forearm or lateral thigh. All of these techniques, however, require microsurgical skills.

The surgeon felt that in this case, due to local trauma to the soft tissues, a random-pattern flap or fasciocutaneous flap would potentially involve a higher risk of failure, so a free flap was chosen, specifically a lateral thigh flap. The decision in favor of the anterolateral thigh flap was based on the surgeon's experience as well as the patient's constitution, pedicle length, congruity of donor and recipient vessels, matching of flap thickness, color, texture, and elasticity with the surrounding tissues and donor-site morbidity (primary closure versus skin grafting). Since there was no bone defect, ie, osseous cavity, a bulky muscle or musculocutaneous flap was not necessary. More complicated flaps such as a free muscle were not indicated because the bulk of the muscle flap might preclude ankle motion or the wearing of regular footwear.

Procedure

An anterolateral thigh flap marked to fit the wound after debridement was chosen to cover this wound (Fig 12.18-3). This flap is based on the descending branch of the lateral femoral circumflex artery and was anastomosed to the posterior tibial artery by microsurgery. The patient was managed postoperatively with bed rest for ~5 days and prophylactic anticoagulation medication. Gradual verticalization was initiated on the fifth postoperative day (chapter 10.7). Progressive weight bearing was started after 2 weeks.

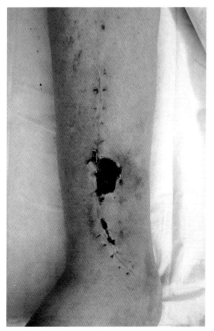

Fig 12.18-1 Circumscribed skin necrosis adjacent to the surgical incision.

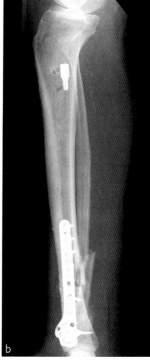

Fig 12.18-2a–b X-rays of the right lower leg 15 days after fracture fixation. The fracture has been adequately stabilized.
a AP view.
b Lateral view.

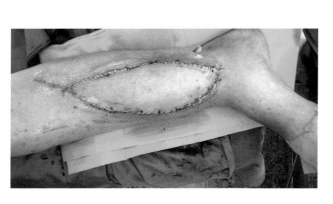

Fig 12.18-3 Well-perfused flap the day after surgery. Some swelling is present.

Follow-up

Follow-up after flap surgery was uneventful. At 3 months the fracture had healed (Fig 12.18-4a–b), the range of motion of the leg was unrestricted and the limb was pain-free. The flap was well integrated within the adjacent skin with a good match of color and texture (Fig 12.18-5a–c). Some swelling still occurs at the end of the day, if no compression stockings are worn.

Points to remember

- While wounds may seem relatively innocuous, the surgeon has to consider the condition of the surrounding tissues, which may previously have healed, but would not be suitable for local transfer.
- Remember that the simplest solution may not necessarily be the best solution, hence the concept of reconstructive modules (chapter 8.2.2).

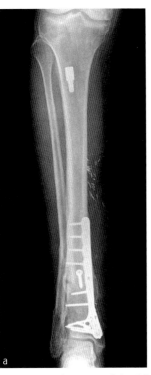
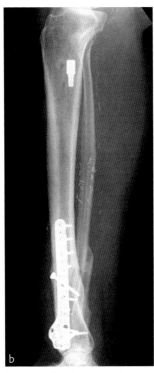

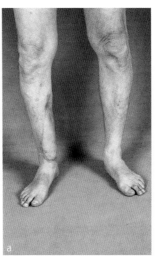
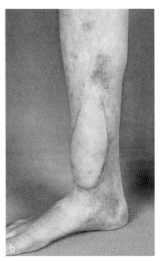

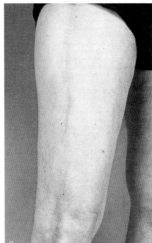

Fig 12.18-5a–c Well-integrated flap.
a   Overview.
b   Medial view showing some swelling of the flap.
c   Donor site with an inconspicuous scar.

Fig 12.18-4a–b X-rays of the right lower leg showing a completely healed fracture with some callus formation 3 months after flap coverage.
a   AP view.
b   Lateral view.

12.19 Skill level **IV**: Case 3

Authors Urs Hug, Elmar Fritsche

Case history

- 48-year-old white female patient
- Security agent
- Divorced
- Nonsmoker
- No other medical problems

The patient was hit by a truck while riding a motorcycle at moderate speed. Her left leg was struck, resulting in an obvious deformity. Despite protective clothing, she sustained a considerable open wound of the left lower leg. Emergency medical personnel in the field applied a clean bandage, a short leg air splint and started intravenous fluids and analgesics. Spine precautions were taken. The patient was initially transported to a local hospital, but rapidly transferred to a level I trauma center within 2 hours after the injury.

In the trauma bay, clinical and radiological findings of the spine, chest, pelvis and abdomen were normal. X-rays of the left hip showed a pertrochanteric hip fracture. The leg was shortened and externally rotated.

Examination of the left leg revealed an open wound at the lateral and posterior aspects of the distal third of the left lower leg that measured 8 × 6 cm and was interrupted by a skin bridge (Fig 12.19-1). There was no evident skin loss.

Bone fragments were exposed. There were palpable pulses distal to the injury, but absence of sensation on the lateral margin and reduced sensation on the lateral dorsum of the foot corresponding to the dermatome of the sural nerve.

Intact sensation of the rest of the sole of the foot was noted. No motor nerve dysfunction was detected clinically. X-rays showed a multifragmentary tibial fracture rather close to the ankle joint as well as a Gustilo type IIIB distal fibular fracture (Fig 12.19-2).

On the day of injury, an external fixator was applied (Fig 12.19-3) and the wound was thoroughly debrided with a scalpel and irrigated with pulsatile lavage until the wound margins showed healthy bleeding (chapter 7.2). Negative-pressure wound therapy was applied (chapter 9.3). The proximal femoral fracture was stabilized simultaneously with a dynamic hip screw.

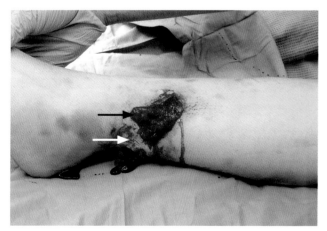

Fig 12.19-1 View of the injury at admission. There is an open wound at the lateral and posterior aspects of the distal third of the left lower leg, interrupted by a skin bridge (white arrow). Note the proximal fibular fragment perforating the skin (black arrow).

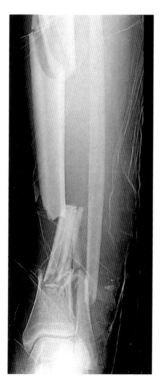

Fig 12.19-2 AP x-ray of the multifragmentary fracture of the left lower leg (Gustilo type IIIA fracture).

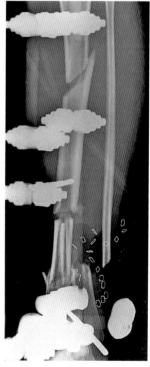

Fig 12.19-3 AP x-ray after temporary fixation with an external fixator.

Wound conditioning: On the second and fifth days after injury, repeated debridement of necrotic soft tissues was performed. On the ninth day, the external fixator on the tibia was removed and exchanged for an unreamed tibial intramedullary nail, respectively a plate fixation of the fibula (Fig 12.19-4a–b). As necrosis of skin and other soft-tissues progressed, definitive coverage was postponed and negative-pressure wound therapy was continued. Three more surgical debridements were necessary on the fifteenth, seventeenth, and twentieth days in order to clearly outline viable tissues. Meanwhile, the patient was treated with systemic antibiotics according to the antibiotic sensitivity test.

Present status

Finally, the extensive defect reached around the entire circumference of the left lower leg exposing both tibia and fibula including implant material on the fibula, the remaining tendons as well as the neurovascular bundles of the anterior tibia. There was extensive damage to the anterior and lateral muscle compartments and viability of the Achilles tendon appeared questionable (Fig 12.19-5).

Decision making

Open questions

- What is a realistic goal for this patient?
- What are definitive treatment options?
- Apart from skin defect reconstruction, is there any need for further reconstruction?
- What are the surgical options for soft-tissue coverage?
- What should the timing of soft-tissue coverage be?

A realistic treatment goal is limb salvage with good motor function and sensation. Multiple surgical procedures are to be expected as well as a long period of recovery.

Options and plan

Large soft-tissue defects in an extensively injured extremity are usually best restored using free flaps, especially at the lower end of the leg where there is a lack of adequate regional options. While fasciocutaneous flaps match the local tissues very well, they may be restricted in size in comparison to large muscle free flaps which, in addition, may fill dead spaces. Thorough preoperative examination of the limb's vascularity—including angiography (ie, angiography, CT angiography, MR angiography)—is indicated in order to exactly assess the recipient vessels (usually the anterior or posterior tibial artery and concomitant veins) (Fig 12.19-6).

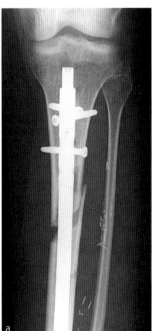
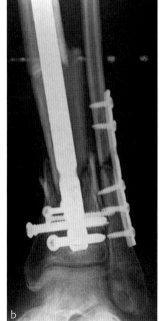

Fig 12.19-4a–b AP x-rays after internal fixation of the tibia (unreamed intramedullary nail with static fixation) and fibula (plate fixation).
a   Proximal lower leg.
b   Distal lower leg.

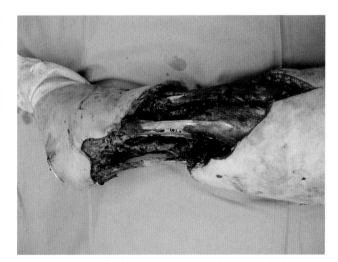

Fig 12.19-5 Considerable circular soft-tissue defect after final debridement of skin, muscles, and tendons, exposing bone and implant material, the remaining tendons as well as the neurovascular bundles.

Procedure

Soft-tissue coverage was planned to consist of a free latissimus dorsi flap and split-thickness skin graft. On the day of surgery, and following exact intraoperative measurement, it became obvious that the latissimus dorsi flap alone would not suffice to cover the entire defect. Therefore, it was decided to increase the size of the flap by adding the lower third of the serratus anterior muscle (Fig 12.19-7), which is supplied by the serratus branch of the thoracodorsal artery.

Accordingly, the initially planned latissimus dorsi flap turned into a chimeric flap, ie, two free flaps supplied by the same vascular pedicle (chapter 10.6). In this case, the subscapular arteriovenous pedicle secured the vascular supply (Fig 12.19-7). The anterior tibial artery and one concomitant vein were chosen as the recipient vessels. End-to-end anastomoses were performed under the microscope. The large latissimus dorsi portion was used to cover the anterior, lateral and posterior aspects of the defect (Fig 12.19-8), whereas the small serratus anterior portion was used to cover the medial aspect of the defect. The well-vascularized muscle flap was finally covered with a meshed split-thickness skin graft harvested from the thigh.

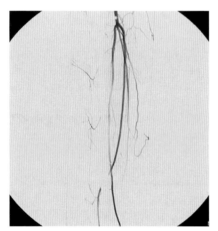

Fig 12.19-6 Arteriography showing normal patency of the lower leg's arteries.

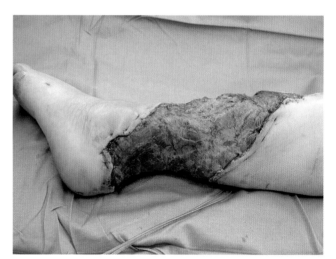

Fig 12.19-8 Intraoperative view after flap insertion and before application of the split-thickness skin graft.

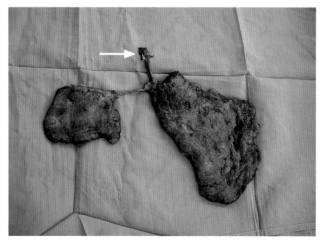

Fig 12.19-7 Chimeric flap consisting of the lower third of the serratus anterior muscle (left) and the latissimus dorsi muscle (right). The pedicle is based on the subscapular artery and vein (arrow).

Follow-up

Two weeks after soft-tissue coverage, revision of the donor site for extensive seroma as well as debridement of the entire necrotic Achilles tendon became necessary. A small split-thickness skin graft covered the remaining defect at the site of tendon excision. Thereafter, healing was uneventful. Intensive in-hospital rehabilitation was followed by outpatient physical therapy. Full weight bearing was allowed at 13 weeks despite a delayed union of the tibia. Five months after soft-tissue coverage, there was a rather good match of thickness, texture, and color (Fig 12.19-9). The fracture had healed without incident (Fig 12.19-10). Presently, the patient shows surprisingly good function of the ankle joint, with a dorsal extension and plantar flexion of 0° respectively 40°

(range of motion E/F 0-0-40°). The knee joint has recovered normal mobility (range of motion E/F 10-0-110°) (Fig 12.19-11a–d). The donor site presents with a discrete scapula alata as a consequence of the serratus flap elevation and some injury to the thoracic longus nerve (Fig 12.19-12), which has not limited shoulder function in daily activities.

Points to remember

- A fracture that is segmental or comminuted is usually associated with a significant soft-tissue injury, even if the extent of that injury is not fully appreciated at first.
- Necrotic tissue must be debrided regardless of the size of the resulting soft-tissue defect.

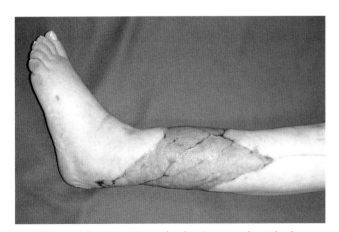

Fig 12.19-9   Follow-up at 5 months showing a good match of thickness, texture, and color. Note the hypertrophic scars at the junction of the skin graft patches.

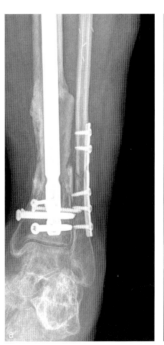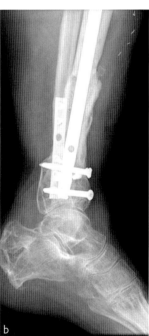

Fig 12.19-10a–b   X-rays showing the fracture to have healed. Note the considerable disuse osteopenia.
a   AP view.
b   Lateral view.

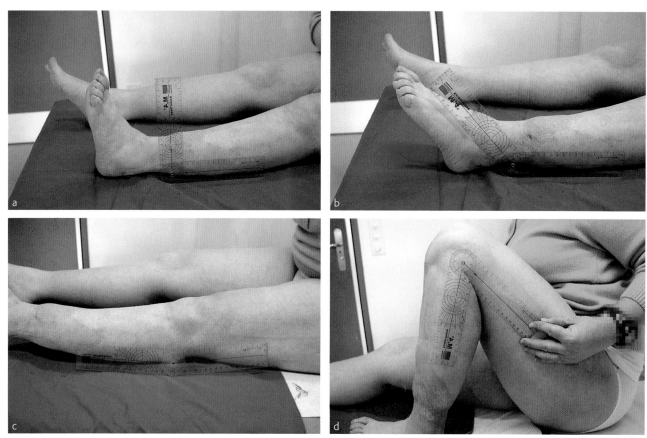

Fig 12.19-11a–d Follow-up at 2 years showing mobility of the ankle and knee joints.
a   Dorsal extension of the left ankle: 0°.
b   Plantar flexion of the left ankle: 40° (range of motion 0-0-40°).
c   Extension of the left knee: 10°.
d   Flexion of the left knee: 110° (range of motion 10-0-110°).

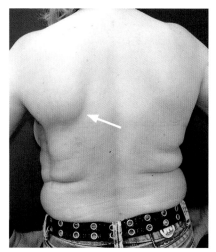

Fig 12.19-12 Clinical photograph of the donor site at 5 months, demonstrating a visible scapula alata on the left side (arrow).

12.20 Skill level IV: Case 4

Authors Themistocles S Protopsaltis, L Scott Levin

Case history

- 27-year-old African American male patient
- Unemployed
- Right hand dominant
- Single
- Smoker
- No other medical problems

The injuries of both forearms were inflicted by low-velocity missiles, fired from a handgun. Paramedics first applied saline-soaked dressings to all wounds and then air splints to both injured forearms.

Examination in the emergency department revealed the following:
- conscious patient
- abdomen, chest, pelvis, spine, and legs uninjured
- gunshot wounds to both forearms
- both hands warm and well perfused.

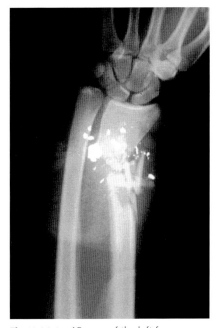

Fig 12.20-1 AP x-ray of the left forearm. Gunshot wound demonstrating a complex metaphyseal distal radius fracture (22-A3) with bullet fragments scattered throughout the soft tissues.

Findings on the left forearm:
- entry wound on the palmar aspect of the distal forearm
- exit wound on the dorsoradial aspect of the middle third of the forearm
- palpable radial pulse and strong ulnar pulse using Doppler ultrasound
- intact motor and sensory function of median and ulnar nerves
- diminished sensation in the distribution of the superficial radial nerve
- preserved motor function of extensor pollicis longus, extensor digitorum communis, and wrist extensors
- exposed flexor tendons on the palmar side
- comminuted extraarticular fracture (22-A3) of the distal third of the radius with many bullet fragments scattered throughout the soft tissues (Fig 12.20-1); Gustilo type IIIA fracture.

Findings on the right forearm:
- entry wound on the dorsal ulnar aspect of the mid forearm
- exit wound on the palmar aspect of the proximal to mid forearm
- preserved motor and sensory function of the radial, median and ulnar nerves
- no fractures.

Management of the right arm will not be discussed in this case.

The patient underwent emergency debridement and irrigation of both upper extremities. The contaminated subcutaneous tissue and the skin edges about the entry and exit wounds were debrided back to healthy tissue.

In more detail, debridement on the left arm consisted of:
- partial excision of the devitalized brachioradialis muscle
- neurolysis of the superficial branch of the radial nerve found to be contiguous but contused
- removal of many bullet fragments and devascularized bone fragments stripped of their soft-tissue attachments.

I
II
III
IV

Wound conditioning: Following the initial debridement, an external fixator was placed on the radius in order to maintain its alignment and length despite the presence of a bone defect of 5–6 cm in length (Fig 12.20-2, 12.20-3a–b). The wound on the left forearm was dressed with a negative-pressure wound-therapy device (chapter 9.3). A window in the dressing was created in order to monitor the radial and ulnar artery pulses postoperatively. After 48 hours, a second look and further debridement of the open fracture was carried out.

Present status

The left forearm was now left with:
- a large bone defect with a diameter of ~6 cm
- an exposed radial artery and flexor tendons on the palmar aspect of the forearm
- a dorsal soft-tissue wound measuring 15 × 7 cm and a palmar wound 6 × 3 cm
- a contused but contiguous superficial radial nerve
- an intact radial artery and median nerve.

Decision making

Open questions
- What type of flap might restore both bone continuity and provide skin coverage?

Options and plan
Treatment could result in a functional hand if the large bone defect and skin defect can be repaired. The ultimate goal is the reconstruction of the skeletal defect and soft-tissue injury of the left forearm in order to restore the anatomical relationships of the forearm that will facilitate functional recovery. This requires restoration of the articular relationship between the radius and ulna in order to regain normal wrist kinematics as well as allow pronation and supination.

In choosing a treatment plan, the surgeon is guided by the principle of selecting the option with the best chance of providing the desired result, which does not necessarily mean the simplest approach (chapter 8.2). Similarly, like should be replaced with like (chapter 8.1).

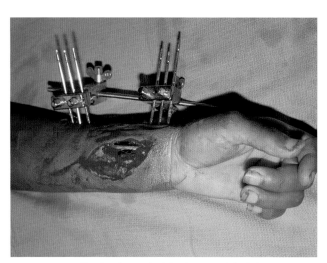

Fig 12.20-2 Following thorough debridement of the left upper extremity, an external fixator is applied in order to gain provisional stability of the distal radial bone defect. Note the exposed tendons on the radiopalmar side.

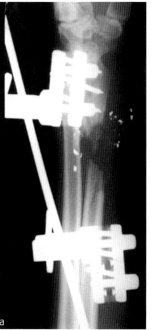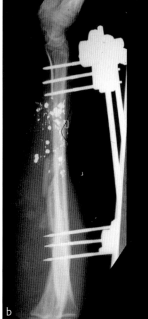

Fig 12.20-3a–b X-rays of the left forearm showing the segmental bone defect after initial debridement and application of an external fixator to the radius.
a   AP view.
b   Lateral view.

The options for managing long-bone defects include conventional bone grafting, bone graft substitutes, distraction osteogenesis, and vascularized bone transfer. For large bone defects greater than 6 cm, the microvascular transfer of a vascularized bone graft is most advantageous. Since a significant soft-tissue defect is also involved on the dorsal and palmar aspect of the forearm, a fibula bone flap that includes cutaneous elements is able to provide vascularized tissues in order to reconstruct the bone defect, fill the dead space, and provide definitive soft-tissue coverage.

Free flaps from the iliac crest, scapula or radius would represent less ideal options with considerable risk of donor site morbidity.

For fixation of the open, contaminated fracture of the radius, external fixation is the preferred method for temporary stabilization. The external fixator facilitates carrying out the multiple debridements and allows for definitive fixation at a later date.

Definitive skeletal fixation in combination with a vascularized free fibula transfer is preferably performed with plates, and only exceptionally with intramedullary devices, either alone or in combination with external fixation.

Inappropriate in this particular case are:
- healing by secondary intention since tendons and neurovascular structures are exposed
- secondary wound closure due to the lack of soft tissues
- rearrangement of local tissues to completely cover vessels, tendons, or bare bone because they are not loose enough and their health is compromised
- local flaps from within the zone of injury (chapter 10.3.3). They are at risk and should therefore not be used to cover a large, contaminated open fracture that will require the reconstruction of a bone defect.
- the transfer of a portion of the radius because the viability of such a bone graft is compromised by the considerable damage to the radius.

Procedure

In the final procedure, an osteoseptocutaneous vascularized free fibula flap was harvested from the right lower extremity. The incision for the fibula flap was outlined to include a skin paddle of appropriate dimension (**Fig 12.20-4**) in order to restore the palmar soft-tissue defect (**Fig 12.20-2**). The fibula with a vascular pedicle of the fibular artery and two concomitant veins was raised under hemostatic control with a thigh tourniquet using loupe magnification (**Fig 12.20-5**).

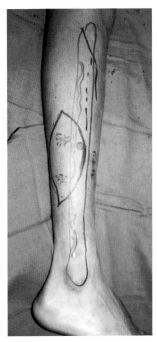

Fig 12.20-4 Outlined skin incision on the lower leg in order to harvest both the fibula and the skin paddle (ie, osteoseptocutaneous fibula flap) as cover for the soft-tissue defect of the forearm.

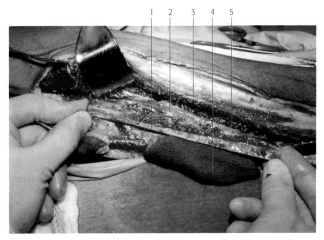

Fig 12.20-5 Raising the osteoseptocutaneous fibula flap based on the fibular artery and its concomitant veins.
1 Fibula segment after proximal and distal osteotomy.
2 Fibular artery and concomitant veins.
3 Fibular muscles.
4 Skin paddle.
5 Flexor hallucis longus muscle.

The external fixator was removed and the recipient site was redebrided. The bone defect of the radius was measured while distracting the proximal and distal bone ends with a bone spreader in order to maintain the correct length of the radius (Fig 12.20-6), this was confirmed radiographically (Fig 12.20-7).

After placement of the segment of vascularized fibula into the radial defect, the distraction was released, resulting in good compression at both proximal and distal interfaces. A long dynamic compression plate was contoured and fixed to the radius under axial compression (Fig 12.20-8). The bone graft itself was held with one monocortical screw alone. Using standard microsurgery techniques, the fibular artery and its two concomitant veins were anastomosed end-to-end to the radial artery, a concomitant vein and the cephalic vein, respectively (Fig 12.20-9). Intraoperative x-rays demonstrated good alignment of the graft, anatomical restoration of the radioulnar relationships and good positioning of the plate and screws (Fig 12.20-10a–b). Implantable ultrasonic Doppler probes were loosely placed around the arterial and venous anastomoses for continuous postoperative monitoring. The skin paddle was sutured into the soft-tissue defect and the wound was closed over a suction drain (Fig 12.20-11).

A split-thickness skin graft was necessary in order to cover the donor site on the right lower extremity. The left upper extremity was protected in a posterior long-arm splint with a window for monitoring the skin paddle (chapter 2, 10.7). The right lower extremity was placed into a posterior long-leg splint in order to maintain the ankle in neutral thereby protecting the skin graft.

The intubated and sedated patient was transferred to the intensive care unit for close overnight monitoring. Postoperatively, buffered aspirin was prescribed for 2 weeks.

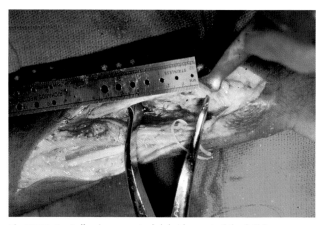

Fig 12.20-6 Following repeated debridement of the left forearm, the skeletal defect of the distal radius is measured with a bone spreader in place.

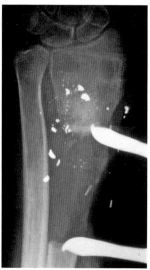

Fig 12.20-7 AP x-ray of the distal radius with a bone spreader in place in order to check the correct anatomical relationship of the distal radioulnar and wrist alignment more accurately and to measure the exact length of the segmental skeletal defect (6 cm).

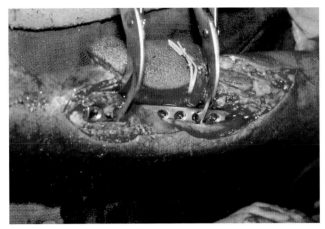

Fig 12.20-8 The fibula flap is placed into the defect of the distal radius and a dynamic compression plate is applied with axial compression.

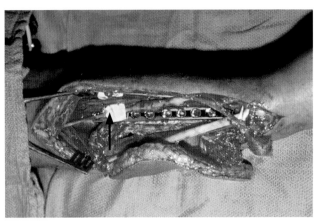

Fig 12.20-9 The fibular artery (arrow) and its two concomitant veins are anastomosed end-to-end under the microscope to the recipient vessels in the forearm.

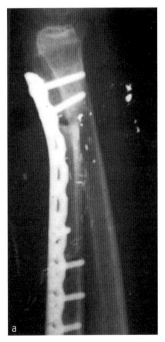 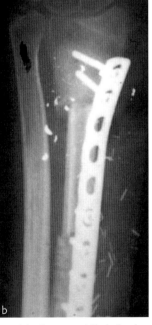

Fig 12.20-10a–b Intraoperative x-rays of the interposed fibula fixed to the radius with a dynamic compression plate. Good bone interfaces between fibula and radius proximally and distally.
a AP view.
b Lateral view.

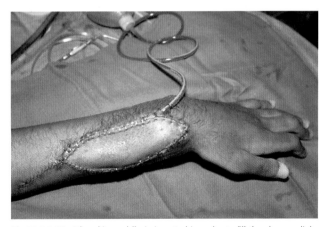

Fig 12.20-11 The skin paddle is inserted in order to fill the dorsoradial soft-tissue defect and the wound is closed over a suction drain. This will provide a reliable means to monitor the viability of the fibula flap.

Follow-up

The postoperative course was uneventful. The patient was discharged after 9 days. Weight bearing on the right lower extremity in a walking boot was permitted after the fourth postoperative day (Fig 12.20-12). The left arm was placed in a long arm cast until bone union was confirmed radiographically at the proximal and distal flap-host-bone interface (Fig 12.20-13a–b).

The patient had symmetrical forearm supination (Fig 12.20-14a) with a slightly reduced pronation (50° compared to 65°

on the left side (Fig 12.20-14b). Wrist flexion was 40° and extension 30°, respectively (Fig 12.20-14c–d). At 9 months postoperatively, function and healing of the forearm wounds on the right side were within normal limits (Fig 12.20-15a–e).

Points to remember

• In any defect, the surgeon has to assess exactly what structures and tissues are missing and, therefore, what must be replaced. In this case, bone and skin were required. The guideline to replace like with like was followed.

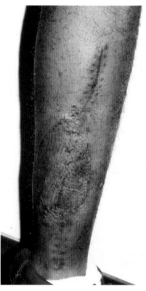

Fig 12.20-12 Healing of the split-thickness skin graft at the donor site on the leg. Hyperpigmentation, but no pathological scarring. Weight bearing on the right lower extremity in a walker boot was allowed after the fourth postoperative day.

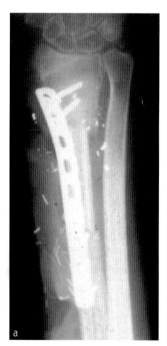
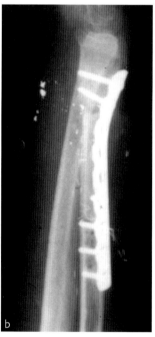

Fig 12.20-13a–b X-rays of the left forearm at 3 months postoperatively demonstrating union of the flap-host-bone interfaces.
a   AP view.
b   Lateral view.

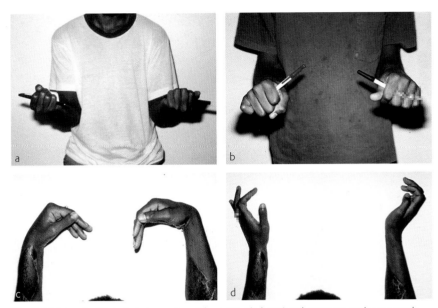

Fig 12.20-14a–d Clinical photographs of the patient's functional outcome at the 3-month follow-up.
a   Supination.
b   Pronation.
c   Wrist flexion.
d   Wrist extension.

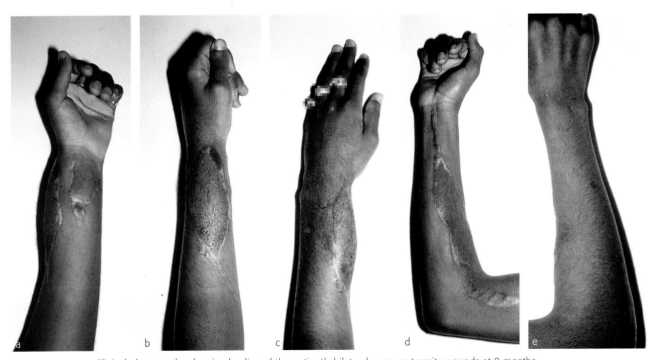

Fig 12.20-15a–e Clinical photographs showing healing of the patient's bilateral upper extremity wounds at 9 months.
a   Palmar view of the left upper extremity with still bulky but healed free fibula flap.
b   Lateral view of the left upper extremity.
c   Dorsal view of the left upper extremity.
d   Palmar view of the right upper extremity with hyperpigmented split-thickness skin graft.
e   Dorsal view of the right upper extremity.

APPENDIX

Credits

Chapter 1.2

Fig 1.2-1a–b modified according to: **Langer K** (1861) Zur Anatomie und Physiologie der Haut I. Über die Spaltbarkeit der Cutis. Sitzungsbericht der Mathematisch-naturwissenschaftlichen Classe der Kaiserlichen Academie der Wissenschaften, 45, 233.

Chapter 1.3

Fig 1.3-2a courtesy of Yves Harder, Munich.

Fig 1.3-4a courtesy of Yves Harder, Munich.

Fig 1.3-5a courtesy of Yves Harder, Munich.

Fig 1.3-7a–c courtesy of David A Volgas, Columbia.

Fig 1.3-8 courtesy of David A Volgas, Columbia.

Fig 1.3-9a–b courtesy of David A Volgas, Columbia.

Chapter 2.2

Fig 2.2-2a–b modified according to both: **Suami H, Taylor GI, Pan WR** (2003) Angiosome territories of the nerves of the lower limbs. *Plastic and Reconstructive Surgery;* 112(7):1794, Lippincott Williams & Wilkins, Wolters Kluwer Health. **Morris S, Tang M, Geddes, CR** (2006) Vascular anatomical basis of perforator skin flaps. *Cirugía Plástica Ibero-Latinoamericana [online];* 32(4):233, Sociedad Española de Cirugía Plástica, Reparadora y Estética (SECPRE), Madrid.

Fig 2.2-3 modified according to: **McCarthy JG** (1990) *Plastic Surgery.* 1st ed. Philadelphia: W.B. Saunders, 282.

Fig 2.2-4a, 2.2-4c–e courtesy of Yves Harder, Munich.

Chapter 3.1

Fig 3.1-2 modified according to: **Järvinen TA, Järvinen TL, Kääriäinen M, et al** (2005) Muscle Injuries: biology and treatment. *American Journal of Sports Medicine;* 33(5):748, The American Orthopaedic Society for Sports Medicine, SAGE Publications.

Fig 3.1-4 courtesy of Colonel (ret) Roman Hayda, Providence, Rhode Island.

Fig 3.1-5 courtesy of David A Volgas, Columbia.

Chapter 3.2

Fig 3.2-1 modified according to: **Bellamy RF, Zajtchuk R** (1991) The physics and biophysics of wound ballistics. *Jenkins DP, Zajtchuk R (eds) Conventional warfare: Ballistic, blast, and burn injuries.* Washington, DC: US Government Printing Office, 118.

Fig 3.2-2 modified according to: **Bellamy RF, Zajtchuk R** (1991) The physics and biophysics of wound ballistics. *Jenkins DP, Zajtchuk R (eds) Conventional warfare: Ballistic, blast, and burn injuries.* Washington, DC: US Government Printing Office, 140.

Fig 3.2-3 modified according to: **Bellamy RF, Zajtchuk R** (1991) The physics and biophysics of wound ballistics. *Jenkins DP, Zajtchuk R (eds) Conventional warfare: Ballistic, blast, and burn injuries.* Washington, DC: US Government Printing Office, 124.

Fig 3.2-4 modified according to: *Emergency War Surgery: 3rd United States Revision of the Emergency War Surgery NATO Handbook,* 2004, Department of Defense, 17.

Fig 3.2-6 courtesy of Colonel (ret) Robert Granville, Fort Lauderdale, Florida.

Chapter 3.3

Fig 3.3-1 modified according to: a sketch by Heather Ficke.

Fig 3.3-2, 3.3-3 courtesy of David A Volgas, Columbia.

Chapter 4.1

Fig 4.1-1a–b modified according to: **Monaco JL, Lawrence WT** (2003) Acute wound healing: an overview. *Clinics in Plastic Surgery;* 30(1):2, Review, Elsevier Science (USA).

Fig 4.1-2a–c, 4.1-3a–c modified according to: **Bruch HP, Trentz O** (2001) *Berchtold Chirurgie.* 4th ed. München Jena: Urban & Fischer, 201.

Chapter 4.2

Fig 4.2-1 to **4.2-3** courtesy of Jonny Huard, University of Pittsburgh, Pennsylvania.

Chapter 4.3

Fig 4.3-5a courtesy of Berton A Rahn, Davos.

Fig 4.3-5b courtesy of Stefan M Perren, Davos.

Chapter 5.1

Fig 5.1-1a–b courtesy of David A Volgas, Columbia.

Fig 5.1-2a–b courtesy of David A Volgas, Columbia.

Fig 5.1-5a–c courtesy of Alexander N Serov, Lausanne.

Chapter 5.3

Fig 5.3-2a–h courtesy of Yves Harder, Munich.

Fig 5.3-2i–j courtesy of Jörn A Lohmeyer, Munich.

Chapter 6.2

Fig 6.2-1 modified according to: **Südkamp NP** (2007) Soft-tissue injury: pathophysiology, evaluation, and classification. *Rüedi TP, Buckley RE, Moran CG (eds), AO Principles of Fracture Management.* 2nd ed. Stuttgart New York: Georg Thieme Verlag, 95.

Chapter 7.1

Fig 7.1-2, 7.1-3 courtesy of David A Volgas, Columbia.

Fig 7.1-6 courtesy of David A Volgas, Columbia.

Chapter 7.2

Fig 7.2-1a–h courtesy of Yves Harder, Munich.

Chapter 8.2

Fig 8.2-1 modified according to **Aston SJ, Beasley RW, Thorne CHM** (1997) *Grabb and Smith's Plastic Surgery.* 5th ed. Philadelphia: Lippincott-Raven, 14.

Fig 8.2-2a–b modified according to: **Wong CJ, Niranjan N** (2008) Reconstructive stages as an alternative to the reconstructive ladder. *Plastic and Reconstructive Surgery;* 121(5):362–363, Lippincott Williams & Wilkins, Wolters Kluwer Health.

Chapter 9.2

Fig 9.2-1a–d courtesy of David A Volgas, Columbia.

Chapter 9.3

Fig 9.3-1a–d courtesy of David A Volgas, Columbia.

Chapter 10.1

Fig 10.1-12a–h courtesy of Yves Harder, Munich.

Chapter 10.2

Fig 10.2-2, 10.2-3 courtesy of Yves Harder, Munich.
Fig 10.2-5a–e courtesy of Dominique Erni, Küssnacht.

Chapter 10.3

Fig 10.3-1a–b modified according to: **Masquelet AC, Gilbert A** (1995) *An Atlas of flaps in limb reconstruction.* 1st ed. London: Martin Dunitz.

Fig 10.3-2a–e modified according to both: **Masquelet AC, Gilbert A** (1995) *An Atlas of flaps in limb reconstruction.* 1st ed. London: Martin Dunitz.
Mathes SJ, Nahai F (1981) Classification of the vascular anatomy of muscles: experimental and clinical correlation. *Plastic and Reconstructive Surgery;* 67(2):178, Lippincott Williams & Wilkins, Wolters Kluwer Health.

Chapter 10.4

Fig 10.4-1a–e, 10.4-2a–c modified according to: **Aston SJ, Beasley RW, Thorne CHM** (1997) *Grabb and Smith's Plastic Surgery.* 5th ed. Philadelphia: Lippincott-Raven, 25.

Fig 10.4-3a–e, 10.4-4a–f, 10.4-5a–f modified according to: **Aston SJ, Beasley RW, Thorne CHM** (1997) *Grabb and Smith's Plastic Surgery.* 5th ed. Philadelphia: Lippincott-Raven, 22.

Fig 10.4-6a–f courtesy of Thomas Fischer, Berne.

Fig 10.4-7a–e modified according to: **Aston SJ, Beasley RW, Thorne CHM** (1997) *Grabb and Smith's Plastic Surgery.* 5th ed. Philadelphia: Lippincott-Raven, 20.

Fig 10.4-7f–h courtesy of Hans-Günther Machens, Munich.

Fig 10.4-8a–b modified according to: **Aston SJ, Beasley RW, Thorne CHM** (1997) *Grabb and Smith's Plastic Surgery.* 5th ed. Philadelphia: Lippincott-Raven, 24.

Fig 10.4-9 modified according to: **Cormack CC, Lamberty BGH** (1986) *The arterial anatomy of skin flaps.* 1st ed. Edinburgh: Churchill Livingstone, 65.

Fig 10.4-11 modified according to: a sketch by Jörg Grünert, St. Gallen.

Chapter 10.5

Fig 10.5-1a–h to **10.5-7a–i** modified according to: **Masquelet AC, Gilbert A** (1995) *An Atlas of flaps in limb reconstruction.* 1st ed. London: Martin Dunitz.

Chapter 10.6

Fig 10.6-2, 10.6-3a–b, 10.6-8, 10.6-9a–c courtesy of Yves Harder, Munich.

Fig 10.6-5a–b, 10.6-6 courtesy of Dominique Erni, Küssnacht.

Chapter 11.1

Fig 11.1-4 modified according to: **Marieb EN, Hoehn K** (2007) *Human Anatomy and Physiology.* 7th ed. San Francisco: Pearson Benjamin Cummings, 498.

Chapter 11.2

Fig 11.2-3a–b modified according to: **Cierny G III, DiPasquale D** (2006) Treatment of Chronic Infection. *Journal of the American Academy of Orthopaedic Surgeons;* 14(10):S108, American Academy of Orthopaedic Surgeons.

Chapter 11.3

Fig 11.3-1a–b, 11.3-2, 11.3-3, 11.3-4a, 11.3-12 courtesy of Yves Harder, Munich.

Fig 11.3-4b courtesy of Reto Wettstein, Solothurn.

Chapter 11.4

Fig 11.4-3, 11.4-4 courtesy of Yves Harder, Munich.

Front and back cover

Front cover photograph courtesy of David A Volgas, Columbia.

Back cover photographs (top to bottom):
Fig 1 courtesy of David A Volgas, Columbia.
Fig 2 courtesy of Yves Harder, Munich.
Fig 3 courtesy of David A Volgas, Columbia.
Fig 4 courtesy of Yves Harder, Munich.
Fig 5 courtesy of Yves Harder, Munich.

Find narrated educational videos about soft-tissue management in orthopaedic trauma online at MediaCenter.thieme.com

Simply visit MediaCenter.thieme.com and, when prompted during the registration process, enter the scratch-off code below to get started today.

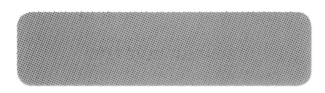

This book cannot be returned once this panel has been scratched off.

Surgical videos/animation of this book available online:

Videos 1.3
Instruments

Video 7.1-1
Debridement

Video 7.2-1
Irrigation

Video 9.3-1
Negative-pressure wound therapy

Video 10.1-1
Suture techniques

Video 10.2-1
Split-thickness skin graft

Video 10.5-1
Sural flap

Video 10.5-2
Gastrocnemius flap

Video 10.5-3
Soleus flap

Animation 11.1-1
Compartment syndrome

System requirements:

	WINDOWS	MAC	TABLET
Recommended Browser(s)**	Microsoft Internet Explorer 8.0 or later, Firefox 3.x	Firefox 3.x, Safari 4.x	HTML5 mobile browser. iPad – Safari. Opera Mobile – Tablet PCs preferred.
	** all browsers should have JavaScript enabled		
Flash Player Plug-in	Flash Player 9 or Higher* * Mac users: ATI Rage 128 GPU does not support full-screen mode with hardware scaling		Tablet PCs with Android OS support Flash 10.1
Minimum Hardware Configurations	Intel® Pentium® II 450 MHz, AMD Athlon™ 600 MHz or faster processor (or equivalent) 512MB of RAM	PowerPC® G3 500 MHz or faster processor Intel Core™ Duo 1.33 GHz or faster processor 512MB of RAM	Minimum CPU powered at 800MHz 256MB DDR2 of RAM
Recommended for optimal usage experience	Monitor resolutions: • Normal (4:3) 1024×768 or Higher • Widescreen (16:9) 1280×720 or Higher • Widescreen (16:10) 1440×900 or Higher DSL/Cable internet connection at a minimum speed of 384.0 Kbps or faster WiFi 802.11 b/g preferred.		7-inch and 10-inch tablets on maximum resolution. WiFi connection is required.